Professional Issues
in Primary Care Nursing

Professional Issues in Primary Care Nursing

Edited by

Carol Lynn Cox
*PhD, MSc, MA Ed, PG Dip Ed, BSc (Hons),
RN, ENB 254, FHEA*

Marie C. Hill
M.H.M., Pg Dip, BSc (Hons), RN

WILEY-BLACKWELL

A John Wiley & Sons, Ltd., Publication

Library of Congress Cataloging-in-Publication Data

Professional issues in primary care nusing / edited by Carol Lynn Cox, Marie Hill.
p. ; cm.
Includes bibliographical references and index.
ISBN 978-1-4051-8755-8 (pbk. : alk. paper)   1. Primary nursing.   I. Cox, Carol Lynn.
II. Hill, Marie, 1959–
[DNLM: 1. Primary Nusing Care.   2. Ambulatory Care.   3. Nurse–Patient Relations.
WY 101 P964 2010]

RT90.7.P76 2010
610.73—dc22
2009028298

A catalogue record for this book is available from the British Library.

Set in 10 on 12.5 pt Sabon by MPS Limited, A Macmillan Company
Printed and bound in Malaysia by KHL Printing Co Sdn Bhd

1   2010

Contents

6 Health education and health promotion

Daryl Evans

Domain 2: The Nurse–Patient Relationship   95

7 Working with individual patients and groups: creating and strengthening relationships   97

Karen Thompson

Foreword

Practice and walk-in-centre nurses are a relatively new addition to the group of advanced practice nurses who deliver high-level care and treatment with the ever-changing NHS. As a fast-growing group of professionals, they have forged new ways of working and addressed many challenges as they strove to establish themselves as key players in the new world of health care and treatment.

Over the past 20 years, practice nurses have become vital partners in the delivery of care and treatment working within the teams that are to be found in any general practice surgery today. It was not always so.

In 1989, as Head of a School of Nursing serving several hospitals and the community of two large Northwest towns, I was asked to ascertain the need for a Practice Nursing Course to be validated by the then English National Board and our partner university. It would form one option within the Community Nursing degree which was at planning stage. I wrote to all GP practices within the catchment area. None had a practice nurse who did any nursing. One or two employed them as receptionists, chaperones or assistants when treating a child and someone who 'saw' relatives; one said he used his wife as a nurse when he needed one and a few said they had 'trained their receptionists' for the role. A few GPs worked single practices without any support other than from a receptionist.

Similar situations across the country led to the introduction of first a module, and then a course, an undergraduate degree, a Clinical Masters and access to doctoral studies. Practice nurses are now prepared and educated to the highest possible standards and are delivering highly competent health promotion and rehabilitative and curative care across the UK. Patients are highly satisfied with their contribution to the care they receive at the surgery, with many choosing to see them instead of the GP when they need immunisations, advice or regular review.

Newer, but no less important to the patients of today are those nurses who head up our walk-in-centres and are the first point of contact for many who want treatment for a minor injury, advice on how to best manage a symptom of ill health that is of concern or guidance on a health or medication query. They give the public the quick, accessible and, most importantly, the safe advice and intervention they need. As a nurse-led service, the nurse working in the centres is a competent, skilled and knowledgeable practitioner who is constantly pushing boundaries as the role becomes more and more complex. In the past few years, the centres have moved to support out-of-hours services and they will surely change further as polyclinics develop and more care is moved from acute, to community settings.

Like practice nurses, they benefit from excellent educational development and experience high levels of patient satisfaction.

As both groups of nurses continue to adapt to the constant ongoing change demanded by both the public and the government paymasters, they will face ever-growing self-questioning about their role and responsibilities and their need to remain competent, knowledgeable and safe practitioners.

This book will guide them through that maze. It has been long awaited and Carol Cox, Marie Hill and their expert contributors are to be congratulated on its quality.

Professor Dame Betty Kershaw, DBE, FRCN
Education Advisor, The Royal College of Nursing
President of the Scholarship Society for
Nurses and Midwives

Preface

This book represents the culmination of several years of planning in order to ensure that the most salient issues associated with professional issues in practice nursing and walk-in-centre nursing are addressed. Each chapter is associated with the Royal College of Nursing's (2008) specific Domain of Practice and Competencies delineated within the realm of advanced practice nursing (refer to Chapter 4, The context of practice nursing and walk-in-centre nursing: differences and similarities relating to the domains of practice – setting the scene, which articulates the RCN (2008) advanced nurse practitioner role and competencies to learn more about the Domains of Practice and Competencies). Part 1 of this text sets the scene of practice nursing and walk-in-centre nursing. It provides the foundation for understanding Part 2 of the text. In addition, Part 1 identifies how practice nursing and walk-in-centre nursing have evolved into advanced practice roles and delineates the new responsibilities associated with these roles. Part 2 of this text explicates each domain of practice and critical issues that the practice nurse and walk-in-centre nurse must consider within their professional practice. For example, in Domain 1, Management of Patient Health/Illness Status, critical thinking and diagnostic reasoning in clinical decision-making are addressed and in Domain 2, The Nurse–Patient Relationship, working with individual patients and groups and creating and strengthening relationships are considered.

As a practice nurse or walk-in-centre nurse, it is imperative to recognise that your practice is evolving. It is evolving at such a rapid pace that it is no longer possible for you to keep up to date with current issues and practice mandates on your own. Therefore, this text will help you to get to grips with the professional issues that affect your practice in primary care.

Reference: RCN (2008) *Advanced Nurse Practitioners – An RCN Guide to the Advanced Nurse Practitioner Role, Competencies and Programme Accreditation.* London: Royal College of Nursing.

Carol L. Cox, PhD, RN
Professor of Nursing
Advanced Clinical Practice
and
Marie C. Hill, MHM, RN
Senior Lecturer in Practice Nursing

Acknowledgements

We wish to thank the many nurses and students who suggested developing this text. Without their ongoing support and enthusiasm, this text would not have reached fruition.

Dedication

This text is dedicated to practice nurses and walk-in-centre nurses who strive to make the very best of their professional practice.

Contributors

Maisie Allen RN, RHV, Cert Project Management
Management Consultant and Managing Director of Mentfor (CIC)

Jane Bickerton MA (Phil), BA (Psych), RN, HV, WHNP
Visiting Lecturer
Nurse Practitioner in Public Health and Primary Care
Department of Public Health, Primary Care and Food Policy
School of Community and Health Sciences
City University
London

Shuling Breckenridge MSc, P.G. Dip Academic Practice, BSc (Hons), BA, RN
Visiting Lecturer in Practice Nursing
School of Community and Health Sciences
City University
London

Carol L. Cox PhD, MSc, MA Ed, PG Dip Ed, BSc (Hons), ENB 254, RN, FHEA
Professor of Nursing, Advanced Clinical Practice
Department of Applied Biological Sciences
City University
London

Daryl Evans MA, BSc (Hons), RN, RNT, Dip N Ed, FHEA
Principal Lecturer in Health Promotion and Nursing
School of Health and Social Sciences
Middlesex University
London

Anjoti Harrington PhD, MBA, MA, Dip Ed, RNT, DPSN, ENB 100, RN
Senior Lecturer
Law and Ethics and Adult Nursing
School of Community and Health Sciences
City University
London

Marie C. Hill M.H.M., Pg Dip, BSc (Hons), RN
Senior Lecturer in Practice Nursing
School of Community and Health Sciences
City University
London

Christopher Johns PhD, RN, PACT
Professor of Nursing
University of Bedfordshire
Bedfordshire

Victoria Lack MSc, Pg Dip (Academic Practice), BN, DN cert, RGN, FNP
Lecturer in Practice Nursing
Department of Public Health and Primary Care
City University
London

Nita Muir MSc, PgCHSCE, BSc (Hons), RN, Specialist Practitioner/DN
Senior Lecturer
School of Nursing and Midwifery
University of Brighton
Brighton

Karen Thompson MA, BSc (Hons), RN, FHEA
Senior Lecturer in Adult Nursing
School of Nursing and Midwifery
University of Brighton
Brighton

Kathryn Waddington PhD, MSc, PGCE(A), BSc (Hons), CPsychol, RN
Director of Interprofessional Practice Programmes
School of Community and Health Sciences
City University
London

Nicola L. Whiteing MSc, BSc (Hons), RN, ANP
Lecturer in Nursing
Department of Adult Nursing
City University
London

Part 1

Setting the Scene of Practice and Walk-in-Centre Nursing

In the chapters that follow in Part 1 of this book, the historical development of practice nursing and walk-in-centre nursing are explicated. The context of practice is delineated in relation to advanced practice, as it is recognised that practice nurses and walk-in-centre nurses are now working at an advanced practice level. Part 1 sets the scene for the professional issues chapters that follow in Part 2 of this book.

The historical development of practice nursing and walk-in-centre nursing 1

Marie C. Hill, Carol L. Cox and Shuling Breckenridge

Introduction

The aim of this chapter is to explore the historical background in the growth of practice nursing (PN) and walk-in-centre (WiC) nursing in the UK. The reasons for growth in these two distinct nursing groups are examined and related to governmental health policy. A critical discussion ensues on the impact that both practice nurses (PNs) and WiC nurses have had on their respective communities.

Learning Outcomes

- To understand the reasons for the growth in practice nursing
- To comprehend the reasons for the introduction of walk-in centres by the National Health Service (NHS)
- To be able to articulate the differences and similarities between practice nursing and walk-in-centre nursing:
  a. the complexities and questions concerning the efficiency of walk-in centres
  b. the possible future evolution of the National Health Service walk-in-centre concept.

Background

In order to place our discussion in the appropriate context, we should begin by looking at the definition of the term primary health care. Unfortunately, there is no universally agreed definition (Peckham and Exworthy, 2003).

For example, in the Alma Ata declaration, the World Health Organization (WHO) defined primary health care as 'essential health care based on practical, scientifically sound and socially acceptable methods and technology, made universally available to individuals and families in the community through their full participation and at a cost that the community and the country can afford to maintain at every stage of their development in the spirit of self-reliance and self-determination' (WHO, 1978:VI:3–4).

Starfield (1998:8–9) indicated that primary care is 'that level of a service system that provides entry into the system for all new needs and problems, provides person-focused (not disease-orientated) care over time, provides for all but very uncommon or unusual conditions, and co-ordinates or integrates care provided elsewhere or by others', while Lakhani and Charlton (2005) argue that the definition of primary care will be dependent upon the identity of the care provider and the location of care provision as well as the type of service provided. Jones and Menzies (1999:3) support this view, that patients present themselves to general practice as the 'first level of professional care, accessed when self-care is seemed inadequate'.

PNs and WiC nurses have cultivated and developed an important role in the provision of both treatment and health promotion services to patients in the context of primary health care. This emphasis is evident in the principles that underpin primary care. Drennan and Goodman (2007) have identified five principles that underpin primary care which are:

1. accessibility to heath services;
2. use of appropriate technology;
3. individual and community participation;
4. increased health promotion;
5. disease prevention.

This concept of primary care, with the associated five principles, is the context within which we will examine, in turn, the development of both PN and WiC nursing in the UK.

Practice nursing

The increasing role of the PN within primary care has seen a significant rise in numbers. In 1983, the numbers of whole time equivalent PNs in England and Wales were 1,729 (Williams, 2000). This figure rose to 7,520 in 1990 (Ross and Mackenzie, 1996) and to 23,797 in 2006 (Robinson, 2007). This meteoric rise in the numbers of PNs made them the largest branch of community nurses in 2001 (Macdougald et al., 2001). What has precipitated this huge growth in PN numbers? In order to understand why this growth has occurred, it is necessary to understand how governmental health policies have influenced this growth. Ham (1992) has argued that there is little agreement regarding the definition of policy. However, other writers have been more specific in defining health policy as having guidelines for organisational action in terms of the implementation of its goals and action plans (Watson and Wilkinson, 2001).

Peckham and Exworthy (2003) argue that governmental policy interest in primary care only began to develop in the 1960s with a keener interest in the role of primary care and its organisation. They identified a number of key factors that have contributed to the growth in this area namely:

- an increase in the availability of medical techniques and technologies;
- the increasing need to provide community-based care for patients with long-term conditions;
- the need to increase access to health care following the introduction of the National Health Service in 1948;
- the shift of care from secondary to primary care (Peckham and Exworthy, 2003).

The general practitioner (GP) *Charter* in 1966 changed the way in which GPs were paid. Furthermore, the *Charter* gave GP incentives for procuring better premises and the reimbursement of ancillary staff, which culminated in the employment of PNs (Macdougald et al., 2001; Hampson, 2002). Although the 1966 charter led to a rise in the numbers of PNs, it was the GP contract of 1990 that significantly increased these numbers. In 1990 alone there was a 60% increase in PN numbers (Luft and Smith, 1994). The main changes in the 1990 contract were:

- an increased emphasis on capitation services, with the payment to GPs being directly related to the number of registered patients;
- the setting of target payments for certain procedures such as the administration of immunisations, cervical cytology and child health surveillance;
- additional incentives to run health promotion services (e.g. a designated hypertension clinic), undertaking minor surgery and working in deprived areas;
- the requirement to provide health checks for certain groups of patients, such as all new patient registration at a general practice, those patients having not attended a practice for 3 years and all those patients over 75 years of age (Ross and Mackenzie, 1996).

Taken together, the changes resulted in GPs being strongly motivated to employ PNs to provide primary health care services not directly requiring a doctor. This increased the throughput of general practices in terms of the number of registered patients they could support, and therefore GP's earning power. The development of a distinct role for PNs, with a generally well-defined remit within primary health care delivery, laid a foundation upon which the concept of the WiC as a nurse-led health care delivery vehicle could be built.

WiC nursing

The Department of Health (DoH, 1997) has stated that the NHS needs to modernise in order to meet patients' expectations for an up-to-date, quicker, more responsive health service. In April 1999, nurse-led WiCs were piloted as part of a bid to modernise health services with improved access to primary care services (DoH, 1999). NHS WiCs are intended to complement other initiatives such as NHS Direct and Healthy Living Centres (DoH, 2001).

Since they were introduced in 2000, NHS WiCs have treated over five million people. There are currently around 90 NHS WiCs in England providing quick and easy access to a range of NHS facilities (www.nhs.uk), with further sites being developed.

As a further development to the WiC scheme, the NHS has contracted with the private health care sector for the provision of a number of commuter WiCs. These are located close to railway stations and focus predominantly on providing services to 'out-of-area' patients, for whom seeing a GP can be difficult to manage within regular office hours.

There are three common themes in the development of WiCs (Salisbury et al., 2002). First is the improvement of accessibility, second is to make the NHS more responsive to modern lifestyles and third is maximising the role of nurses as more cost-effective health care providers in the majority of cases.

The concept of WiCs can be traced to other developments in the UK and abroad. For example, the minor injuries units, entirely staffed by nurses, replacing small casualty departments as services are rationalised within larger centralised accident and emergency (A&E) departments, offer a safe, effective and popular service (Dolan and Dale, 1997; Heaney and Paxton, 1997). Another example is the telephone helpline, NHS Direct, that has been implemented nationally. The positive evaluation of NHS Direct has led to the suggestion that nurses working with decision support may be able to provide similar advice face-to-face. The research work of Kinnersley et al. (2000) and Venning et al. (2000) has supported the notion that nurses with additional training can manage most patients presenting with acute minor illness. These results, which build upon the foundation laid by PNs, led more or less directly to the concept of the NHS nurse-led WiC.

Note that the notion of the WiC as a nurse-led health care delivery vehicle within the NHS is very different from those that exist in other countries, even though WiCs in other countries predate those of the NHS by many years. For example, the first WiCs in the USA opened in the early 1970s and were termed 'emergency centres', 'ambulatory care centres' or 'urgent care centres'. During the 1980s, walk-in medical clinics were also developed in Canada. These walk-in clinics in other countries are, however, doctor-led and can therefore provide full GP services, whereas NHS WiCs are nurse-lead, treating only acute minor ailments. This reflects an important difference in aim between the NHS and the health systems of these other countries. The main aim of these clinics in other countries is to provide care outside normal office hours for important sectors of society, such as affluent working professionals (Borkenhagen, 1988). Whereas, the NHS WiC can be construed as an attempt to deflect the care of patients with minor ailments away from A&E departments, thus increasing the global cost effectiveness of the NHS.

As there has been controversy over the role and impact of walk-in clinics on primary health care in other countries for over two decades, NHS WiCs have been one of the most controversial initiatives within the NHS in recent years.

As one would expect, some aspects of the NHS WiC concept have been relatively successful, while other aspects have been less so. According to Salisbury's Final Report of the National Evaluation of NHS WiCs (Salisbury et al., 2002), WiCs have been generally successful in four basic areas: patient satisfaction, access to care, quality of care and patient appropriateness.

Patient satisfaction was consistently identified by WiCs as a success. This was mainly judged by verbal feedback from patients as well as some letters of appreciation. Few centres had the resources to carry out formal surveys of patients' views, and in light of this, one must take into account the tendency for dissatisfied patients to be less vocal and to simply seek care elsewhere rather than complain. No statistics on repeat patients at NHS WiCs are available at this time.

Access to care was identified as the second successful aspect. The general conclusion is that WiCs, with their extended hours of operation, improve access for those whose situation makes access to their regular GP difficult on a day-to-day basis. For example, the increasing numbers of people who commute long distances to work all potentially fall into this category, with the commuter centres specifically targeted towards this group. The WiCs provide a new avenue to health care services which is highly valued by those who use the service.

Thirdly, we have quality of care. The quality of the organisation, interpersonal care, advice and treatment provided in WiCs has been generally excellent. Of course, there is always room for improvement, for example, the use of Patient Group Directions (PGDs).

And lastly, the fourth success to result from the introduction of WiCs is seen to be appropriateness of clients. With any health care service which has a limited remit, i.e. not all health care services are available, there is a risk that a substantial fraction of patients seeking to make use of the service have needs which fall outside the remit of care. There was a general consensus among WiC health care professionals that the overwhelming majority of presenting cases were appropriate to be seen at a WiC. This tends to indicate that the remit of WiC service is broad enough to be generally useful, as well as indicating that communication to the public of the role and services available from WiCs has been effective.

On the other hand, it is far from clear that the introduction of NHS WiCs has been an overall success, in spite of the four points noted above. Central in this debate has been the impact of the WiC initiative on other health care providers. The results of the study tend to indicate that the only significant impact of WiCs has been to reduce workload growth somewhat on local GP practices, with no statistically significant impact at all found on A&E departments (Salisbury et al., 2002).

If NHS WiCs are particularly efficient at providing health care services, then they could have a net positive impact on the efficiency of the overall health care system. According to Salisbury et al. (2002), the direct cost of an NHS WiC consultation is less than that of a consultation in A&E departments, but remains more expensive than consultations undertaken through the main alternative providers such as GPs, PNs, pharmacists and NHS Direct. Therefore, the fact that WiCs seem to draw most of their clients from less expensive health care providers would support the conclusion that the NHS WiC is having a negative impact on the efficiency of the overall health care system. If these results are confirmed by further studies, then there will be an important question as to whether the current WiC model is the right one, or whether there is perhaps a more efficient way of achieving the same aims.

Future NHS developments, such as those outlined in the *High Quality Care for All: NHS Next Stage Review*' by Lord Darzi (DoH, 2008), may result in the current NHS concept of the WiC evolving significantly. It may be possible, for example, to recast the nurse-led WiC as a component within a more general health care access avenue which combines the improved access of existing WiCs with the general-purpose nature of GP and hospital outpatient services.

Extended role in PN and WiC nursing

The development and evolution of PN and WiC nursing as distinct disciplines has led inevitably to an expansion in nurses' scope of practice and responsibilities. Along with this naturally comes a demand for greater training and skills development. The implementation of legislation which has served to formalise the role of PGDs and independent nurse prescribers, in conjunction with the continued growth in PN, has led to substantial increases in demand for nurses with these skills. This growth in demand has been further fuelled by the NHS WiC initiative. Both PN and WiC nursing are a natural fit for PGD and/or independent prescribing skills.

The development of PGD skills amongst nurses is not, however, encouraged by the lack of a national model, leaving many decisions to the local Primary Care Trust (PCT). Principal amongst which are the basic PGD definitions, and in particular the PGD training requirements, which make PGD skills difficult to transfer from one PCT to another.

Less formal, but no less important for the development of nursing in the practice and WiC settings is improvement in patient first-contact and triage skills. These can be considered important sub-disciplines as well as advanced nursing skills, making them suitable areas for specialised training. However, the lack of such specialised training creates challenges for nurses to improve their skills in these areas. Informal learning from colleagues, seminars and conferences, and the professional literature are some of the ways in which PNs and WiC nurses make themselves more competent practitioners.

Conclusion

Changes in NHS policy led to the development of PN as a more formal distinct nursing sub-discipline. This led more or less directly to two related developments, the first being the implantation of nurse-led minor injury units within some A&E departments, and further to the development of the nurse-led WiCs. The WiC was intended to improve access to NHS, as well as to absorb some of the minor ailment workload from A&E departments, and improve the overall efficiency of the NHS. While there is some evidence that WiCs have improved access, there is no evidence that NHS efficiency has improved with their introduction.

The impact of the development of practice and WiC nursing on nursing skills has been very positive. This is despite certain difficulties such as a lack of national standardisation for PGDs and a lack of formal training for other advanced nursing skills like triage and first-contact.

The future of the WiC nurse, unlike that of the PN, is not assured. Changes in NHS policy, e.g. as a result of the report by Lord Darzi, may imply that the WiC becomes a more full-featured health service, but it also could be absorbed into a new structure yet to be defined.

References

Borkenhagen, R. (1988) Walk-in-clinics. Medical heresy or pragmatic reality? *Canadian Family Physician*, 42; 1879–1883.

DoH (1997) *The New NHS: Modern, Dependable*. London: DoH.

DoH (1999). *Up to £30 Million to Develop 20 NHS Fast Access Walk-in Centres*. Press release 1999/0226. London: DoH.

DoH (2001) *NHS Walk-in Centres – Questions and Answers* (online). DoH. http://www.doh.gov.uk/nhswalkincentres/questions.htm (accessed 21 March 2008).

DoH (2008) *High Quality Care for All: NHS Next Stage Review Final Report*. London: DoH.

Dolan, B. and Dale, J. (1997) Characteristics of self referred patients attending minor injury units. *Journal of Accident & Emergency Medicine*, 14; 212–214.

Drennan, V. and Goodman, C. (2007) *Oxford Handbook of Primary Care and Community Nursing*. Oxford: Oxford University Press.

Ham, C. (1992) *Health Policy in Britain*. 3rd edn. Basingstoke, Hampshire: MacMillan.

Hampson, G. (2002) *Practice Nurse Handbook*. 4th edn. Oxford: Blackwell Science.

Heaney, D. and Paxton, F. (1997) Evaluation of a nurse-led minor injuries unit. *Nursing Standard*, 12; 35–38.

Jones, R. and Menzies, S. (1999) *General Practice – Essential Facts*. Abingdon: Radcliffe Medical Press.

Kinnersley, P., Anderson, E. and Parry, K. (2000) Randomised controlled trial of nurse practitioner versus general practitioner care for patients requesting 'same day' consultations in primary care. *British Medical Journal*, 320; 1043–1048.

Lakhani, M. and Charlton, R. (2005) *Recent Advances in Primary Care*. London: Royal College of General Practitioners.

Luft, S. and Smith, M. (1994) *Nursing in General Practice. A Foundation Text*. London: Chapman and Hall.

Macdougald, N., King, P., Jones, A. and Eveleigh, M. (2001) *A Tool Kit for Practice Nurses*. Chichester: Aeneas.

Peckham, S. and Exworthy, M. (2003) *Primary Care in the UK. Policy Organisation and Management*. Basingstoke: Palgrave McMillan.

Robinson, F. (2007) A decade of change. *Practice Nurse*, 33(10); 11, 13.

Ross, F. and Mackenzie, A. (1996) *Nursing in Primary Health Care*. London and New York: Routledge.

Salisbury, C., Chalder, M., Manku-Scott, T., et al. (2002) *The National Evaluation of NHS Walk-in-Centres Final Report*. Bristol: University of Bristol.

Starfield, P. (1998) *Primary Care: Balancing Health Needs, Services and Technology*. New York: Oxford University Press.

Venning, P., Durie, A., Roland, M., Roberts, C. and Leese, B. (2000) Randomised controlled trial comparing cost effectiveness of general practitioners and nurse practitioners in primary care. *British Medical Journal*, 320; 1048–1053.

Watson, N. and Wilkinson, C. (2001) *Nursing in Primary Care. A Handbook for Students*. Basingstoke Hampshire: Palgrave.

Williams, A. (2000) *Nursing, Medicine and Primary Care*. Buckingham: Open University Press. www.nhs.uk (accessed 30 August 2008).

World Health Organization (1978) *Primary Health Care. Report of the International Conference on Primary Health Care*, Alma-Ata, USSR, 6–12 September (Health for All Series, No. 1). Geneva.

Practice nursing: the unique nature of practice nursing 2

Marie C. Hill

Introduction

The aim of this chapter is to explore the unique nature of practice nursing in the UK. The main areas of responsibility of the practice nurse (PN) will be critically explored, as well as other areas of responsibility that PNs undertake in the primary care setting. The influence of the new General Medical Services (new GMS) contract will be examined and how this has influenced the role of the PN will be discussed. After an in-depth review of the diversity of the PN role, there will be a critical discussion on how education and training needs to be centred on the service needs of a practice to meet this varied role of today's increasingly autonomous PN.

Learning Outcomes

- To identify and examine the diverse role of the PN
- To critically explore and evaluate how the new GMS contract has influenced and changed the role of the PN
- To appraise how education and training needs to be tailored to prepare the PN for their diverse role.

Background

Chapter 1 provided a framework on how these nursing groups have developed and how governmental health policies have been a catalyst for this change. A question the reader may ask is 'What is the role of the PN'? Hampson (2002:7) has described the title PN as generally applying 'to a qualified nurse employed directly by a general practitioner (GP) or by a GP partnership'. Whilst a vast majority of PNs are indeed direct employees of a GP or a GP partnership, some PNs are employed by Primary Care Organisations (PCO). This separates the majority of PNs in terms of their employer from other groups of Nurses and Specialist Community Public Health Nurses working in primary care, such as District Nurses, Health Visitors and School Nurses. In addition, GP employers of PNs adhere to UK employment law; thus, a PN's terms and conditions of employment may be different compared to their PCO-employed counterpart (Hill, 2006).

Drennan and Goodman (2007) have categorised the PN's main areas of responsibility as:

- audit, particularly relating to the Quality and Outcome Frameworks;
- child and adult immunisation, including catch-up programmes (e.g. *Haemophilus influenza* type B) and the influenza and pneumococcal programmes;
- chronic disease management, including asthma, chronic obstructive disease management, diabetes mellitus, hypothyroidism, heart failure and hypertension;
- clinical procedures, such as cerumen removal using either ear irrigation or (depending on the PN level of expertise) instrumentation;
- family planning, including cervical cytology;
- health promotion, providing smoking cessation services and running weight reduction clinics;
- minor surgery;
- new patient registration;
- travel health;
- wound care, for example, four-layer compression bandaging.

Other writers such as Hampson (2002) have considered the role of the PN to fall under a number of areas such as that of management, clinical, communication, audit and research.

- Management. This role includes day-to-day organisation of self and others, and ensuring that protocols are contemporary and reflect best evidence-based practice.
- Clinical. This role includes assessing patients' health needs and chronic disease management.
- Communication. This role includes counselling and health promotion, teaching patients and liaising with other members of the Primary Care Team.
- Audit and research. This role includes evaluating effectiveness of clinics and self-audit (e.g. assessing a PN's cervical cytology adequacy rate).

However, these lists are by no means exclusive. In Martin and Lucas' (2004) *Handbook of Practice Nursing*, the roles undertaken by the PN as well as some of those included in Hampson (2002) are expanded. See Table 2.1.

Macdougald et al. (2001) have commented on the fragmented role that many PNs have as their employing organisation dictates the services required. In a focused rapid review of the role and impact of the general PN and health care assistant (HCA) within general practice by Stafford University, there was conclusive evidence that PNs operate at different levels depending on their experience and

Table 2.1   The Role of the Practice Nurse

Health promotion and education	Breast screening
Disease management	Epilepsy Depression Arthritis Dermatology Anticoagulation monitoring User involvement in primary care
Health maintenance and clinical procedures	Clinical procedures Taking swabs Venepuncture Recording an electrocardiogram
Management and professional issues	Using information technology in primary care Accountability The law of negligence Consent Complaints Record keeping Employment issues Health and safety

Martin and Lucas (2004).

the needs of the practice (Longbottom et al., 2006). In addition to many of the roles identified by Hampson (2002) and Drennan and Goodman (2007), Longbottom et al. (2006) have added the administration and supervision of other staff such as HCAs.

What does the future hold for the PN role? It would seem that there is capacity for further growth. A review has suggested that up to 70% of the work undertaken by a GP might be undertaken by a PN. Furthermore, approximately 90% of all patient journeys commence and end in primary care (DoH, 2002). These factors alone have significant implications for the expansion of the PN role.

It can be argued that the role of the PN has changed since the new GMS contract was agreed by the UK Department of Health in April 2004 (Twomey and Pledger, 2008). The impact of the new GMS contract and how this has affected the day-to-day working life of the PN will be explored in detail in Chapter 15. Furthermore, the implementation of the new GMS contract has led to an increase in the number of PNs, making them the largest branch of primary care nurses (Macdougald et al., 2001). This role evolvement includes some PNs acquiring advanced skills in assessment, diagnosis and prescribing, whilst others have developed entrepreneurial skills and have become practice partners with their GP colleagues (Derrett and Burke, 2006). To understand this role change and evolvement, it is necessary to briefly explore the new GMS contract and how these changes have occurred and consequently affected the PN.

The GMS contract

Some of the key drivers for the new GMS contract were a national shortage of GPs and an ageing primary care workforce, one-third of the primary care nursing workforce being aged 50 years and over (Storey et al., 2007). According to the Royal College of Nursing (RCN) membership survey of 2002, whilst the nursing population is ageing, PNs have an increasingly older profile with almost half aged 45 years or more (RCN, 2004).

The new GMS contract came into effect on 1 April 2004 after a period of consultation between the NHS Confederation and the devolved administrations across the UK (White et al., 2004). The key features of the new GMS contract included that the contract would be more practice based, with greater control of the workload and funding arrangements (White et al., 2004). The new GMS contract has incorporated a new formula that is a radical departure from the traditional way in which GP practices have previously been funded (RCN, 2004). The focus has shifted away from the number of patients on a GP list to a framework that takes account of the health needs of patients, the practice workload and the quality of care provision. Practice has greater freedom to design services to meet the local population's needs (White et al., 2004). However, not all have welcomed the new GMS contract, which has been seen as divisive by some.

> The new contract imposes changes that will service to accelerate the fragmentation and privatisation of primary care and leave it open to commercial pressure in a manner unprecedented since the inception of the NHS in 1948. (Heath, 2004:320)

The contract provides not only financial security, in the form of a minimum practice income guarantee (i.e. the provision of essential services), but also practices with the opportunity to generate additional income by delivering additional services and enhanced services. The 'needs-based' formula has been developed to ensure that funding is no longer based simply on the number of GPs within a practice. Instead, allocation is founded on local patient needs and practice workload. Resources are made available whether or not a GP is in post, as long as the agreed range of services continues to be provided. Therefore, this opens a window of opportunity for PNs to provide these services, if, for example, some practices decide to opt out of providing certain services. However, this would not apply to services that fall into the essential category.

Practice nursing: a roller-coaster ride

The new and challenging environment of practice nursing can be both exciting and daunting for the new PN. This is regardless of the level of expertise that the nurse has had previously. Many PNs come from an acute background and with expertise in their area of practice. It can be argued that many skills are transferable (e.g. clinical skills and chronic disease management). Initially, the diversity of the role of a PN can be overwhelming for a practitioner new to this area, for example, critically understanding and applying to practice the UK childhood immunisation schedule. The previous 'expert nurse' now becomes a 'novice'. Benner (2001) has explored the different levels of nursing expertise from novice to expert. Benner (2001:31–32) defines the expert nurse as a practitioner not reliant on rules or guidelines (e.g. analytical principles) to connect 'her understanding of the situation to an appropriate action. The expert nurse, with an enormous background of experience, now has an intuitive grasp of each situation and zeros in on the accurate region of the problem without wasteful consideration of a large range of unfruitful, alternative diagnoses and solutions'. A clear example of this role transition relating to a perceived greater autonomy and accountability in practice is given by a newly employed PN.

> While, in essence, the principle of accountability should be the same wherever you work within healthcare, it certainly feels different in primary care. I have always been aware of my own professional accountability and responsibility, but within the acute sector it feels like there are more people around to ask for advice and you are more likely to be working within a team. It is therefore easy to feel like the responsibility is shared. That isn't to say that I have no one to approach for help in the surgery where I work, but it's harder to interrupt people when they are with a patient. Not only that, but coming from a more specialised area (post-operative care) which I knew very well, the transition to primary care has, at times, been hard. This is particularly the case because I had been out of clinical nursing for two years beforehand and was 'out of practice'.
>
> Practice-nursing is an extremely varied role which means that you need to develop a sound knowledge-base in a wide number of different areas and it can therefore take some time to feel both competent and confident. It is a much more autonomous role which, although there are protocols for everything, can feel daunting at first. It is just you and your patient and, ultimately, you are responsible for all the decisions you make and are accountable for all your actions. I have never been more aware of this and the importance of knowing your own limitations than I am now. It can be difficult to admit if you are unsure about something, both to your colleagues and your patients, but the ability to do this is essential in such an autonomous role.
>
> My transition to practice-nursing has been a rollercoaster of sorts. I believe that practice-nursing is the way forward and there is so much scope to develop your knowledge and skills and influence public health. There are so many opportunities. I started on a real high but experienced quite a dip when I realised how much there is to learn and how important your own accountability is. I think it is normal to experience a certain lack of confidence for a while and this can be a bit scary when you are used to knowing your area and you realise how accountable you are. The importance of documentation has, for example, been emphasised strongly to me. However, I'm now on the upward climb again. I am lucky to be working in a place where I am being offered

training left, right and centre. It has been a bit overwhelming at times but I feel invested in and this gives me confidence. (Rebecca Cosgrave, PN in London).

Education and training: are today's PNs equipped for their role in primary care?

This chapter has explored the multifaceted role of the PN in the primary care setting. A question for both employers and Higher Education Institutions (HEIs) is how this diverse role can be supported in terms of education and training to develop a nursing force that is fit for purpose. At present, there is no nationally recognised qualification to prepare PNs for their unique role. However, there are training programmes available from module to degree level throughout the UK, which have responded to local need for training, rather than developing nationally (Longbottom et al., 2006). This has implications for PNs entering the new environment of practice nursing, as some PNs will be more supported to develop their role and the transition to working within a primary care setting in comparison to others where educational initiatives are not so developed.

Although PNs along with other nurses, midwives and specialist community public health nurses are clearly professionally accountable for their nursing practice as per guidance from their regulatory body, which is the Nursing and Midwifery Council (NMC, 2008), they are accountable and managerially responsible to their GP employers. Here lies the quandary: although regulation meets one of the tenets of being affiliated to a professional group, many nurses are professionally accountable to another professional group (i.e. the medical profession).

The NMC (2008) provides clear guidance for each nurse, midwife and specialist community public health nurse (hereafter referred to collectively as practitioners) on the standards that are expected with regard to a range of areas such as respecting clients as individuals and ensuring training is up to date and evidence based. The aforementioned list is by no means exhaustive (NMC, 2008). Furthermore, the NMC (2008) emphasises the responsibility of practitioners to ensure that education and training needs are both appropriate and specific to the task and/or clinical area being undertaken.

You must have the knowledge and skills for safe and effective practice when working without direct supervision. . . . You must keep your knowledge and skills up to date throughout your working life. You must take part in appropriate learning and practice activities that maintain and develop your competence and performance. (NMC, 2008:7)

However, in a recent commentary by Young (2008) '*Incompetence and empty pockets: all in a day's work*', it is indicated that a significant number of PNs report that they are asked by their employers to carry out procedures which they feel incompetent to perform. Clearly, this practice is unacceptable for both the practitioner who agrees to undertake such procedures and the employer, as it contravenes

The Code (Standards of Conduct, Performance and Ethics for Nurses and Midwives) (NMC, 2008) in which it is stated: 'You must take part in appropriate learning and practice activities that maintain and develop your competence and performance' (NMC, 2008:4). In addition, the safety of the client is in jeopardy. These PNs may have a criminal charge brought against them for negligence, as well as their employer who would be vicariously liable for this practice. Questions could be raised on the validity of the consent (written or verbal) that a client had given. A PN must be aware of the implications of The Mental Capacity Act 2005 (Cressey, 2008), which came into full effect from October 2007, as this has raised important factors related to obtaining consent. These are whether a client can understand the information given to them, retain the information from the health care provider long enough to make an informed decision, evaluate the information to make a decision and finally communicate their decision (Cressey, 2008). Indeed, how could a client give valid consent if the PN undertaking the procedure was incompetent to perform such a task? This certainly questions whether the employers or the PNs in the Young (2008) commentary fully comprehend the significant legal implications of their uninformed decision-making.

Longbottom et al. (2006) undertook a review of the role and impact of the general PN and the HCA within general practice. The summary of their findings with the involvement of employing organisations and HEIs in the training and development of PNs and HCA is as follows:

- Access to training and education for general PNs and HCAs varies across the country.
- HCAs have difficulty in accessing National Vocational Qualification (NVQ) courses that provide the appropriate mix of units for general practice.
- Some Primary Care Trusts (PCTs) have developed their own assessment centres or agreed with local training providers such as Further Education (FE) colleges' common units for HCAs in general practice to undertake.
- Commitment to the delivery of training by PCTs varies across the country.
- Evidence from the application forms shows that practices value support from PCTs that take an active role in the commissioning, design and delivery of education and training for nurses and HCAs in general medical practice.
- Development of a PN 'bank' in one PCT allows for backfill, freeing PNs to attend training.
- There are no set educational requirements for nurses in general practice. Each HEI develops courses according to demonstrated needs, for example, introduction to practice nursing, in accordance with professional body guidance.
- There are certain courses that are recognised nationally for specific disease processes such as the Warwick course for diabetes.
- Access to funding for courses varies across the country.
- Funding for training is included within the global sum for general practice.
- Central funding for non-professionally qualified staff (NHS Learning Accounts) has now stopped.
- In-house training accounts for a large part of personal and professional development that takes place (Longbottom et al., 2006:10).

PNs are professionally responsible to ensure that they are fit for the purpose of their role, along with other practitioners. This is a mandatory requirement of the nursing and midwifery regulatory body (NMC, 2008). However, it would seem from the Longbottom et al. (2006) review that educational opportunities to develop the PN role are fragmented in some areas and certainly more robust in others. One of the principle findings of this paper was the development of education and training for PNs that had been driven by local service needs. A local initiative for PN development was undertaken by the author in 2001. In 2000, three local PCTs approached City University London to develop a stand-alone introductory module for newly employed PNs. This module is still available at degree level, with an award of 15 credits on successful completion of a 3,000-word assignment.

The emphasis from the PCTs, prior to 2001, was that the module must be flexible so that it could be delivered either on site of the commissioning PCT or on site in City University London. Another key requisite was that the module would be available throughout the year, rather than fitting into a semester pattern. The principal aim was that newly employed PNs would be able to access this module – ideally as soon as employed, thus ensuring that they were exposed to relevant theory in order to apply this theory to their new clinical environment.

The challenge for the author and indeed for the educational commissioners of the PCTs was designing a module for newly employed PNs, considering the diversity of this role. There was agreement that the four-day module would be clinically focused on the following topics: immunisation programmes, dealing with unknown immunisation histories, managing and treating anaphylaxis, an introduction to travel health, ear care (including ear examination and ear irrigation), assessment guidelines and the implementation of theory to the new practice setting. In addition to the theoretical input, a 12-chapter pack was developed on a range of topics, some of which supported the taught element of this module, whilst others covered areas such as health policy relating to the role of practice nursing to employment law (Hill, 2006). The author's vision was that a new PN development would be moulded by the specific service needs of the practice (e.g. chronic disease management) and that the local HEI would meet the educational needs for this. However, it can be argued that national drivers (i.e. the new GMS contract) would constitute a driver for HEI to develop educational programmes, be it at a module or at degree programme level for their PNs. A key assumption here was that employers would support their employees to have a lengthy period of training, such as a degree programme, when the main emphasis for the providers would be on service delivery and improving access to services. Therefore, a newly employed PN must be mindful and adhere to their regulatory board's guidance that: 'As a Professional, you are personally accountable for actions and omissions in your practice and must always be able to justify your decisions' (NMC, 2008:1). However, with the diversity of the PN role as identified at the beginning of this chapter, it may be difficult for some PNs to be even aware of what education and training they require to develop into their new role. Nevertheless, the onus of professional responsibility to develop competence in practice ultimately lies with the PN.

Young (2008) argues that nurses (i.e. PNs) are key to the success of general practice and should be both encouraged and enabled to receive the requisite training and education. A philosophy such as a supportive and enabling environment will assist and promote development of competence and retention of staff. The findings of Longbottom et al. (2006) have revealed that there is variability in the provision of education for PNs across the country. Therefore, it could be argued that there seems to be a postcode lottery system in operation where PNs in one area would be more educationally supported than those in others. In response to the new GMS contract, a programme was developed in 2004 to support general practice. The launch of the Working in Partnership Programme (WiPP) was developed to support general practice with capacity-building resources and strategies. The WiPP designed, developed, tested and delivered a range of tools, working in collaboration with NHS and lay organisations (www.wipp.nhs.uk; WIPP, 2008).

The WiPP programme which concluded in 2008 consisted of 13 initiatives. Key to the development of these initiatives was the input of the Working in Partnership Programme Advisory Group (WiPPAG). The constituents of the WiPPAG were diverse with representation from the Department of Health, the British Medical Association, NHS Direct, the RCN and The Patients Association (www.wipp.nhs.uk, 2008). One of the 13 initiatives of the WiPPs was the General Practice Nursing Toolkit which set out to develop a range of core principles to support the PN. The Toolkit was developed around a number of key areas such as:

- employment practice;
- education and professional development;
- competence;
- integration with the wider community health care workforce;
- career development;
- quality improvement and evaluating practice.

The Toolkit explored each of the areas described above from a variety of perspectives, such as those of a PN, an employer, a PCT, a patient or an educational provider. Each section included tools that could be downloaded to provide practical help towards improving practice. A key drive for this development was to improve standards across England and diminish anomalies in roles, skills and remuneration in general practice nursing. One of its central aims was to ensure that support for general practice became embedded into primary care and that the initiatives of the WiPP continue. Herein lies the question: will these initiatives such as the General Practice Nursing Toolkit continue, taking into consideration that the Toolkit was developed to support PN in England solely? Another issue for consideration is that general practices can opt out of such initiatives, as these are not mandatory.

Carpe Diem

The role of the PN is expanding in tandem with the expansion of primary care. Certainly, this is reflected in the growing numbers of PNs and the reported job satisfaction of many PNs (Young, 2008). There are increasing opportunities for PNs to professionally develop their practice through relevant education and training. However, as noted, there is a disparity on how some PNs can access educational opportunities. However, PNs have the opportunity to 'seize the day' in proactively providing services that are relevant to their practice populations. Practice-based commissioning (PBC) has been defined as commissioning that takes place locally for practice populations to ensure that services provided meet the needs of the population (Sawbridge, 2007). Of course, PBC is not solely the premise of the PN, as this process is intended to be multidisciplinary. Nevertheless, it raises the issue of how important the role of the PN could be in commissioning local services.

Conclusion

The number of PNs has risen meteorically since 1990 due to changes in governmental health policy and the way primary care services are funded. Governmental health policies have driven changes in primary care, more recently with the new GMS contract. The role of PNs has expanded to meet the diverse and challenging health needs within primary care. It has been noted that the role of PNs will continue to evolve and change due to the expansion of the Quality and Outcome Framework. Threats exist for some PNs due to the lack and/or reduced educational opportunities in some areas, leading to some PNs not being 'fit for practice'. This has serious implications for both patient safety and the professional accountability of the PN. Therefore, education and training are essential for PNs to 'seize the day' and make a difference in today's health economy.

References

Benner, P. (2001) *From Novice to Expert: Excellence and Power in Clinical Nursing Practice*. Upper Saddle River, NJ: Prentice Hall Health.

Cressey, S. (2008) Understanding consent. *Practice Nurse*, 35(2); 38–41.

Derrett, C. and Burke, L. (2006) The future of primary care nurses and health visitors. *British Medical Journal*, 331(December); 1185–1186.

DoH (2002) *Liberating the Talents: Helping Primary Care Trusts and Nurses deliver the NHS Plan*. London: Department of Health.

Drennan, V. and Goodman, C. (2007) *Oxford Handbook of Primary Care and Community Nursing*. Oxford: Oxford University Press.

Hampson, G. (2002) *Practice Nurse Handbook*. 4th edn. Oxford: Blackwell Science.

Heath, I. (2004) The cawing of the crow . . . Cassandra-like, prognosticating woe. *British Journal of General Practice*, 54(501); 320–321.

Hill, M. (2006) *The Practice Nurse Distance Learning Programme*. 3rd edn. London: St. Bartholomew School of Nursing and Midwifery, City University.

Longbottom, A., Chambers, D., Rebora, C. and Brown, A. (2006) *A Focused Rapid Review of the Role and Impact of the General Practice Nurse and Health Care Assistant within General Practice*. Staffordshire: Staffordshire University.

Macdougald, N., King, P., Jones, A. and Eveleigh, M. (2001) *A Tool Kit for Practice Nurses*. Chichester: AENEAS.

Martin, J. and Lucas, J. (2004) *Handbook of Practice Nursing*. 3rd edn. Edinburgh: Churchill Livingstone.

NMC (2008) *The Code. Standards of Conduct, Performance and Ethics for Nurses and Midwives*. London: Nursing and Midwifery Council.

RCN (2004) *Nurses employed by GPs. RCN Guidance on Good Employment Practice*. London: Royal College of Nursing.

Sawbridge, Y. (2007) Getting to grips with practice based commissioning. *Nursing Management*, 14(4); 14–15.

Storey, C., Ford, J., Cheater, F., Hurst, K. and Leese, B. (2007) Nurses working in primary and community care settings in England: Problems and challenges in identifying numbers. *Journal of Nursing Management*, 15(8); 847–852.

Twomey, P. and Pledger, D. (2008) Different DCCT-aligned HbA1c methods and the GMS contract. *International Journal of Clinical Practice*, 62(2); 202–205.

White, E., Singer, R. and McQuarrie, R. (2004) An opportunity for community nurses? *Community Practitioner*, 77(4); 129–130.

WIPP (2008) http://www.wipp.nhs.uk/about-us/AboutWipp (accessed 17 February 2008).

Young, L. (2008) Incompetence and empty pockets: All in a day's work. *British Journal of Nursing*, 17(1); 6.

Walk-in-centre nursing: the unique nature of walk-in-centre practice

3

Jane Bickerton

Introduction

The aim of this chapter is to explore the nature of nursing in a National Health Service (NHS) walk-in-centre (WiC) and its relation to first contact primary urgent care nursing in the UK. The chapter will explore the main areas of responsibilities of the WiC practitioner, as well as the role of management in a nurse-led service. WiCs over the past decade have offered a unique opportunity for experienced nurses to develop clinical skills for the completion of a complete episode of patient care, including diagnosis and treatment. In the primary care setting, this opportunity was previously associated with general practitioners (GPs). A nurse-led setting also provides an opportunity to develop leadership skills along with clinical skills in corporate management. The educational and training needs of nurses in this context will be discussed and, after an overview of the WiC nurse alongside the first contact practitioner in the urgent care, the chapter will consider if these services are meeting goals set by an NHS patient-led service.

Learning Outcomes

- To identify and examine the role of the WiC nurse
- To critically explore and evaluate how the role of the WiC nurse is being influenced by the changing primary urgent care environment
- To examine educational and training needs for WiC nurses developing autonomous primary care practitioners' skills in practice
- To explore professional issues concerning corporate leadership and management in a nurse-led service
- To consider patient-led NHS consumers and their evaluations of health care in the nurse-led WiC setting.

Background

NHS WiCs were set up as nurse-led primary care health services at the beginning of the millennium to complement GP primary care services. Nearly a decade on there has been a rapid expansion of WiCs that have become part of a growing variety of primary care and first contact services for health care that are an alternative form of care from the GP general practice. A single WiC provides more than 36,000 consultations each year (DoH, 2006a).

When WiCs first opened in 2000, the aim was to provide primary care to health consumers whose lifestyles prevented them from easy access to a GP near their home. Nine WiCs opened in London and they included free-standing community-based centres such as Soho WiC, hospital-based WiCs where there were no Accident and Emergency (A&E) Departments such as Barnet, London, and hospital-based WiCs co-joined with A&E such as Whitechapel, London. More recently, walk-in commuter clinics have opened, operated by private firms such as Liverpool Street, London, and nurse-led Primary Urgent Care Centres (PUCC) such as Homerton, Hackney, based in Emergency Departments. The next wave of WiCs can be expected to be based in the planned GP-led polyclinics in London (Darzi, 2007).

What is the clinical role of the nurse in the WiC setting?

The first national evaluation of WiC (Salisbury et al., 2002) found WiC nurses had a diverse profile of skills and abilities and that clinical skills needed for WiCs and first contact care depended on local needs for the area. The nursing role extended from treating primary care minor injuries to minor ailments offering treatment, as well as health and education and, if necessary, referring on to other services. The Department of Health required nurses to complete episodes of first contact care that included 'acute assessment, diagnosis, treatment, discharge and/or referral' (DoH, 2002:8). This meant in reality that in some WiCs, clinicians needed more clinical skills than the following (NHS, 2008):

- blood pressure checks;
- contraceptive advice;
- coughs, colds and 'flu-like' symptoms;
- dressing care;
- emergency contraception;
- hay fever, bites and stings;
- health promotion: diet and exercise;
- information on staying healthy/local services;
- minor cuts and wounds – care and dressings;
- muscle and joint injuries – strains and sprains;
- skin complaints – rashes, sunburn and head lice;
- smoking cessation support;
- stomach ache, indigestion, constipation, vomiting and diarrhoea;

- suturing (stitching);
- women's health problems, for example, thrush and menstrual advice.

Although minor ailments and injuries are listed as the normal case load for the WiC nurse, the nurses may also need competence in other health areas. Some WiCs expect nurses to see and treat children as part of their local patient directive and to be knowledgeable about children's health and development as well as protection issues. At some sites minor injuries may be seen by an adjacent Minor Injuries Unit (MIUs), whereas at others nurses have the clinical knowledge and may be able to provide services such as reading X-rays and suturing. The nurse must always be ready to identify the patient with more severe or multiple health problems (Rosen and Mountford, 2002). At the very least, nurses need to be competent to identify signs and symptoms of 'red flags' that require immediate referral to A&E such as meningitis, appendicitis, pelvic inflammatory disease (PID), myocardial infarction (MI) and transient ischaemic attacks (TIAs).

These health presentations emphasise the importance of critical thinking skills for the first contact nurse. But for nurses working in the WiC environment, this does not necessarily equate with advanced practitioner education as the management 'cannot afford to send nurses on a two and a half year nurse practitioner course. There would be no one left to run the service' (Hatchett, 2003:32). It is arguable, however, that where nurses are completing episodes of care, they should meet or be working towards meeting most if not all of the advanced nurse practitioner (ANP) competencies outlined by the Royal College of Nursing (RCN, 2008). To accomplish this without the combination of a formal education and practice-based learning is challenging because the scope of practice for a practitioner providing first contact care is broad and demanding.

A study carried out in acute and primary care trusts in the north-east of London found that many of the health consumers attending a WiC believed their health complaint to be an emergency (Procter et al., 2008). The first contact practitioner is required to calculate the health risk of a client's reported emergency and identify 'red flags'. In this way, they are able to differentiate between signs and symptoms that they are able to diagnose safely and those that they need to refer on to specialty services and/or emergency care. Thus, in order to complete an episode of care, a practitioner needs clinical skills outlined by the Nursing and Midwifery Council (NMC, 2006; RCN, 2008) and that includes the ability to undertake the following tasks:

- Take a comprehensive patient history and carry out physical examinations;
- Use expert knowledge and clinical judgement to decide whether to refer patients for investigations and make diagnoses;
- Decide on and carry out treatment, including the prescribing of medicines, or refer patients to an appropriate specialist;
- Use their extensive practice experience to plan and provide skilled and competent care to meet patients' health and social care needs, involving other members of the health care team as appropriate;
- Ensure the provision of continuity of care including follow-up visits;

- Assess and evaluate, with patients, the effectiveness of the treatment and care provided and make changes as needed;
- Work independently, although often as part of a health care team that they will lead;
- Make sure, as a leader of the team, that each patient's treatment and care is based on best practice.

The unprecedented expansion of the non-medical autonomous practitioner in the UK over the past decade has meant that training and development of autonomous nursing practice has not necessarily kept pace with the competencies and required standards. In fact, a review of the literature examining the substitution of doctors by nurses found that, although appropriately trained nurses do provide a high standard of care, there is no agreement on the level of training nurses should receive. Experienc ed nurses, such as health visitors (HVs) and midwives, although trained to a high standard in their own area of expertise, do not necessarily have the competencies relevant to first contact practice (Laurant et al., 2005), as the Association of Advancing Nursing Practice Educators (AANPE) highlight in their assessment of nurses studying advanced nursing skills:

> . . . that, whilst they are experienced nurses, they also have significant learning needs. As they progress through the course they broaden and deepen their knowledge and experience and so become aware of the depth and breadth of patient's social holism, pathology, presenting symptoms and clinical care management needs. (AANPE, 2008:7)

However, where these experienced nurses have access to experienced ANPs and GPs for training and development, their knowledge enables them to acquire clinical skills more readily than less qualified nurses as they usually already fulfil some of the domains of practice for ANPs listed as follows (AANPE, 2008; RCN, 2008):

- assessment and management of patient health/illness status;
- the nurse/patient relationship;
- the education function;
- professional role;
- managing and negotiating health care delivery systems;
- monitoring and ensuring the quality of advanced health care practice;
- respecting culture and diversity.

These domains of practice (RCN, 2008) are related to the Knowledge and Skills Framework (KSF). Managers are asked to include no more than four specific dimensions of practice with the six core components. The four specific dimensions chosen will vary from service to service but will usually include Health and Wellbeing (HWB) six and seven at level four and one at level 3, General (G) two at level four and Information and Knowledge (IK) three at level four. Advanced practice nurses (PNs) are expected to work at level four for all the core dimensions except for service improvement which is required at level three. The domains of practice for the advanced practitioner include all but HWB nine at level four, G1 at level descriptor three and G2 at level descriptor four. The IK dimensions at IK1 and 2 at level three and IK3 at level four are included.

As early as 2002, nurses in WiCs were asked to identify challenges in the WiC setting for their practice and they highlighted two in particular:

> . . . first, the requirement to combine clinical assessment – a core part of the nursing role – with diagnosis and formation of a treatment and management plan, and secondly, the diversity of the patient case-mix in walk-in centres. (Rosen and Mountford, 2002:243)

'Nurses are trained to listen and be with patients as they empathetically and caringly are making sense of a patient's life' (Schickler, 2004:184). However, because until recently, advanced nursing practice skills were GP skills, a core training programme has been needed for first contact and WiC nurses across the NHS in order to learn these skills.

Communication interactions

Interactions between practitioners and health consumers in the first contact and WiC environment are qualitatively different from those in the primary care GP practice setting. Practitioners do not have access to previous history on clients and clients are attending because in many cases they consider their problem an emergency and do not have ready access to their GP. Clients want the condition resolved, for example, through a prescription, reassurance and advice or a specialist referral (Procter et al., 2008).

Patients expect a different experience with a nurse from other health professionals. Research identified nurses' communication skills as tending to be mediated by patients' contributions and explanations and found the consultation interaction began from the viewpoint of a patient's responsibility and behaviour (Collins and Britten, 2006). Collins and Britten (2006) found that doctors tend to take a biomedical intervention approach providing an overarching point of view to consultation interactions and that allied health professionals (AHPs) have good listening skills. Research examining different nurse practitioners' (NPs') consultation styles in the WiC environment found that NPs adapt their consultation styles to help resolve tensions between a patient's reasons for attending the WiC and their clinical assessment outcomes, and that these styles were influenced by five patient presentation styles (Barratt, 2005), namely:

■ seeking treatment;
■ presenting clinical histories;
■ checking severity of illnesses;
■ patients who initially seek treatment but change to a confirmatory style;
■ patients who anticipate their need for treatment.

A WiC consultation presents its own unique problems as the consultation is expected to take place between two people meeting for the first time. The nurse is without any documentation of the patient's previous medical history and is dependent on the information shared by the patient in this patient-led relationship. The RCN Nurse Practitioner Association (NPA) in 2006 found that 1 in 20 NPs work in WiCs. Their research identified NPs as typically highly qualified with nearly three-quarters (72%) holding a degree and a further 10% currently studying for one and that in 35% of cases study is at master's level (Ball, 2006). However, there is no official number of qualified NPs in the UK. Mike Walsh, a board member for the AANPE at the AANPE 2008 conference, reported that a survey sent to its members identified approximately 3,000 qualified NPs in the UK.

In primary care and GP practices when the nurse provides first contact consultations, the patient's records would normally be available. Nurses in the urgent care GP practice role may be qualified NPs with perhaps a master's level advanced practice qualification (ANP qualification). There are, however, far fewer master's level nurses working in the WiC setting. As yet, the NP role in the UK is not formally protected (AANPE, 2008) and so WiC nurses calling themselves NPs, with considerable nursing experience and often qualified in other specialist fields such as District Nursing, Midwifery and Health Visiting, are expanding their primary care clinical practice through embedded practice-based learning and continuing practice development outside an academic advanced nurse practice programme.

Promoting health and well-being in a WiC setting

An important part of any health consultation is the promotion of health and practitioners look for ways to encourage well-being while respecting culture and diversity. WiC patient populations are often at risk for problems associated with smoking (e.g., mouth cancer) obesity, diabetes mellitus, hypertension and heart disease (Salisbury et al., 2002). WiC nurses find creative ways to include health messages in culturally appropriate patient-centred ways within the consultation as well as sharing health and well-being messages through the provisions of smoking cessation sessions, the supply of condoms and emergency contraception, blood pressure, diabetes mellitus and lipid checks.

WiC nurses have considerable experience in many nursing specialities such as Midwifery, District Nursing, A&E Nursing, Health Visiting and Mental Health (Gallacher and Garlick, 2008). This provides many opportunities for collaboration between nurses when diagnosing and treating some of the common health presentations related to mental health, reproductive and sexual health, child health, child protection, domestic violence, etc. Clinical skills in these areas are essential as are clinical management skills, knowledge regarding health issues common to refugees and immigrants, as well as self-limiting minor illnesses and injuries and self-care.

Clinical decision-making support

When WiCs first opened in 2000, they used NHS Direct clinical decision support software (Hanlon et al., 2005). This software was developed by Stanford

University in the USA and was algorithmic rather than protocol driven. The NHS had full control over the clinical content and it was regularly updated. It provided clinical support to WiC nurse clinicians, but had no diagnostic component. However, it was a useful aid to help novice nurses consider aspects of the subjective history that might raise concern over medical history and a 'red flag' to discuss the case with a more advanced practitioner colleague. This software has since been removed in most English WiCs because, as more nurses developed first contact competencies, the decision software was used less. Today more on-line websites are used by nurses such as NICE (NHS, 2008) and Patient UK (EMIS and PIP, 2008), but none of these sites provide the same step-by-step algorithmic learning process of the Clinical Assessment System (CAS) from AXA.

Non-medical prescribers

WiCs usually have their own trust protocols that are used for prescriptions supplied under Patient Group Directions (PGDs) and/or guidelines that provide the steps needed to deliver care or treatment. These PGDs are prescriptive and so do not always give the practitioner the opportunity to be patient centred when they prescribe medicine. Trusts develop integrated care pathways (ICP) (NLH, 2008) that embed these guidelines, protocols and local evidence-based practice. Often clinical books and references used by GPs prove as useful as any for the NP working in the first contact environment.

A recent change in UK legislation has meant that nurses, AHPs and health scientists can qualify as non-medical prescribers. This means that non-medical practitioners now have the possibility to provide prescriptions and pharmaceuticals, previously only available through GPs (DoH, 2006a,b). Qualified nurses and pharmacists are able to prescribe as independent prescribers from all of the British National Formulary (BNF, 2008) and physiotherapists, chiropodists/podiatrists and radiographers as supplementary prescribers are able to prescribe medicines using management plans agreed in partnership with a physician. The ability to prescribe is far less prescriptive for non-medical prescribers than supplying medicines under PGDs and allows for more appropriate patient-centred concordant care (Haynes, 2002). This is evident from the following comment:

> As a qualified NP I found the PGDs incredibly restrictive, and felt this encouraged employment of GPs just to be there to sign prescriptions. Nurse prescribing streamlined the whole process for me enabling more efficient use of my time and knowledge and experience. (Siobhan Hicks, NP)

Autonomous practice and completing episodes of care with prescribing has led to concerns amongst NPs about possible negligence claims. NHS Trusts cover nurses through their indemnity insurance as long as nurses work within the job description requirements as the RCN states 'it is generally the employer who is sued if things go wrong and that an organisation usually provides full indemnity' (RCN, 2008:6).

Clinical supervision

Clinical supervision is an essential component of nursing practice when nurses are extending and developing new roles, especially as first contact nurses are often working under considerable stress. Clinical supervision as described by Proctor (1986) is divided into three distinct areas related to practice that include:

- The formative educative process of developing skills is provided through university education and clinical days.
- The normative development of competent practice occurs through the internalisation of clinical practice in work-based learning.
- The restorative supportive help for professionals working constantly with stress and distress is usually provided through individual or group clinical supervision where issues are shared in confidence.

The WiC training and development budgets have been generous. It is not only NHS WiCs, but also privately owned WiCs that have access to funding sources for clinical supervision and education. The formative and normative clinical supervision can be covered through formal university education integrated with practice-based learning. Restorative supervision is usually provided in house and is essential in the WiC learning environment.

Educating nurses in a WiC

There is no national model of training for WiC nurses, and this means that in practice each centre develops its own unique training package. Some WiCs develop their programmes in tandem with local universities such as Nottingham WiC with Trent Deanery (Nottingham NHS PCT, 2008) and Whitechapel WiC with City University London (City University London, 2004). City University London in partnership with the North East London Strategic Health Authority (Abbott et al., 2004) went as far as to map skills required for the WiC practitioner against education offered in London. The domains of practice used to map the skills included the following individual areas:

- leadership and management;
- clinical background knowledge;
- consultations;
- management of self-limiting conditions and non-life-threatening conditions;
- management of different patients' groups/specialist areas;
- out-of-hour's service provision.

These domains of practice consider practical aspects of WiC nursing care and differ from the ANP competencies. Gallagher and Garlick (2006) developed a three-tier model for unscheduled care training in Lothian and emphasised that new competences and learning were required by all nurses at all three levels of unscheduled care skills. They found nursing competencies that were transferable to unscheduled care from the competencies of the PN and district nurse (DN) at level one, but that necessary competencies were lacking. Gallagher and Garlick (2006:5) view their framework as a way to offer nurses a 'career pathway through levels one to three whilst developing a high level of knowledge and skills'. The three levels they outline are:

- level 1 – a practitioner working under supervision;
- level 2 – a practitioner working with clinical decision-making support;
- level 3 – ANP.

There are courses available all over the UK that meet the requirements of a first-level practitioner working in a WiC setting. Most courses can be taken as individual modules or as part of a broader programme. The first contact course at City University London offers training for the novice first contact clinician and provides 30 level 3 credits (City University London, 2004) and is included as the first successful step on a three-level skills escalator programme using Benner (2001) to differentiate nursing competencies from the novice, proficient and ANP (NELSHA, 2005; NMC, 2006). The following sections differentiate the three different levels.

The novice urgent care practitioner

The novice urgent care practitioner is taught through structured university education dovetailed with structured practice-based learning. The novice first contact practitioner is expected to take from nine months to a year to complete successfully the first contact course that includes physical assessment, biological foundations as well as mentored practice. The WiC provides embedded training through individualised induction, mandatory training, a personal development plan and essential competencies.

As a WiC nurse describes:

> I have been working at the walk-in-centre for just over a year now. Prior to this I was nursing predominantly in a variety of acute medical wards, having qualified 35 years ago. During the last year I have gone through the steepest learning curve I can remember and I am still climbing! The transition from secondary to primary care has been facilitated through completion of the first contact course; work based shadowing and supervised practice, together with private study. More recently giving case presentations and receiving, regular teaching sessions from nurse practitioners and medical colleagues have all contributed towards developing my ability to work autonomously. Although many of the conditions patients present with have similarities, there is a constant need to be alert, for the sometimes more subtle and possibly more serious diagnosis. This requires ongoing reflection during practice and constant updating of my knowledge and skills. (Liz Annun, WiC nurse)

The novice practitioner works with a mentor, attends case presentations and shadows ANPs and GPs as well as attends clinical away days. Clinical supervision and mentorship are essential components of this learning process. The importance of communication skills, understanding of the nursing role as well as the ethical and legal implications when working in a nurse-led service, such as a MIU, cannot be underestimated when trying to develop and implement changes in clinical practice (Gledhill, 2003).

Proficient urgent care practitioner

The second level of training in a WiC is usually based on nursing needs. The nurse develops practice through practice-based and embedded learning. The nurse identifies along with their mentor as well as through clinical supervision areas of development. Nurses may choose to extend their knowledge and study advanced health assessment and extend their paediatrics knowledge. One-day master classes on respiratory, cardiac, abdominal and ear, nose and throat (ENT) systems offered by Practitioner Development UK Ltd. and Practitioner Associates Ltd. provide the appropriate level of skills. Nurses often begin to enquire about taking the independent prescriber qualification at this stage.

Nurses may attend an ANP programme. A typical programme takes two years part time and is intensive, so nurses working full time in practice often find they take longer than the two-year period. There are many programmes run in the UK that are delivered by a number of Higher Education Institutions. The majority of nurse academics involved in the design of these programmes are members of the AANPE, with some programmes accredited by the RCN.

Primary care ANP

As an ANP, a nurse consolidates coursework in practice and takes continuing education courses to maintain and extend clinical skills. Whereas the ANP course focuses on providing the nurse with knowledge of the well person, in practice the nurse will begin to distinguish clearly between health, illness and disease.

Educational provision in a WiC setting can be provided through the skills escalator approach, beginning with knowledge and clinical skills appropriate for a novice first contact nurse developing their clinical skills and competencies to the level of expert practitioner through competency standards outlined in the KSF (DoH, 2004; RCN, 2008).

Future education

Daly and Carnwell (2003:158) state that: 'Nursing practice is becoming more diverse than ever before and the boundaries of inter and intra-professional practices are becoming increasingly blurred'.

In the future, WiC training might be expected to start with pre-registration training on the first contact access and urgent care pathway described in *Modernising Nursing Careers: Setting the Direction Consultation* (DoH, 2007a) with nurses developing their skills further with post-registration training. With the introduction of KSF (DoH, 2004), the NHS is now able to compare competencies across professions with the result that in the future a health consumer might realistically expect to experience greater professional skill mix in the first contact care working environment (DoH, 2004). The AANPE has already compared other professional competencies against ANP competencies and there are some professional titles where it does find substantial overlap. The competency framework of the ANP compares well with the community matron (CM), the physician's assistant and the emergency care practitioner (ECP; AANPE, 2008). Experienced WiC nurses find their knowledge and skills transfer to many other specialist areas including working as NPs in GP practices, CMs, A&E lead nurses, other WiCs both private and NHS run, Diabetes Specialist Nurses and PNs.

A nurse-led service

The RCN vision for the future of nursing (RCN, 2004) viewed nurses who lead teams as expert nurses working at the level of advanced practice, and who are able to understand the local health context, managerial change and uncertainty while enabling the clinical team to provide flexible person-centred care. For nurses working in a WiC setting, this definition includes two further principles, namely:

- Enabling practitioners to reach their potential;
- A systematic approach to practice development (Bryar and Griffiths, 2003).

The above two principles are essential to a nursing team which is developing new autonomous practice skills. The following leadership competencies were outlined by the government in liberating the talents of NHS workers (DoH, 2002):

- Act on good ideas that meet the needs of local people and that are based on best available evidence.
- Provide clinical and professional leadership to front line nurses, midwives and HVs.
- Corporate leadership for nursing and not rely on the lead nurse alone.
- See a leadership role for everyone wherever they work.
- Encourage nurses to be part of clinical leadership on the Professional Executive Committee.
- Identify, nurture and encourage potential leaders and champions through leadership programmes ensuring access to Black and minority ethnic groups.
- Think and plan the future of nursing in the primary care trust.
- Promote networks and forums that bring together staff across the wider health and social care community.

More importantly, as Bellman (2003) argues in her book on nurse-led change and development in clinical practice, a nurse-led service is best placed to empower nurses. This is an essential part of the role, as in the past nursing leadership in the UK developed a system of oppressing its own because the nursing hierarchy could not cope with anything that was outside of command and control (Ashbridge, 2001 cited in Bellman, 2003). The WiC then is an opportunity for nurses to develop and advance clinical skills in an empowering team-building environment with organisational support. Contextual factors have been identified to improve both patient and practitioner outcomes (Wallin et al., 2006). These factors include:

- supporting skills development and staff learning by developing a learning and professionally supportive environment;
- establishing performance feedback at individual, group and organisation levels involving staff in decision-making at the unit level;
- supporting professional authority and autonomy;
- increasing staff retention and evidence-based practice by indicating the following areas for leadership initiatives.

WiCs are working towards this goal, but many of the nurses leading the service are still not necessarily nurses working at an advanced practice nursing level, although a WiC may employ ANPs, ENPs, nurse consultants (NCs), PNs and NPs (Hatchett, 2003). Many of these new expanded roles, such as the NP, ANP and the NC role, are still not well understood in practice (Daly and Carnwell, 2003). Issues that are barriers for nurses in the WiC role are organisational factors, training and prescribing issues, lack of a professional register and cultural issues, including tensions, boundaries and responsibility (Main et al., 2007).

Nurses can take many years to work through the banding levels outlined in Band 7 that meet the different levels of clinical competencies required for the novice to expert practitioners' competency standards in the KSF (DoH, 2004; RCN, 2008). The clinical and management leadership roles are normally banded 8.

Where a NC role exists, it should be considered as individual to each service (Abbott, 2007). The NC plays a complementary role to the lead nurse focusing on promoting an understanding of advanced clinical practice as well as research and education more than a focus on operational management (Guest et al., 2004). Kotter (1990) makes a clear differentiation between management and leadership for management focusing on planning and budgeting, organising and staffing, controlling and problem solving, and predictability and order. Leadership includes establishing direction, aligning people, motivating and inspiring and producing change often in a dramatic degree.

Establishing a WiC

The NHS provides a Web page that explains opportunities for establishing new WiCs (NHS, 2007). The average WiC has at least three treatment rooms and a triage area. A WiC expects to see approximately 2,500 patients a month and to employ on average 12 full time equivalent (FTE) nursing staff. The staff employed fulfil the competencies found in Bands 3–8 (NHS, 2007). The staff includes receptionists and administrative staff usually employed at Band 3, or 4 for health care assistants (HCAs). A recent innovative approach to health care is extending HCAs' practice to include work previously carried out by nurses. This is one of the innovative practice additions that are part of the new NHS that was proposed by the Wanless Report (2004). Nurses fulfil many competencies previously considered a GP role and are banded through 8 in Agenda for Change. GPs' salaries are outside the banding. The NHS Web page suggests that nursing competencies fall in Bands 6–7 for experienced practitioners and that senior nurses do not necessarily have advanced nurse practice qualifications (NHS, 2007). A recent study identified large variations between NP salaries with the majority ranging between Bands 7 and 8 (Ball, 2006).

The lead nurse role involves operational and line management responsibility for the team of staff working in the WiC and they would normally be expected to hire the new team that will be working under them when a WiC is being developed. The centre may be managed by a project or manager and/or a lead nurse. At the time of setting up a new WiC, the issues a lead nurse will be considering are:

- resources;
- bands;
- skills and knowledge;
- professional background;
- case mix and range of services provided.

Other WiC staff includes receptionists and other staff depending on local area needs. WiC staff may include patient advocates, HCAs, interpreters, a NC and AHP such as physiotherapists, ECPs and health scientists (e.g. pharmacists). Most WiCs have ICPs so that clinicians can refer to more experienced GPs if the clinical problems are outside the clinician's competence. The budget of a WiC tends to be dictated by staff salaries rather than physical costs of the clinical area.

Urgent care environment

WiCs are included by the Healthcare Commission in their review of urgent and emergency care services (DoH, 2007b). The review has addressed criteria associated with 'urgent care centres'. These criteria are:

- They are WiCs, minor injury units and other similar facilities that provide unscheduled care (i.e. care which does not require a booked appointment).
- Patients do not need to be registered with them.
- They are open outside usual office hours (but are not open *only* out of hours, as these centres, usually called primary care centres, are picked up as part of out-of-hours' GP services).

- They have a reception and clear point of access for walk-in patients.
- They have over 50 attendances per week.

As early as 2004, a national evaluation of WiCs emphasised the importance of developing a coherent vision for urgent care services (WiC, GPs, pharmacists and A&Es) and how they fit together (Salisbury et al., 2007). Research carried out found there was little agreement amongst practitioners when streaming patients to A&E or a WiC in London (Bickerton et al., 2005). A follow-up study found similar results (Procter et al., 2008).

Patient satisfaction with WiC health care

Patients attend WiCs for a variety of reasons. A Cochrane review found no real differences between doctors and nurses in health outcomes for patients, process of care, resource utilisation or cost. In five studies looking at urgent and first contact care, outcomes were similar between GPs and nurses but satisfaction was higher with nurse-led care because nurses tended to give patients more information and take longer with client consultations (Laurant, 2008). Nurses provide appropriate triage in first contact care in GP surgeries (Reveley, 1998). Research has shown that patients were very satisfied with NP care and were able to make appropriate choices in a GP urgent care situation to see either a NP or GP (Myers et al., 1997). More recently, a study by Seale et al. (2006) identified holistic care and information given by nurses provided more patient satisfaction than the GP who quickly focused on gathering information, diagnosing and treating the presenting complaint.

Conclusion

The first 40 WiCs opened in the UK in 2000 and the number has now more than doubled. WiCs see and treat about 5,000,000 patients a year. The first contact WiC nurses are developing clinical skills that extend their role to include some of what was traditional practice for GPs and are receiving both university and practice-based learning to meet the competencies of advanced nurse practice. The role of the first contact WiC nurse is being developed in other urgent care primary care services and the skills being developed are relevant for roles such as the PN, the CM, ECP, HV and the paediatric nurse.

Patients' presenting with health complaints at WiCs require advanced practice skills. More primary care nurses are meeting the advanced practice criteria through MSc nursing programmes. Overall, NHS WiCs are a very positive addition to local health service provision and achieve valuable results (RCN, 2007) and patients express satisfaction with nurse-led services.

References

AANPE (2008) *Briefing on Advanced Clinical Education and Prospective Professional Regulation.* http://www.aanpe.org/ConsultationsResponses/AANP EDoHExtendingProfessionalRegulation08/tabid/1320/language/en-US/Default. aspx (accessed 2 June 2008).

Abbott, S., Bickerton, J., Daly, M.L. and Procter, S. (2008) Evidence based primary health care and local research: A necessary but problematic partnership. *Primary Helth Care Reserch and Development*, Vol 9, 191–198.

Abbott, S. (2007) leadership across boundaries: a qualitative study of the nurse consultant roal in English primary care. Journal of Nursing Management, 15(1); 703–710.

Abbott, S., Berry, T., Bickerton, J., Bryar, R., Davies, H., Hostettler, M., Lack, V., Lee, B., Loudon, C. and Procter, S. (2004) *Scoping Education Needs and Provisions for Walk-in-centres in North East London.* London: NELSHA.

Ball, J. (2006) *Nurse Practitioners: The Results of a Survey of Nurse Practitioners conducted on behalf of the RCN Nurse Practitioner Association.* http://www.rcn. org.uk/__data/assets/pdf_file/0005/78764/003183.pdf (accessed 8 July 2008).

Barratt, J. (2005) A case study of styles of patient self-presentation in the nurse practitioner primary health care consultation. *Primary Health Care Research and Development*, 6(4); 329–340.

Bellman, L. (2003) *Nurse-led Change and Development in Clinical Practice.* London: Whirr.

Benner, P. (2001) *From Novice to Expert: Excellence and Power in Clinical Nursing Practice.* New Jersey: Prentice Hall.

Bickerton, J., Dewan, V., Procter, S. and Coats, T. (2005) Streaming A&E patients to walk-in centre services. *Emergency Nurse*, 13(3); 20–23.

BNF (2008) *British National Formulary.* http://www.bnf.org/bnf/bnf/current/ 104945.htm (accessed 8 July 2008).

Bryar, R. and Griffiths, J. (Eds.) (2003) *Practice Development in Community Nursing: Principles and Processes.* London: Hodder & Stoughton.

City University London (2004) *First Contact Programme boosts Unscheduled Care.* http://www.city.ac.uk/sonm/news/connected/first_contact.html (accessed 7 June 2008).

Collins, S. and Britten, N. (2006) *Conversation Analysis.* Malden, MA/Williston, VT: Blackwell Publishing/BMJ Books.

Daly, W. and Carnwell, R. (2003) Nursing roles and levels of practice: A framework for differentiating between elementary, specialist and advancing nursing practice. *Journal of Clinical Nursing*, 12(2); 158–167.

Darzi, A. (2007) *Our NHS, Our Future: Interim Report.* London: Department of Health.

DoH (2002) *Liberating the Talents: Helping Primary Care Trusts and Nurses to deliver the NHS Plan.* London: Department of Health.

DoH (2004) *The NHS Knowledge and Skills Framework (NHS KSF) and the Development Review Process.* London: Department of Health.

DoH (2006a) *Chief Executive's Report to the NHS. Statistical Supplement.* www.dh.gov.uk/assetRoot/04/13/58/41/04135841.pdf (accessed 1 July 2008).

DoH (2006b) *Mechanisms for Nurse and Pharmacist Prescribing and Supply of Medicines.* London: Department of Health.

DoH (2007a) *Modernising Nursing Careers: Setting the Direction.* London: Department of Health.

DoH (2007b) *Urgent Care Update: Key Areas highlighted by the Direction of Travel Consultation and Other Work.* http://www.dh.gov.uk/Consultations/Responsestoconsultations (accessed 15 November 2007).

EMIS and PIP (2008) *Patient UK.* http://www.patient.co.uk/ (accessed 8 July 2008).

Gallacher, T. and Garlick, E. (2006) *Lothian Unscheduled Care Service: Nursing Competency Framework.* http://www.nes.scot.nhs.uk/OOH/mapping/documents/ProjectReportLothianUnscheduledCareService.pdf (accessed 8 July 2008).

Gledhill, H. (2003) Local guidelines: Development and implementation in minor injury units. In Bryar, R. and Griffiths, J. (Eds.) *Practice Development in Community Nursing Principles and Processes.* London: Hodder & Stoughton.

Guest, D., Pecked, R., Rosenthal, P., Redfern, S., Wilson-Barnett, J., Dewed, P., Caster, S., Evans, A. and Sudbury, A. (2004) *An Evaluation of the Impact of Nurse Midwife and Health Visitor Consultants.* http://www.kcl.ac.uk/content/1/c6/01/69/94/NCFullReport.pdf (accessed 10 July 2008).

Hanlon, G., Strangleman, T., Goode, J., Luff, D., O'Cathain, A. and Greatbach, D. (2005) Knowledge, technology and nursing: The case of NHS Direct. *Human Relations,* 58(2); 147–171.

Hatchett, R. (2003) *Nurse-led Clinics: Practice Issues.* New York/London: Routledge.

Haynes, R. (2002) Physicians' and patients' choices in evidence based practice: Evidence does not make decisions, people do. *BMJ,* 324; 674.

Kotter, J. (1990) *A Force for Change: How Leadership differs from Management.* New York: Free Press.

Laurant, M., Reeves, D., Hermens, R., Braspenning, J., Grol, R. and Sibbald, B. (2005) *Substitution of Doctors by Nurses in Primary Care.* http://www.update-software.com/Abstracts/ab001271.htm (accessed 10 July 2008).

Main, R., Dunn, N. and Kendall, K. (2007) 'Crossing professional boundaries': Barriers to the integration of nurse practitioners in primary care. *Education for Primary Care,* 18(1); 480–487.

Myers, P., Lenci, B. and Sheldon, M. (1997) A nurse practitioner as the first point of contact for urgent medical problems in a general practice setting. *Family Practice,* 14(1); 492–497.

NELSHA (2007) *Second DRAFT PCT Walk in Centre Project Plan framework NHS. Establishing an NHS Walk-in-Centre.* http://www.dh.gov.uk/en/Healthcare/PatientChoice/Waitingbookingchoice/DH_4087369 (accessed 10 June 2008).

NICE guidelines (2009) http://www.library.nhs.uk/pathways/ (accessed 15 September 2009).

NHS (2007) *Walk-in Centre Services.* http://www.nhs.uk/AboutNHSservices/walkincentres/Pages/Walk-incentresFAQ.aspx (accessed 4 June 2008) .

NHS (2008) Establishing an NHS walk-in-centre. http://www.dh.gov.uk/en/Helthcare/patient/choice/waitingbookingchoice/DH_4087369 (accessed 10 June 2008).

NMC (2006) *Framework for the standard for Post Registration Nursing.* http://www.nmc-uk.org/aArticle.aspx?ArticleID=2038 (accessed 2 June 2008).

Nottingham NHS PCT (2008) *Nottingham City PCT Board Meeting*, May 2008, B 85/08. www.nottingham+PCT+NHS+First+Contact+Programme (accessed 3 February 2009).

Procter, S., Bickerton, J., Allan, T., Davies, H. and Abbott, S. (2008) *Streaming to Streaming Emergency Department Patients to Primary Care Services: Developing a Consensus in North East London.*

Proctor, B. (1986) Supervision a cooperative exercise in accountability. In Marken, M. and Payne, M. (Eds.) *Enabling and Ensuring.* Leicester: Leicester National Youth Bureau and Council for Education and Training in Youth and Community Work.

RCN (2004) *The Future Nurse: The RCN Vision.* http://www.rcn.org.uk/_data/assets/pdf_file/0008/78614/002302.pdf (accessed 10 July 2008).

RCN (2007) *RCN Wales welcomes Call for Nurse-led Facilities.* http://www.rcn.org.uk/newsevents/news/article/wales/article2290 (accessed 11 June 2008).

RCN (2008) *RCN Competencies: Advanced Nurse Practitioners: An RCN Guide to the Advanced Nurse Practitioner, Competencies and Programme Accreditation.* http://www.rcn.org.uk/_data/assets/pdf_file/0003/146478/003207.pdf (accessed 2 June 2008).

Reveley, S. (1998) The role of the triage nurse practitioner in general medical practice: An analysis of the role. *Journal of Advanced Nursing*, 28(3); 584–591.

Rosen, R. and Mountford, L. (2002) Developing and supporting extended nursing roles: The challenges of NHS walk-in centres. *Journal of Advanced Nursing*, 39(3); 241–248.

Salisbury, C., Chalder, M., Manku-Scott, T., Ruth, N., Deave, T., Noble, S., Pope, C., Moore, L., Coast, J., Anderson, E., Weiss, M., Grant, C. and Sharp, D. (2002) *National Evaluation of NHS Walk in Centres.*

Salisbury, C., Hollinghurst, S., Montgomery, A., Cooke, M., Munro, J., Sharp, D. and Chalder, M., (2007) The impact of co-located NHS walk-in centres on emergency departments. *Emergency Medicine Journal*, 24(4); 265–269.

Schickler, P. (2004) Lay perspectives and stories – Whose health is it anyway? In Smith, P., James, T., Lorentzon, M. and Pope, R. (Eds.) *Shaping the Facts: Evidence-based Nursing and Health Care.* Edinburgh: Elsevier Science Publishers.

Seale, C., Anderson, E., Kinnersley, P., Seale, C., Anderson, E. and Kinnersley, P. (2006) Treatment advice in primary care: A comparative study of nurse practitioners and general practitioners. *Journal of Advanced Nursing*, 54(5); 534–541.

Wallin, L., Ewald, U., Wikblad, K., Scott-Findlay, S. and Arnetz, B.B. (2006) Understanding work contextual factors: A short-cut to evidence-based practice? *Worldviews on Evidence-based Nursing*, 3(4); 153–164.

Wanless, D. (2004) *Securing Good Health for the Whole Population: Final Report.* London: HMSO.

The context of practice nursing and walk-in-centre nursing: domains of practice and competencies – setting the scene

4

Carol L. Cox

Introduction

The aim of this chapter is to delineate the context of practice nursing (PN) and walk-in-centre (WiC) nursing within the domains of advanced practice. It was identified in Chapter 2 that practice nurses (PNs) are working at an advanced practice level. This is also evident amongst WiC nurses as noted in Chapter 3. Therefore, what is considered advanced practice within PN and WiC nursing and its importance in the provision of health care are explicated in the narrative that follows in this chapter. This chapter begins by describing advanced nursing practice in general. It outlines the events associated with the evolution of advanced nursing practice and reflects on its origins in order to ground the practice and WiC nurse's perspective. It follows with the definition, role, educational preparation and Domains of Practice and Competencies (RCN, 2002, 2008; NMC, 2005) related to advanced nursing practice. This chapter concludes by considering the profession of advanced PN and its expanding role.

Learning Outcomes

- To describe advanced nursing practice
- To consider skills associated with advanced nursing practice

▨ To reflect on the Domains of Practice and Competencies associated with advanced nursing practice
▨ To acknowledge the holistic approach of practice and WiC nursing.

Background

In 2008, Griffith delineated advanced nursing practice in Hinchliff's and Rogers' (2008) text on *Competencies for Advanced Nursing Practice*. Griffith (2008:1) indicated that 'clarifying the concept of 'advanced nursing practice' will facilitate further innovation. However, despite the decision (by the Nursing and Midwifery Council in 2005 to regulate advanced nursing practice) it will have profound repercussions'. In publications such as Hinchliff and Rogers (2008), Marsden and Shaw (2007), Mayberry and Mayberry (2003) and McGee and Castledine (2003), it has been noted that advanced practice roles have enabled the delivery of the policy agenda with high-quality outcomes. It has been further noted that whilst advanced practice roles in nursing are diverse, they continue to respond to service need.

Social trends, advances in technology and an ageing population are placing increased demands on health care. It can be seen that changes are occurring rapidly in the National Health Service (NHS) throughout the UK in response to service need and in line with Government policy initiatives. In relation to advanced practice roles in nursing, development has been partially due to the *New Deal for Junior Doctors* (National Health Service Management Executive, 1991) resulting in the reduction in junior hospital doctors' clinical hours and restructuring of the NHS as delineated in *Making a Difference* (DoH, 1999) and the *NHS Plan* (DoH, 2000) so that health care becomes seamless and more orientated towards care in the community.

Recently, with spiralling costs in the NHS and cutbacks and reductions in the workforce, the need for nurses to advance their clinical practice has become acute. Medical and allied health professionals are diminishing in numbers and in some instances no longer available to provide this care. The reduction of medical and allied health professionals has direct implications for extension of practice by nurses and assumption of advanced clinical practice roles.

Because the provision of health care is changing, it is important to consider how PNs and WiC nurses working in primary care can provide more complex/sophisticated care to patients and promote health. This is particularly relevant in relation to the recommendations made by the British Medical Association (BMA, 2002) in which the first point of call for most patients should be an advanced PN rather than a doctor. It is also relevant in relation to the mandates put forward by the Chief Nurse for England in her consultation document of July 2004 (DoH, 2004a) and the Nursing and Midwifery Council (NMC) decision following conclusion of its consultation on advanced practice (NMC, 2005) to open a second part of the register to record an advanced practice qualification as an advanced nurse practitioner. This NMC initiative is presently sitting in Privy Council where consideration is being given to standardisation and regulation of advanced practice across nursing, midwifery, the allied health professions and optometry.

It is important to consider that the NMC initiative, which delineates the title of advanced nurse practitioner, is intended to regulate all advanced nursing practice roles. Therefore, although nurses may be working as advanced PNs in practice and WiC nursing, they will be required to hold a registration on the second part of the register, under the title of advanced nurse practitioner, unless the Privy Council recommends otherwise.

Origins of the advanced practice role in the UK

It may be argued that advanced PN and educational programmes associated with advanced practice arose not from specific planning efforts or consensus within the profession, but as a response to a demand in health care. The impetus for introducing advanced PNs in the UK was economic. It has been viewed that nurses are key to achieving cost savings (SEHD, 2005). They evolved out of the economic necessity of service providers, who were experiencing a shortage of doctors in primary and secondary care. Generally, it is postulated in the UK that advanced practice in nursing became legitimised with the reduction in junior hospital doctors' hours in acute care (Cox, 2001) and the paper published by the BMA (2002).

It can be seen, overall, that an emphasis on advanced nursing practice occurred in the context of a post-modern culture, with increased professionalisation of health care, a fundamental emphasis on interprofessional working, an increasing consumerist approach to health and a move away from the traditional biomedical model of health care towards a more holistic approach that has an increased emphasis on improving the health care experience for patients (Colyer, 2004). McGee and Castledine (2003) indicate that the early definition of advanced practice published by the United Kingdom Central Council for Nursing, Midwifery and Health Visiting (UKCC, 1994) arose from the recognition that modern health care was placing new demands on nurses that required them to extend their practice. The definition provided recognition and subsequent opportunities to develop new roles and assume responsibilities that were 'undreamt of by earlier generations of the profession' (McGee and Castledine, 2003:1).

It is recognised that although advanced practice has been primarily medically driven, nurses have been at the forefront of advanced practice, facilitating cost-effective care and positive patient outcomes (Czuber-Dochan et al., 2006) for a number of years. This can be evidenced by the professional autonomous decisions in which they made a differential diagnosis of a patient's previously undiagnosed problem(s) and developed with the patient an ongoing plan for health that has an emphasis on preventative measures.

Globally there has been a desperate attempt to promote health. With this demand has come the need for nurses to extend their practice. This demand has been followed by a response throughout the UK for educational institutions to provide the knowledge, and in some instances generate the knowledge that addresses the need for appropriately trained advanced PNs/advanced nurse practitioners (Horrocks et al., 2002). It is evident from the systematic review undertaken by Horrocks et al. (2002) that nurses working in primary care provide equivalent care to that of doctors. Horrocks et al. (2002) examined randomised controlled trials and observational studies. Their research indicates that nurses working as advanced PNs provide care that leads to increased patient satisfaction as well as having similar health outcomes compared to the care provided by a doctor. On the whole it can be seen that once the advanced practice role is established, nurses drive the role forward and continue to expand their practice.

Over the past decade, many nurses in the UK have extended their practice and assumed advanced practice roles. In the present political and professional climate, it is appropriate to provide PNs and WiC nurses with the opportunity to acquire the formal academic education and clinical practice experience that empowers them to take a lead role in advanced nursing practice. However, in order to do this, advanced practice as a function and role must be clarified.

Delineation of advanced practice

In the early 1990s, the UKCC (1994:20) defined advanced PN as:

> adjusting the boundaries for the development of future practice, pioneering and developing new roles responsive to changing needs and with advancing clinical practice, research and education to enrich professional practice as a whole.

McGee and Castledine (2003) indicate that this was the first attempt in the UK to clarify the nature of practice beyond initial registration.

According to Hickey et al. (2000), many definitions of advanced practice in nursing have been proposed. The key components in all of the definitions that have been published by organisations such as the International Council of Nurses (ICN, 2002), the Chief Nurse for England (DoH, 2004a), the NMC (2005) and the Royal College of Nursing (RCN, 2002, 2008) are the requirement for education at master's degree level or the ability to demonstrate master's level knowledge, patient/family focused practice and an expanded role. In the UK, advanced practice is associated with competencies articulated in the RCN (2008) and the NMC (2005) Domains of Practice.

In February 2006, the NMC expanded its definition of advanced nursing practice and published 12 core skills that can be expected from an advanced PN (refer to Box 4.1).

The NMC has published a definition of the ANP that patients and the public can understand. The definition as delineated by the NMC (2006:1) is:

> Advanced nurse practitioners are highly experienced, knowledgeable and educated members of the care team who are able to diagnose and treat your health care needs or refer you to an appropriate specialist if needed.

Box 4.1   Skills of the Advanced Nurse Practitioner (NMC, 2006)

- Undertakes a comprehensive patient history
- Undertakes physical examinations
- Uses expert knowledge and clinical judgement to identify the potential diagnosis
- Refers patients for investigations where appropriate
- Makes a final diagnosis
- Decides on and carries out treatment, including the prescribing of medicines, or refers patients to an appropriate specialist
- Uses extensive practice experience to plan and provide skilled and competent care to meet patients' health and social care needs, involving other members of the health care team
- Ensures the provision of continuity of care including follow-up visits
- Assesses and evaluates, with patients, the effectiveness of the treatment and care provided and makes changes as needed
- Works independently, although often as part of a health care team
- Provides leadership
- Makes sure that each patient's treatment and care is based on best practice.

However, Mayberry and Mayberry (2003:38) provide a more specific definition of advanced PN which is:

> Advanced nursing practice can be defined as a set of skills that involve the undertaking of: taking a clinical history, performing a physical examination, performing appropriate investigations including, for example, proctoscopy and endoscopy, prescribing treatments following agreed protocols based on research or consensus and providing advice and counselling on prognosis and management.

According to the RCN (2008:3), an advanced nurse practitioner is:

> A registered nurse who has undertaken a specific course of study of at least first degree (Honours) level and who practices according to the defining role shown in Box 4.2.

Box 4.2   Definition of the Advanced Nurse Practitioner (RCN, 2008:3)

A registered nurse who has undertaken a specific course of study of at least first degree (Honours) level and who:

- makes professionally autonomous decisions, for which he or she is accountable;
- receives patients with undifferentiated and undiagnosed problems and makes an assessment of their health care needs, based on highly developed nursing

(Continued)

> knowledge and skills, including skills not usually exercised by nurses, such as physical examination;
> ▨ screens patients for disease risk factors and early signs of illness;
> ▨ makes differential diagnosis using decision-making and problem-solving skills;
> ▨ develops with the patient an ongoing nursing care plan for health, with an emphasis on preventative measures;
> ▨ orders necessary investigations, and provides treatment and care both individually, as part of a team, and through referral to other agencies.

Therefore, it is apparent that:

> advanced practice nurses work alongside doctors, practice autonomously and are legally responsible for the care they provide. They make clinical decisions based on investigations and subsequently can treat patients independently. (Cox, 2004:Foreword vii–viii)

Role of the advanced practice nurse

According to Jacobs (1998), Rolfe (1998) and McGee and Castledine (2003), advanced nursing practice includes physical examinations, diagnosis and treatment of illnesses, ordering and interpreting tests independently of the doctor, establishing preventive health care through health promotion and education, prescribing medications, managing caseloads based on a population perspective that ideally includes individuals, families and/or communities and using business and management strategies for the provision of quality care and efficient use of resources. Their practice includes cooperative and/or collaborative practice arrangements with other health care disciplines as well as working in interdisciplinary health care teams. Advanced PNs are accountable as direct providers of services. Clinical decision-making is based on critical thinking, diagnostic reasoning and research.

They can have either an acute care (secondary) or a primary care focus which means they can work anywhere. They provide comprehensive health and illness management, consultancy and primary care in a variety of clinical settings (Cox, 2000) and work with doctors and other health professionals in expanded collaborative relationships that influence the care provided by other health professionals. It is seen more often now than ever before that the advanced PN works independently managing a caseload of patients without supervision or may work in a team that is consultant led (Brush and Capezuti, 1997). The model of care provided by the advanced PN has been identified as making an important contribution to quality, cost-effective care (Cox and Hall, 2007).

To summarise, articulation of the remit of an advanced PN according to recent literature and the definitions published by the RCN (2008) and NMC (2005) indicates that the advanced PN possesses advanced assessment, diagnostic, prescriptive and technological skills with a hospital-based acute health/illness perspective and transitional points of health/illness management focus or a community-based primary care focus. The advanced PN provides comprehensive health/illness management, consultancy and primary care in a variety of clinical settings. Within the context of advanced practice in PN and WiC nursing, most nurses are directly accountable to other nurses, to a manager who is not a nurse or directly to a general practitioner (GP). What is evident within these advanced practice roles is that the advanced PN works with doctors and other health care professionals in expanded collaborative relationships and influences the care provided by all health care professionals.

Educational preparation

According to the Chief Nurse for England (DoH, 2004a), advanced PNs should be educated at Master's degree level or above. According to the NMC (2005), they should possess master's level knowledge and advanced assessment, diagnostic, prescriptive and technological skills as well as research acumen. In their education, which is interprofessional in nature, the central core knowledge, skills, competencies and values of advanced professional and clinical practice experience are acquired in:

- addressing the determinants of health and working with others in the primary, secondary and tertiary care setting to integrate a range of activities that promote, protect and improve the health of the patient/client population served;
- functioning in new health care settings and interdisciplinary teams that are designed to meet the primary, secondary and tertiary health care needs of the public, with an emphasis on high-quality, cost-effective integrated care;
- managing and continuously using scientific, technological and patient information that leads to the maintenance of professional competence throughout clinical practice life;
- gaining advanced assessment skills used in the provision of care in primary, secondary and tertiary health care settings;
- diagnosing, screening, treatment and case management of care in primary, secondary and tertiary health care settings;
- prescribing and supplying drugs, independently and/or according to patient group directions, in primary, secondary and tertiary health care settings;
- providing emotional support, counselling, referral and discharge in primary, secondary and tertiary health care settings (NMC, 2005).

Learning outcomes within advanced practice programmes are pre-set with clearly defined objectives for the core competencies that must be achieved as specified by the RCN (2008) and the NMC (2005). The outcomes identify what a nurse will know and be able to do at the end of the programme of study. Additional aspects of learning can be individually negotiated through learning contracts. In the main, the programmes are competency based and focus on the knowledge, skills, attributes and outcomes that are informed by practice (Masterson and Mitchell in McGee and Castledine, 2003). Competencies are informed by theories and hierarchies of skills and knowledge.

With the delineation of the RCN (2008) and NMC (2005) Domains of Practice and Competencies, universities throughout the UK have restructured their programmes to ensure that the essential components of advanced practice are addressed. A variety of advanced practice programmes are now available for nurses who want to become advanced PNs. The key component within all of the programmes is a clear emphasis on clinical practice that initially builds and then extends as the nurse gains confidence and competence.

RCN (2002, 2008) and NMC (2005) Domains of Practice and Competencies

The RCN (2002, 2008) and NMC (2005) Domains of Practice and Competencies were adapted from the National Organization of Nurse Practitioner Faculties (NONPF, 1995, 2001). It is interesting to note that in the UK, in addition to the NONPF (1995, 2001) Domains of Practice and Competencies informing advanced nursing practice, a number of the competencies are evident in the Standards of Proficiency for some of the advanced roles in the allied health professions such as orthodontists and biomedical scientists (HPC, 2006) (Box 4.3). The Domains of Practice as specified by the NMC (2005) are:

- the nurse–patient relationship;
- respecting culture and diversity;
- management of patient illness/health status;
- education function;
- professional role;
- managing and negotiating health care delivery systems;
- monitoring and ensuring quality of health care practice.

The Domains of Practice which have been linked to the NHS Knowledge and Skills Framework (DoH, 2004b) dimensions by the RCN (2002, 2008) are:

- assessment and management of patient illness/health status;
- the nurse/patient relationship;
- the education function;
- professional role;
- managing and negotiating health care delivery systems;
- monitoring and ensuring quality of advanced health care practice;
- respecting culture and diversity.

Box 4.3   Reflections of an Advanced Practice Nurse (APN) caring for a 74-year-old Patient

Doreen Brown is a 74-year-old lady who has lived alone in a sixth-floor council flat since her husband died three years ago. She has a daughter in Australia and a son who lives about 20 miles away. She has smoked for the past 40 years and as a result of this has chronic obstructive pulmonary disease (COPD).

The National Institute of Clinical Excellence (NICE) guidelines on the management of COPD (National Institute of Clinical Excellence, 2004) identify the need for confirmation of COPD as a diagnosis so that appropriate care can be provided. To achieve this, the advanced practice nurse will need to be competent in the following.

Management of patient health/illness status (NMC, 2005, Domain 3; RCN, 2008, Domain 1)

Management of patient illness

Doreen's history was taken by the advanced practice nurse, who identified that she had risk factors for developing COPD as she was in the correct age group and had smoked for the past 40 years. Doreen's smoking history identified that she was currently smoking 10 cigarettes per day and had smoked a total of 50 pack years which means Doreen had smoked the equivalent of one pack a day for 50 years. Doreen also reported that she suffered from regular chest infections (three to four per year). A physical examination was then undertaken by the APN who, on inspection, identified:

1   Breathlessness at rest with a respiratory rate of 24 breaths/min and grade 4 using the MRC dyspnoea scale:
   - use of accessory muscles of breathing;
   - chronic productive cough;
   - presence of central cyanosis which is supported by oxygen saturation of 84% on air;
   - severe finger clubbing caused by prolonged hypoxemia;
   - body mass index of 19.
2   Palpation and percussion:
   - bi-lateral reduction in lung expansion;
   - increased resonance due to hyperinflated lungs.
3   Auscultation:
   - bi-lateral crackles;
   - bi-lateral wheeze.

Based on the history and symptoms, the APN decided to perform spirometry to confirm the provisional diagnosis of COPD. The best of three results was recorded: FEV_1 0.89 (28% predicted), FVC 2.74 (67% predicted) and FEV_1/FVC ratio 0.32. The APN nurse interpreted the results as showing obstructive lung disease as the FEV_1 was reduced (<80% predicted) and the FEV_1/FVC ratio was reduced (<0.7). Subsequently, the APN made a firm diagnosis of severe COPD based on clinical history and spirometry.

The APN then reviewed Doreen's treatment plan, using evidence-based practice to inform her decision-making. Doreen was already using an inhaled long-acting bronchodilator, so her inhaler technique was checked and recorded. Following assessment the APN felt that Doreen was symptomatic and that, in line with the NICE COPD guidelines

(Continued)

(National Institute of Clinical Excellence, 2004), Doreen should have her treatment changed. Inhaled corticosteroids were to be added to Doreen's treatment and therefore the APN, who is a non-medical prescriber, provided Doreen with a prescription for a combination inhaler which contained a long-acting bronchodilator and corticosteroid. Doreen was given a review appointment where an assessment of symptoms (e.g. breathlessness, wheeze and cough) and repeat spirometry would be made. As recommended by the NICE COPD guidelines, inhaled corticosteroids should be prescribed for a four-week trial period and should only be continued if there is clinical improvement.

During the assessment, the pulse oximetry showed that Doreen was in respiratory failure, as her oxygen saturation level was less than 92%, and therefore the APN identified that Doreen required an assessment for long term oxygen therapy (LTOT). The British Thoracic Society (2006) clinical guidance on home oxygen was used to guide the decision to prescribe LTOT. As Doreen's arterial blood gases demonstrated a $PaO_2 < 7.3\,kPa$, home oxygen was ordered by the APN for Doreen, and she was provided with an oxygen concentrator, which evidence has shown as the most acceptable way to deliver LTOT in home. It was also identified that she may benefit from ambulatory oxygen; however, Doreen did not want to be seen outside wearing oxygen and therefore a note of this was made in her records so that this could be revisited at a future consultation as and when it was thought to be appropriate.

Management of patient health/illness status (NMC, 2005, Domain 3; RCN, 2008, Domain 1)

Health promotion/health protection and disease prevention
The APN identified the need for Doreen to be provided with smoking cessation advice, as this would prevent disease progression and thereby reduce disability. In addition, as there had been a decision to provide Doreen home oxygen, the risk of fire associated with oxygen and smoking needed to be addressed. The APN explained to Doreen how stopping smoking would halt the progress of the disease which would prevent her becoming more breathless and outlined the risk of fire if she smoked whilst using oxygen. Doreen's feelings about smoking were then explored and whether she would consider quitting smoking. As Doreen showed interest in quitting smoking, she was provided with a booklet about smoking cessation and given a follow-up appointment to discuss this further in the level II smoking cessation clinic that the APN runs. The fact that Doreen attended this appointment suggested that she was motivated and may be contemplating quitting smoking. During the consultation, it was decided that this was an appropriate time for her to quit smoking with the assistance of nicotine replacement therapy (NRT), as this doubles the chance of successfully quitting. The APN is a non-medical prescriber and therefore supplied Doreen with a prescription for NTR patches for six weeks when she was reviewed.

The education function (NMC, 2005, Domain 4; RCN, 2008, Domain 3) and the nurse–patient relationship (NMC, 2005, Domain 1; RCN, 2008, Domain 2)

The APN recognised that Doreen would require considerable education so that she could feel empowered to self-manage her illness and to know when she requires health care support and advice. Information on her disease process, medication and signs of exacerbation was provided, and at subsequent appointments this was built upon, so that there was no overload of information. The APN also discussed the Expert Patient Programme (EPP) with Doreen, as she felt this would assist her with developing self-management skills. An information leaflet about the local programme was provided so that Doreen could decide if and when this may be appropriate for her.

As the nurse–patient relationship developed, the APN became more aware of the impact that Doreen's breathlessness was having on her daily life and how she was becoming socially isolated. Doreen was beginning to describe signs associated with anxiety and depression as a consequence of the impact of her breathlessness on her life. The APN used the Hospital Anxiety and Depression Scale (HADS) (Zigmond and Snaith, 1983) as an assessment tool so that future interventions, such as pulmonary rehabilitation, could be evaluated. As Doreen had described that she had a degree of functional disability, and this was quantified by a score of 4 on the MRC dyspnoea scale (Fletcher, 1960), Doreen was referred to the community pulmonary rehabilitation programme run by a respiratory physiotherapist. However, as there is usually an eight-week waiting list for the programme, the APN provided advice on exercise, nutrition and coping with breathlessness, which would be built upon during the rehabilitation programme. It was also evident that Doreen's circle of friends had decreased and she felt they did not understand how the breathlessness and exacerbations prevented her planning social events in advance. The APN discussed the benefit of peer support and provided her with details of the local Breathe Easy Club which is a patient support group for those with respiratory diseases.

Managing and negotiating health care delivery systems (NMC, 2005, Domain 6; RCN, 2008, Domain 5)

When Doreen's social circumstances were assessed by the APN, it became apparent that her circumstances were having a negative impact on her quality of life. She was finding it very difficult to cook as she became very breathless when preparing food. As a result, she was showing signs of malnutrition which was supported by a body mass index of 19. Her daughter-in-law does her shopping on a weekly basis, but she can only visit Doreen at weekends, as she and her son, who live 20 miles away, both work and have two children. This is also the only time Doreen gets out of her flat as she is living on the sixth floor and she is too frightened to travel in the lift on her own as it frequently breaks down. The APN referred Doreen to the social worker, who arranged for her to receive home help, meals-on-wheels during the week and made an urgent housing application for ground floor accommodation. The APN also arranged for an occupational therapy (OT) assessment so that equipment and adaptations could be identified to assist Doreen to remain as independent as possible by maximising her ability to undertake activities of daily living.

Practice and WiC nursing and future directions of advanced clinical practice nursing

The Department of Health has mandated the expansion of nursing roles and delineated ways in which knowledgeable experienced advanced PNs can contribute to the NHS by providing leadership in nursing and service delivery (DoH, 2000, 2001, 2006). Health care provision is evolving (BMA, 2002; Horrocks et al., 2002; DoH, 2004a, 2006; Griffith, 2008). In the UK, advanced PN programmes maintain a commitment to educating nurses who will make substantial contributions to the evolution of health care. Although the BMA (2002) indicated in its publication *The Future Health Care Workforce (A Future Model for the Health Care Workforce)* that nurses at advanced practice level would provide expert practice, it is not enough to produce expert nurses. The nurses must be prepared, through appropriate educational programmes, to meet the changing needs of a reformed health care system. In addition, it must be remembered that nursing is more than and different to the sum of its parts and must articulate its unique nature and professional perspective within advanced practice. 'It is more than an aggregation of tasks captured and/or recaptured from other professionals' (Fralic, 1985:292). Acquiring and executing tasks that have been traditionally within the purview of medicine does not make nursing more professional as a practice discipline. It is the fact that nurses approach a patient care situation from a perspective very distinct and different to that of medicine. Medicine's approach has always been to diagnose and eradicate a particular disease process. Nursing's perspective, and particularly that of PN and WiC nursing, is holistic in its approach to caring. In advanced PN, PNs and WiC nurses approach the patient care situation from a perspective which addresses the total constellation of care needs of the patient.

Conclusion

In this chapter, advanced nursing practice in association with PN and WiC nursing and their importance in the provision of health care have been discussed. The events associated with the origins and evolution of advanced nursing practice have been considered. The definition, role, educational preparation and Domains of Practice and Competencies (RCN, 2002, 2008; NMC, 2005) related to advanced nursing practice have been presented. This chapter has concluded with a consideration of the profession of advanced PN and its expanding role. The nature of nursing, as being more than and different to the sum of its parts, was recognised and the requirement to articulate its unique nature and professional perspective within advanced practice was stressed.

It was emphasised that advanced practice in PN and WiC nursing is more than an aggregation of tasks captured and/or recaptured from other professionals. Therefore, the acquisition and execution of tasks that have been traditionally within the purview of medicine does not make PN and WiC nursing more professional than practice disciplines. Within the practice context, it is seen that nurses working at an advanced practice level in primary care approach a patient care situation from a perspective distinct and different than that of medicine. They approach the patient care situation from a perspective that addresses the total constellation of care needs of the patient. The skills and knowledge associated with this approach are explicated in the Domains of Practice and Competencies of advanced practice published by the NMC (2005) and the RCN (2002, 2008).

References

British Medical Association (2002) *The Future Health Care Workforce: Discussion Paper 9*. http://web.bma.org.uk/public/pols (accessed 8 March 2002).

British Thoracic Society (2006) *Clinical Component for the Home Oxygen Service in England and Wales*. www.brit-thoracic.org.uk (accessed 3 February 2009).

Brush, B. and Capezuti, E. (1997) Professional autonomy: Essential for nurse practitioners' survival in the 21st century. *Journal of the American Academy of Nurse Practitioners*, 9(6); 265–270.

Colyer, H. (2004) The construction and development of health professions: Where will it end? *Journal of Advanced Nursing*, 48(4); 406–412.

Cox, C. (2000) The nurse consultant: An advanced nurse practitioner. *Nursing Times*, 96(13); 48.

Cox, C. (2001) Advanced nurse practitioners and physician assistants: What is the difference? Comparing the USA and UK. *Hospital Medicine*, 62(3); 169–171.

Cox, C. (2004) *Physical Assessment for Nurses*. Oxford: Blackwell Publishing.

Cox, C. and Hall, A. (2007) Advanced practice role in gastrointestinal nursing. *Journal of Gastrointestinal Nursing*, 5(4); 26–31.

Czuber-Dochan, W., Waterman, C., Waterman, H. (2006) Atrophy and anarchy: third national survey of nursing skill-mix and advanced nursing practice in opthalmology. *Journal of Clinical Nursing* 15(12); 1480–1488.

DoH (1999) *Making a Difference*. London: The Stationery Office, Department of Health.

DoH (2000) *The NHS Plan: A Plan for Investment. A Plan for Reform*. London: The Stationery Office, Department of Health.

DoH (2001) *Implementing the NHS Plan: Modern Matrons, strengthening the Role of Ward Sisters and introducing Senior Sisters*. Health Service Circular 2001/10. http://www.doh.-gov.uk/hsc.htm.

DoH (2004a) *Framework for developing Nursing Roles: Consultation*. London: The Stationery Office, Department of Health.

DoH (2004b) *The NHS Knowledge and Skills Framework (NHSKSF) and its Use in Development Review*. London: The Stationery Office, Department of Health.

DoH (2005) *Liberating the Talents: Helping Primary Care Trusts and Nurses deliver the NHS Plan*. London: Department of Health.

DoH (2006) *Caring for People with Long Term Conditions: An Education Framework for Community Matrons and Case Managers*. Department of Health. http://www.dh.gov.uk/PublicationsAndStatistics (accessed 18 April 2009).

Fletcher, C. (1960) Standardized questionnaire on respiratory symptoms: A statement prepared and approved by the MRC committee on the etiology of chronic bronchitis; MRC breathlessness score. *British Medical Journal*, 2; 665.

Fralic (1985) Commentary. *Journal of Professional Nursing*, 1(9); 292.

Griffith, H. (2008) What is advanced nursing practice? In Hinchliff, S. and Rogers, R. (Eds.) *Competencies for Advanced Nursing Practice*. Chapter 1, pp. 1–20. London: Hodder Arnold.

Hickey, J., Ouimette, R. and Venegoni, S. (2000) *Advanced Practice Nursing: Changing Roles and Clinical Applications*. 2nd edn. New York: Lippincott.

Hinchliff, S. and Rogers, R. (2008) *Competencies for Advanced Nursing Practice*. London: Hodder Arnold.

Horrocks, S., Anderson, E. and Salisbury, C. (2002) Systematic review of whether nurse practitioners working in primary care can provide equivalent care to doctors. *British Medical Journal*, 324(April); 819–823.

HPC (2006) *Health Professions Council Standards of Proficiency*. http://www.hpc-uk.org/publications/standards/index.asp.

ICN (2002) *ICN announces Position on Advanced Nursing Roles, Geneva*, 31 October. Geneva: International Council of Nurses, http://www.icn.ch/pr19_02.htm.

Jacobs, S. (1998) Advanced nursing practice in New Zealand: 1998. *Nursing Praxis in New Zealand*, 13(3); 4–11.

Marsden, J. and Shaw, M. (2007) The development of advanced practice roles in ophthalmic nursing. *Practice Development in Health Care*, 6(2); 119–130.

Mayberry, K. and Mayberry, J. (2003) The status of nurse practitioners in gastroenterology. *Clinical Medicine*, 3(1); 37–40.

McGee, P. and Castledine, G. (2003) *Advanced Nursing Practice*. 2nd edn. Oxford: Blackwell Publishing.

National Health Service Management Executive (1991) *Junior Doctors: The New Deal*. London: NHSME.

National Institute of Clinical Excellence (2004) *Chronic Obstructive Pulmonary Disease: Management of Chronic Obstructive Pulmonary Disease in Adults in Primary and Secondary Care*. London: National Institute of Clinical Excellence.

NMC (2005) *Annex 1: Domains of Practice and Competencies, NMC Consultation on a Proposed Framework for Post-registration Nursing*. London: Nursing and Midwifery Council.

NMC (2006) *A Revision of the Definition of Advanced Nurse Practice so that it can be accessible to Patients and the Public*. www.nmc-uk.org (accessed 3 February 2009).

NONPF (1995) *Advanced Nursing Practice: Curriculum Guidelines & Programme Standards for Nurse Practitioner Education*. 2nd edn. Washington, DC: NONPF.

NONPF (2001) *Revised Advanced Nursing Practice: Curriculum Guidelines & Programme Standards for Nurse Practitioner Education*. Washington, DC: National Organization of Nurse Practitioner Faculties Education Committee.

RCN (2002) *Nurse Practitioners – An RCN Guide to the Nurse Practitioner Role, Competencies and Programme Accreditation.* London: Royal College of Nursing.

RCN (2008) *Advanced Nurse Practitioners – An RCN Guide to the Advanced Nurse Practitioner Role, Competencies and Programme Accreditation.* London: Royal College of Nursing.

Rolfe, G. (1998) Advanced practice and the reflective nurse: Developing knowledge out of practice. In Rolfe, G. and Fulbrook, P. (Eds.) *Advanced Nursing Practice.* pp. 219–228. Oxford: Butterworth.

SEHD (2005) *Framework for developing Nursing Roles.* Edinburgh: Scottish Executive Health Department.

UKCC (1994) *The Future of Professional Practice – The Council's Standards for Education and Practice following Registration.* London: United Kingdom Central Council for Nursing, Midwifery and Health Visiting.

Zigmond, A. and Snaith, R. (1983) The Hospital Anxiety and Depression scale. *Acta Psychiatrica Scandinavica,* 67(1); 361–370.

Part 2

Domains of Practice

In the chapters that follow, exemplars of professional issues which influence best practice in practice nursing and walk-in-centre nursing are presented. Each chapter is associated with a specific Domain of Practice and its associated competencies. The Domains of Practice as delineated by the Royal College of Nursing (2008) are:

Domain 1: Assessment and management of patient health/illness status

Domain 2: The nurse/patient relationship

Domain 3: The education function

Domain 4: Professional role

Domain 5: Managing and negotiating health care delivery systems

Domain 6: Monitoring and ensuring the quality of advanced health care practice

Domain 7: Respecting culture and diversity

Practice and walk-in-centre nurses are encouraged to review the RCN (2008) publication on the competencies associated with advanced practice.

Reference

RCN (2008) *Advanced Nurse Practitioners – An RCN Guide to the Advanced Nurse Practitioner Role, Competencies and Programme Accreditation*. London: Royal College of Nursing.

Domain 1

Management of Patient Health/Illness Status

Critical thinking and diagnostic reasoning in clinical decision-making 5

Nita Muir

Introduction

The aim of this chapter is to explore critical thinking with an emphasis on diagnostic reasoning and clinical decision-making; throughout the chapter, there will be case studies from practice to illustrate key points and reference to the 'so what' element that is often not considered when exploring this theory. This is very topical, particularly as nurses are increasingly working autonomously and are expected to undertake a range of complex activities and utilise their high-level decision-making skills for the benefit of the patient and to supplement services provided by medical practitioners (Paniagua, 1997; DoH, 2002; NMC, 2006).

The Nursing Midwifery Council (NMC) review identified the range of domains and competencies required by the advanced nurse practitioner (ANP). These highlight that critical thinking underpins all activities both at a patient and at an organisational level with Domain 3 (Management of Patient Health/Illness Status), stressing the fact that ANPs need to be competent in managing the patients' health and illness status. Note that the NMC have identified Domain 3 as Management of Patient Health/Illness Status and the Royal College of Nursing (RCN, 2005) has delineated this as Domain 1. It is evident from the current literature that this means nurses such as practice nurses (PNs) and walk-in-centre (WIC) nurses need to be competent in assessing and evaluating patients with a range of illnesses and within a range of specialties and of varying acute to chronic conditions. The nurse then is required from this assessment to be able to establish a reliable diagnosis and implement an appropriate intervention or plan of care that is responsive and timely to the clinical situation. In order for nurses to be able to achieve this domain, they require a sound knowledge and experience base that is informed by clinical standards and research evidence, an ability to exercise sound critical thinking and diagnostic reasoning skills in addition to the ability to develop the therapeutic relationship with the patient.

Learning Outcomes

- To describe the essential nature and main characteristics of critical thinking.
- To understand the types of knowledge and theory that are exercised within critical thinking.
- To understand the different approaches to clinical decision-making theory and models of use.
- To review how you make a diagnosis and to be able to describe how some of your decisions are made.
- To become more aware of how your critical thinking skills can develop through reflection.

Background

Frequently, the following question is asked: What is meant by the term critical thinking? The word critical comes from the Greek word *Kritikos* meaning 'critic'. To be critical means to question or analyse and by being critical you examine your thinking. This is an active process. It involves specific cognitive skills and a reasoning process, and is context driven (Miller and Babcock, 1996). Clearly it is a broad term that encompasses both reasoning and decision-making.

Bandman and Bandman (1995) identify commonalities within critical thinkers. First, the thinkers need to be able to assimilate information or interferences from a range of data and ensure that this is plausible and reliable data. Second, they need to be able to examine the nursing assumptions made through corroborations, beliefs, conclusions and action. Third, they need to be able to justify their judgements and analyse their arguments to develop their actions and conclusions and finally, they need to evaluate their conclusions for bias and effectiveness. Therefore, the critical thinker will exercise clinical reasoning (or thinking and decision-making processes associated with clinical practice), autonomy, cognitive skills, personal attributes and deliberate activity to be able to function in a professional context. Higgs and Jones (2000) and Rubenfeld and Scheffer (1995) further suggest the following elements are integral and influential to the process:

- the patient and their health beliefs, cultural, socioeconomic frames of references and their perceived needs in relation to their clinical problem;
- context of the health care setting and wider care environment as this can impact on the decisions made;
- personal and professional framework of the clinician and their own beliefs, values and cultural context;
- scientific, technical and personal knowledge of the clinician and understanding of problem solving;
- the thinking skills of the clinician and their levels of expertise.

Table 5.1 The Six Steps of Clinical Decision-making

1. Defining the problem – clarifying the specific nature of the problem from both objective and subjective data and consider differential diagnosis. It is during this phase in diagnosis that cues are sought by the clinician from the patient
2. Defining the outcome goal
3. Considering/generating alternative solutions; here the process focuses on how to modify behaviours, alter biological functioning or facilitate change in the environment
4. Selecting the best 'fit' for the situation – this not only involves reviewing the problem with the patient, but also considers the order of priority with which various problems or presenting cues should be addressed
5. Implementing the solution
6. Evaluating the outcome – against the outcome criteria which should be observable and quantifiable

Advanced PNs may consider that the majority of activity within critical thinking is the exercising of diagnostic skills. Certainly, whilst this is an important aspect of their activity, this is only one aspect of critical thinking.

What is a decision?

Often decision-making appears such a common activity that rarely any thought is devoted to discovering what a decision is. The word decision relates to the activity – to decide (Matteson and Hawkins, 1990).

The actual decision made is the final point of the decision-making process that has involved complex processes of problem solving (McGrew and Wilson, 1982). This often occurs in an environment of uncertainty which is an inescapable fact of decision-making within modern health care (Thompson and Dowding, 2001). Sahler and Carr (2003) identify that the six steps of clinical decision-making given in Table 5.1 are taught to physicians when developing their diagnostic skills. These capture some of the commonalities identified within a critical thinker and can be likened to the nursing process as a structure for problem solving (Rubenfeld and Scheffer, 1995).

Whilst this structure may offer one problem-solving perspective to decision-making, there are a range of other models that are espoused from numerous studies on human judgement and decision-making analysis.

Theories of decision-making

It is important that when attempting to describe decisions, the starting point should be in some form of conceptual framework or model (McGrew and Wilson, 1982). In fact, there are numerous models used to interpret and explain the process of clinical reasoning and the diversity of explanation has often masked common themes between them. There is a topical debate about how best to achieve a 'middle ground' between the various theories that are espoused (Harbison, 2001; Thompson, 2001).

In order to understand this necessary debate, the two key opposing conceptual frameworks that underpin the decision-making process need to be reviewed. These are described by Hamm (1988) as:

1. analysis;
2. intuition.

Analysis is a step-by-step, conscious, logically defensible decision-making process, with characteristics including use of roles and organisation, whereas intuition is the immediate recognition of the key elements of the situation which is characterised by the use of an unconscious process.

The analytical stance on decision-making

When using an analytical approach to decision-making, the decision-maker (the nurse) relates the presented situation to a set of guiding principles or follows some rules. There have been various proponents of this stance and the suggested rules/ guidance are often expressed in information-processing terms (Fonteyn and Ritter, 2000).

Information Processing Model

A key assumption within this model is that the decision-makers store relevant information within their memory and that effective decision-making or problem solving occurs when the problem solver (the nurse) retrieves information from both short- and long-term memory. Fonteyn and Ritter (2000) discuss how information gained from education and experience is stored throughout life in long-term memory and whilst this can take longer to access than short-term memory, there is more storage capacity. They also suggest that clinical experts use information stored in their short-term memory to stimulate retrieval of long-term memory information.

These fundamentals are incorporated in a model suggested by Carnevali and Thomas (1993). The model describes a seven-stage process of 'diagnostic reasoning' or clinical decision-making (Figure 5.1).

Within this model, the clinician starts at the bottom and moves upwards to the diagnosis and discards irrelevant information along the way and increases the focus. In other words, the nurse meets the patient and gathers cues or information; this could be signs and symptoms, patient's history, etc. Either during or following the interaction, the nurse begins to identify the key cues or important aspects of the data from both the patient and the nurse's long/short-term memory. The nurse may then begin to make inferences from this information, as the nurse begins to cluster the cues together and begins to identify patterns. The word

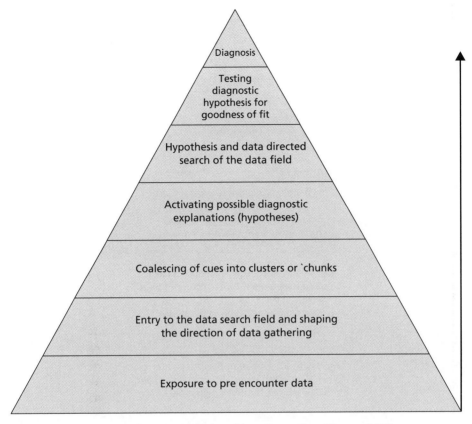

Diagnosis

Testing diagnostic hypothesis for goodness of fit

Hypothesis and data directed search of the data field

Activating possible diagnostic explanations (hypotheses)

Coalescing of cues into clusters or `chunks

Entry to the data search field and shaping the direction of data gathering

Exposure to pre encounter data

Figure 5.1   Information Processing Model adapted from Carnevali and Thomas (1993)

hypothesis is used in this model; this is not defined in the true scientific sense but rather as potential explanations for the situation that uses the information gathered. A hypothesis is thus generated and this then guides the nurse into either gaining more information/cues or interpreting the cues gathered to either confirm or refute the hypothesis that is made. The hypothesis evaluation is suggested to be a key component in the decision-making processes in nursing practitioners (Offredy, 2002). Following these processes, a diagnosis can be made and the process of this for nurse practitioners (NPs) is indicated in Figure 5.2 as applied to a situation where the nurse is assessing a young woman who is referred to the nurse's clinic with lower abdominal pain and profuse, white, offensive vaginal discharge. This approach to decision-making is prevalent within medical literature and is the focus of much discussion with the formulation of differential diagnoses using probability theory to further understand the processes.

Eddy (1988) discusses that to select the most probable diagnosis, a practitioner such as a PN or a WiC nurse needs to calculate and compare the probabilities of various diseases that could have caused the patient's signs and symptoms. To select the most likely diagnosis, one must estimate this probability for all the

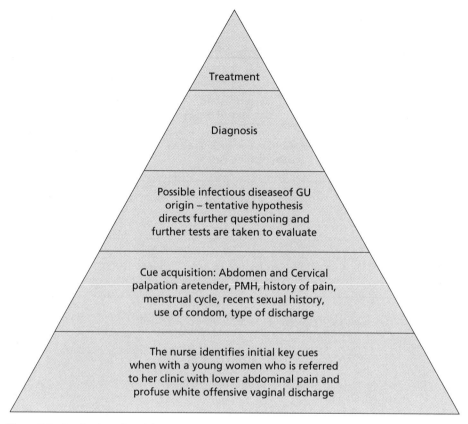

Figure 5.2 Application of model to patient situation

possible diseases, taking into account all the signs and symptoms that are present. The practitioner can face obstacles when making a diagnosis such as the amount of information to be considered, the need to interpret signs and symptoms and the weighing up of probabilities of the likelihood that the diagnosis is correct. Interestingly, Offredy (2002) compared NP's and general practitioner's (GP's) diagnostic hypothesis generation with the same scenario. The results showed that there were more similarities than differences in the abilities of the two groups to identify relevant information. The key differences were that the NPs selected more cues to enable them to reach a diagnosis in comparison with the GPs and the differences in the knowledge base of the NP with the GP. The GP's method of decision-making was determined by the amount of prior knowledge held and their ability to 'chunk' larger pieces of information together.

In these approaches, reasoning is considered to be conscious, speculative and evaluative where the practitioner is solving problems. However, nurses generally manage this process with varying degrees of attention; often if the process occurs frequently, then less attention is paid to the process but if there are new problems or different circumstances with larger risks, then the nurses may undertake more detailed conscious and consultative reasoning.

There is also some evidence that this hypothetico-deductive method is not always the best way to understand the process of clinical decision-making in cases which are straightforward. For example, during routine encounters involving non-complex cases, experienced practitioners appear not to use a hypothesis generation; rather they rely on knowledge of the situation and of other similar cases they may have seen. White and Stancombe (2003) suggest that rather than generating unnecessary sets of competing hypotheses, clinicians rely on pattern recognition. Pattern recognition is the process of making a judgement on the basis of a few critical pieces of information. The primary feature of pattern recognition suggests that each new case is compared to previous cases that are stored in an individual's memory and categorised according to similarity. Offredy (1998) argues that it can be viewed from two levels: analytically where the whole situation is grasped (in this case) and intuitively where pattern matching is linked with intuition and other terms such as gestalt and 'gut feeling'. Experience has a great influence on pattern recognition as once the nurse becomes more experienced, the patterns expand and modify; then the nurse moves to a more refined recognition pattern where key cues are automatically clustered together. Here, positive pattern recognition increases the decision-maker's confidence and as the knowledge base increases, so does a sense of competence (O'Neill et al., 2005).

Critiques of these approaches suggest that this leads to a heavy reliance on the cognitive capacity of the clinician in two ways: first by what is available in memory and second by commitment to the first hypothesis. White and Stancombe (2003) further suggest that this is confounded by the fact that the clinician has a tendency to confirm a hypothesis rather than searching for alternative cues. Therefore, diseases or diagnoses that are most memorable are most easily recalled.

Activity

Identify when you have used analysis in your decision-making.

The intuitive stance
This is the opposing end of hypothetico-deductive model with Polanyi (1983) referring to the 'art' of diagnosing which uses skilful testing and expert observation but cannot be explicitly accounted for. Schön (1988) accepts that some problems can by solved using the scientific application of deduction and defines this as the 'high hard ground'; however, the most important decisions arise in the 'swampy low lands' (Schön, 1988:67). Practitioners in this 'swamp' do not rely on external knowledge, rather they draw upon something within themselves such as intuition. The roots for understanding intuition in nursing were initially identified by Carper (1978), and intuition is regarded as an alternative explanation for how nurses make decisions.

Intuition is defined as:

Understanding without rationale. (Benner and Tanner, 1987)

This is often described in abstract ways such as gut feeling, insight, instinct and hunches. Pyles and Stern (1983) were one of the first researchers to consider that critical care nurses, when identifying cardiogenic shock, used 'gut feelings' in their critical thinking in addition to the objective presenting patient cues.

Benner's (1984) well-known work argues that intuition is an essential part of clinical judgement and is linked clearly with the nurse's expertise. These researchers found that the judgements of expert nurses were different to those of nurses with less expertise. Novice nurses rely on analytical principles to understand the current situation and to guide their actions, whereas the expert nurse no longer relies on an analytical principle to connect with the situation and uses intuition instead.

An alternative approach to understanding intuition is offered by Cioffi (1997) and Buckingham and Adams (2000a,b). They offer the term 'heuristics' as explaining intuition. Heuristics are often referred to as 'rules of thumb' and are strategies the problem solver uses to deal with large amounts of information, where shortcuts are created so that only certain cues are identified amongst huge amounts of information. Cioffi (2001) suggests from her research that these shortcuts are based on past experiences, for example, nurses may recall the usual pattern or presentation of patient with a particular condition and compare this to the presenting patient's progression. Buckingham and Adams (2000a,b) further argue that intuition is rather a function of experience and pattern recognition and may occur at an unconscious level whereas more analytical reasoning may occur at a conscious level.

Activity

Identify when you have used intuition in your decision-making.

The middle ground

How nurses make decisions has incited much debate, and many authors suggest that nurses tend to use a combination of the above strategies when making a decision. As neither single framework offers an exclusive explanation for how decisions are made in nursing practice (Harbison, 2001; Thompson, 2001; Kennedy, 2002), Hamm's cognitive continuum (adapted from Hamm, 1988) is offered as an alternative explanation to consider decision-making in nursing; this acknowledges the differences between analysis and intuition. The key features of this continuum are that the mode of cognition utilised by the clinician is determined by the structure of the task they are undertaking, the time and the amount of information cues that are available. Cognition is viewed along a continuum with analytical thinking opposed to intuition. Hamm (adapted from Hamm, 1988) divided this continuum into six modes of

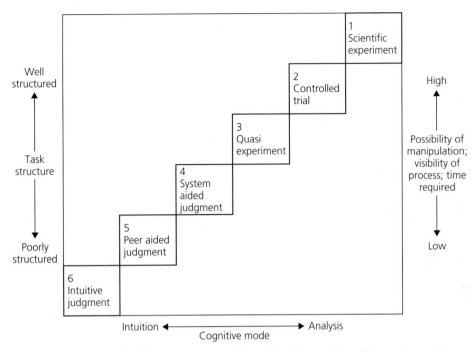

Figure 5.3 Hamm's cognitive continuum (adapted from Hamm, 1988). Reprinted with permission from Cambridge University Press

cognitive practice. For example, when the task is well structured with high degrees of control and more time, it induces an analytical approach – for example, when a nurse is deciding on the significance of an X-ray and if it takes time to compare it with a normal X-ray, then she may use a more analytical approach (this would certainly increase the certainty of her decision). The opposite end of the continuum occurs when the task is unstructured with very little control and with little time to analyse; then the intuitive mode of cognition is utilised and leads the decision-maker to an intuitive judgement (action) (Figure 5.3).

Nurses often work under time constraints with decisions being made from every 30 s to every 10 min and the tasks they undertake are often unstructured with numerous cues. Therefore, the modes of cognitive practice utilised do not merit judgements made within modes 1–3 but neither, argues Thompson (2001), do they merit utilising intuitive guesswork. For example, a nurse prescribing a wound care product for the patient they are currently treating may utilise cognitive practice modes 4–6. A system-aided judgement may occur if the nurse refers to a decision framework (where all statistical probabilities/outcomes have been considered) or a clinical pathway when making their decision. A peer-aided judgement may occur if the nurse arrives at a treatment plan through discussion with peers and review of literature pertaining to the treatment. An intuitive judgement may occur if the nurse relies on intuition to guide their judgement. Hamm (1988) suggests most clinicians make decisions within modes 5 and 6 due to the context of their work.

Cader et al. (2005) argue that understanding the Cognitive Continuum Theory helps nurses in two ways. First, it helps them predict which modes of cognition are relevant to the appropriate nursing decision depending on the context of the decision; this thus increases the accuracy of the nurses' decision-making. Second, this theory can help nurses explain the rationale underpinning their professional decisions. Certainly with Hamm's support for equity, the analytical cognition is not always superior to intuitive stances.

Knowledge within decision-making

We still do not know whether valid and reliable information leads to optimal decision-making and recent studies have demonstrated how clinicians rarely access and use overt research evidence (Thompson, 2001; Gabbay and le May, 2004). Thompson et al. (2001a,b) found in their research that very few sources of information accessed were research based and the strongest piece of anything remotely evidenced based that influenced the nurses' decision-making was human sources such as the clinical specialist and link nurses associated with the specialism under investigation.

Knowledge is often operationalised through decision-making and it is prudent to consider what constitutes knowledge and certainly the effects of knowledge and experience have been identified as significant influences in decision-making (Muir, 2000; Fleming and Fenton, 2002). Of course, the more experience a nurse has, the more patients they will assess and the patterns of illness and common conditions are stored within their memory; eventually the experienced nurse or 'expert' has a store of memorable cases which can be accessed quickly based on cue presentation from the patient. However, experience does not always deliver expertise and the knowledge of experts is constructed from a range of sources.

Luker and Kenrick (1992) acknowledge that nursing knowledge is operationalised through clinical decision-making but whilst nurses demonstrate high levels of skill, often their work is unsubstantiated by any rationale. Their research identified that community nurses' clinical decisions were informed by:

a. knowledge based on research and tested theories;
b. knowledge based on practice and arising out of nursing experience:
   i. clinical experience,
   ii. situational variables;
c. knowledge that is common sense and current.

The majority of nurses in their study identified that clinical experience (82%, $n = 39$) and situational variables (76%, $n = 36$) were the major influences on their decisions. Whilst this research is over 10 years old, the findings are still prevalent in more recent research (see Watson, 1994; Lauri et al., 2001; Kennedy, 2002).

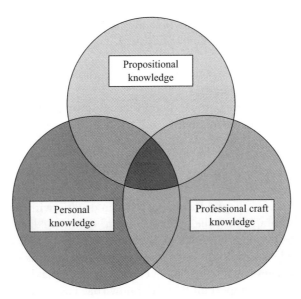

Figure 5.4 Knowledge utilised in clinical decision-making. This article was published in Higgs and Titchen (2001, p. 15). Reprinted with permission from Elsevier

Therefore, to consider what knowledge is utilised in decision-making, it is worth considering the types of knowledge already identified that underpin current thinking in the Western world. Higgs and Titchen (2001) suggest the framework shown in Figure 5.4.

Propositional knowledge is the scientific knowledge, the public objective knowledge of the field. Thompson (2002a,b, 2003) terms this the 'know what' knowledge and Carper (1978) terms this empirical knowledge and that it is the 'science' of the profession. This knowledge can be tested and is open for scrutiny. It is highly valued in current clinical practice through schools of evidence-based practice and quantitative research. However, controlled experiments are rarely the sole basis on which clinical decisions are made and when this knowledge is applied to the patient, other knowledge often overrules this scientific logic (as demonstrated by Luker and Kendrick, 1992).

This scientific knowledge differs from professional craft knowledge. This knowledge can be the practical element that guides everyday activities. Thompson (2002a,b) terms this professional expertise (know-how knowledge) and Carper (1978) terms this aesthetic knowledge which is a tacit knowledge and incorporates the intuitive side of nursing.

Diagnosis and decision-making are affected by the clinician's personal knowledge and experience and are not just a matter of using propositional and nonpropositional knowledge. Personal knowledge has particular reference to the nurses' individual self and is a consequence of the individual's personal experiences, reflections and internal frame of reference and held beliefs. This personal frame of reference also encapsulates the individual personal ethical framework and moral reasoning and would involve an understanding and experience of the following widely accepted principles (Edwards, 1996):

1. autonomy which means the ability to make choices, and is concerned with control and self-governance;
2. beneficence which means doing good through positive acts, and is aligned to the caring perspective in nursing;
3. non-maleficence which means doing no harm, and this principle is implicit within informed consent;
4. justice which means being fair.

Personal knowledge is integral to the nurse when dealing with the patient holistically and should complement the other two forms of knowledge.

These three forms of knowledge as identified by Luker and Kendrick (1992) constitute the individual's knowledge base and it is this that is exercised through a range of approaches when undertaking clinical decision-making. Higgs and Jones (2000) suggest that it is important that this knowledge base be continually critiqued and updated through self-evaluation. The most effective mechanism to do this is through reflection both in and on practice. This ensures that the knowledge that is developed and that which informs professional practice is scrutinised and then able to be articulated.

Activity

Pause for a moment and consider when you have used scientific, aesthetic and personal knowledge in your critical analysis of a situation and decision-making.

Errors within clinical decision-making

Consider the following example: an experienced nurse working in a WiC assesses a patient who is presenting with a red eye that is streaming and the patient articulates that they want to rub this all the time. Other useful contextual cues are that it is a warm sunny spring day with a high pollen count and the patient says that he has been sneezing a lot recently; there are also a lot of other patients waiting to be seen and the air conditioning is not working, thus resulting in a very warm environment. You assess the patient and prioritise the cues that are presented. You know from propositional knowledge that allergic conjunctivitis is the most common problem within all eye problems presented within a GP practice and out of these cases you know that seasonal allergic conjunctivitis accounts for half of allergic conjunctivitis cases. From your professional knowledge, you know that this is easy to treat and that it is likely the patient will respond well to information given. You have also treated this problem before and know the procedure very well.

Table 5.2 Sources of Error in Decision-making

1. Professional and theoretical biases and personal experiences that influence what information is received and how this was interpreted (knowledge-based performance)
2. Diagnosis by formula – trying to fit patients into pre-conceived categories based on previous experience of likelihood of outcome
3. Optimism/pessimism – the clinician's desire to seek to help the patient may result in the optimistic perception or alternatively may over-emphasise the probability of the diagnosis for the worst case scenario; this is related to knowledge-based performance
4. Too many differential diagnoses or hypotheses, so the clinician rules out the least probable quickly (this is based on knowledge performance)
5. Over-simplification – the clinician may assume a simple result based on a misinterpretation of the cues and the probability of the diagnosis and their ability to access their memory of previous similar situations
6. Clinician and patient interaction such as dislike and distrust can affect objective clinical judgement
7. Skill-based failure, where the clinician fails to pay attention at crucial information-gathering situations or is influenced by other contextual situations such as interruptions and environment

You perform the basic assessment and your information seeking and questioning reflects your differential diagnosis.

You make a final diagnosis of seasonal allergic conjunctivitis and implement the recommended plan of care. However, the patient returns to the GP the next day and contact dermatoconjunctivitis is diagnosed which has a risk of ulceration of the cornea and potential visible impairments.

So what went wrong? Clearly the situation at the time influenced the final decision particularly during the rapid nature of the assessment undertaken and the assumptions made throughout the patient/nurse interaction.

Thompson (2002a,b) suggests that the sources of error given in Table 5.2 are commonly seen in decision-making.

Activity

Recall a situation in which you made an error in your clinical decision-making. Analyse this error and identify what influencing factors caused the error. What might you do differently in your practice now if confronted with this situation again?

Systems that improve decision-making

Clinical problems are sometimes constructed as a decision tree and attached to the decision tree is the probability or chance of that event occurring. Studies have shown that these decision trees will aid decision accuracy when used in practice and Dowding and Thompson (2002) suggest that they could be useful for the practice situations shown in Figure 5.5.

Within the tree, each branch point has to compete with another decision based on the previous outcome and a range of consequences are presented. This presentation

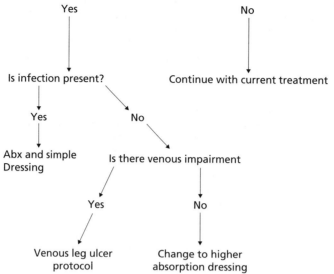

Is wound leaking serous fluid that is not contained in current dressing?

Yes   No

Is infection present?   Continue with current treatment

Yes   No

Abx and simple
Dressing   Is there venous impairment

Yes   No

Venous leg ulcer
protocol   Change to higher
absorption dressing

Figure 5.5   Illustration in relation to the decision to change a wound dressing to respond to a change of circumstances within a chronic wound

offers the measured decisions that can be made and the above framework can be used to guide the clinician in their decision-making. These are particularly popular within the use of protocols in NHS Trust settings; however, these are always applied with the caveat of being a framework only and should be applied using clinical judgement!

If we accept that the propositional knowledge is the only knowledge that has public scrutiny, then this can be aided and developed through support systems and through reading and education.

Clinical decision support systems

These are defined as computer software that employ a knowledge base designed for use by a clinician involved in patient care as a direct aid to clinical decision-making (Johnston et al., 1994). These technologies take the form of algorithms, flow charts or expert systems and in modern clinical decision support systems the medical knowledge that is used by the system is separate from the mechanism using this knowledge. The essence of the knowledge is essentially medical litera-ture and expert opinions. Currently within primary care clinical knowledge sum-maries are being advocated. These are a source of clinical knowledge for the NHS about the common conditions managed in primary and first contact care.

Practical and reliable, these summaries help health care professionals confi-dently make evidence-based decisions about the health care of their patients and provide the know-how to safely put these decisions into action. The intended function for this active system is to assist with forming diagnosis and selecting treatment. The summaries respond to data entered by the clinician and use up-to-date medical knowledge to construct a solution to a problem along with simple decision trees and probability theory. As a system, it is integrated with computerised patient records and covers about 70% of GP consultations. User proficiency is developing with this system.

There is, however, a curious paradox in these statistical programme approaches. Whilst they seek to aide or even replace the judgements of clinicians, they rely on the acceptance that the values within the tools are fully known and are neutrally interpreted. Clearly clinical practice is not this clear and gaining a patient's history is often complex and thus applying these prognostic tools again requires some clinical judgement by the clinician.

Reflective practice

Critical reflection on practice is a process by which knowledge and awareness can be developed. A range of reflective models are available to structure this (Boud et al., 1988; Johns, 2002). Reflection requires critical thinking about situations encountered and considering different options and ways of thinking. Rolf (1998) suggests that this provides the experts with the ability to justify clinical decisions and provide reasoned arguments. Consequently, a reflective practitioner will always be developing their clinical decision-making skills.

Conclusion

The aim of this chapter was to review critical thinking and associated areas of nursing practice. This chapter is only an introduction and further reading is encouraged. However, it is hoped that this has given the reader an insight into the complexity of critical thinking and decision-making and how the nurse can be aware of how mistakes occur and implement strategies to overcome these. The following key points surmise the elements of this chapter:

- Nurses make a range of decisions in their everyday practice, often within time constraints.
- There are different stances or perspectives to explain decision-making. These differ on their account of influencing factors and the extent to which decision-making is analytical or intuitive. Heuristics is offered as an alternative to intuition.
- A case can be made for the middle ground, that nurses use different approaches at different times depending on the context of the clinical situation.
- A variety of knowledge fuels decision-making and is used to varying degrees. Propositional knowledge is the most visible of all; however, this is often filtered through personal knowledge.

- Mistakes can occur within these processes of decision-making and critical thinking and the nurses have a responsibility to be aware of how these occur. Reflective practice and clinical supervision is suggested as a mechanism to improve decision-making skills.
- Primary care nursing is utilising a computerised decision support system to aid the decisions and treatments that nurses are making.

Clinical decision-making is an integral aspect to the nurses' role. When nurses make reasoned judgements, in times of uncertainty, the decisions that are made generally lead to positive patient outcomes. Understanding the basic theory behind the decisions that nurses make can only enhance this process and thus further improve patient outcomes. Furthermore, by being able to identify what types of decisions are made in their every single day, PNs can begin to identify knowledge and/or skill deficits and devise strategies to overcome these.

References

Bandman, E. and Bandman, B. (1995) *Critical Thinking in Nursing*. 2nd edn. Connecticut: Appleton and Lange.

Benner, P. (1984) *From Novice to Expert: Excellence and Power in Clinical Nursing*. California: Addison-Wesley.

Benner, P. and Tanner, C. (1987) Clinical judgement: How expert nurses use intuition. *American Journal of Nursing*, 87(1); 23–31.

Boud, D., Keogh, R. and Walker, D. (1988) *Reflection: Turning Experience into Learning*. London: Kogan Page.

Buckingham, C. and Adams, A. (2000a) Classifying clinical decision making: A unifying approach. *Journal of Advanced Nursing*, 32(4); 981–989.

Buckingham, C. and Adams, A. (2000b) Classifying clinical decision making: Interpreting nursing intuition, heuristics and medical diagnosis. *Journal of Advanced Nursing*, 32(4); 990–998.

Cader, R., Watson, S. and Watsons, D. (2005) Cognitive Continuum Theory in nursing decision making. *Journal of Advanced Nursing*, 49(4); 397–405.

Carnevali, D. and Thomas, M. (1993) *Diagnostic Reasoning and Treatment: Decision Making in Nursing*. Philadelphia: Lippincott.

Carper, B. (1978) Fundamental patterns of knowing in nursing. *Advances in Nursing Science*, 1(1); 13–23.

Cioffi, J. (1997) Heuristics, servants to intuition, in clinical decision-making. *Journal of Advanced Nursing*, 26(1); 203–208.

Cioffi, J. (2001) A study of the past experiences in clinical decision making in emergency situations. *International Journal of Nursing Studies*, 38(5); 591–599.

DoH (2002) *Liberating the Talents*. London: Department of Health.

Donald Schon, (1984) *The Reflective Practitioner: How Professionals think in Action*. New York: Basic Books.

Dowding, D. and Thompson, C. (2002) Using decision trees to aid decision-making in nursing. *Nursing Times*, 100(21); 36–39.

Eddy, D. (1988) Variations in physician practice: The role of uncertainty. In Dowie, J. and Elstein, A. (Eds.) *Professional Judgement: A Reader in Clinical Decision Making*. Chapter 1. Cambridge: Cambridge University Press.

Edwards, S. (1996) *Nursing Ethics: A Principle based Approach*. Basingstoke: Macmillan.

Fleming, K. and Fenton, M. (2002) Making sense of research evidence to inform decision making. In Thompson, C. and Dowding, D. (Eds.) *Clinical Decision Making and Judgement in Nursing*. Edinburgh: Churchill.

Fonteyn, M. and Ritter, B. (2000) Clinical reasoning in nursing. In Higgs, J. and Jones, M. (Eds.) *Clinical Reasoning in the Health Professions*. Oxford: Butterworth-Heinemann.

Gabbay, J. and le May, A. (2004) Evidence based guidelines or collectively constructed 'mindlines'? Ethnographic study of knowledge management in primary care. *British Medical Journal*, 329(7473); 1013–1019.

Hamm, R. (1988) Clinical intuition and clinical analysis: Expertise and the cognitive continuum. In Dowie, J. and Elstein, A. (Eds.) *Professional Judgment: A Reader in Clinical Decision Making*. Cambridge: Cambridge University Press.

Harbison, J. (2001). Clinical decision making in nursing: Theoretical perspectives and their relevance to practice. *Journal of Advanced Nursing*, 35(1); 126–133.

Higgs, J. and Jones, M. (Eds.) (2000) *Clinical Reasoning in the Health Professions*. 2nd edn. Oxford: Butterworth-Heinemann.

Higgs, J. and Titchen, A. (2001) *Practice Knowledge and Expertise in the Health Professions*. Oxford: Butterworth-Heinemann.

Johns, C. (2002) *Guided Reflection; Advancing Practice*. Oxford: Blackwell Science.

Johnston, M., Langton, K., Haynes, B. and Mathieu, A. (1994) The effects of computer-based clinical decision support systems on clinician performance and patient outcome. A critical appraisal of research. *Annual Internal Medicine*, 120; 135–142.

Kennedy, C. (2002) *British Journal of Community Nursing*, 7(10); 505–512.

Lauri, S., Salantera, S., Chalmers, K., Ekman, S., Hesook, S., Kappeli, S. and Macleod, M. (2001) An exploratory study of clinical decision-making in five countries. *Journal of Nursing Scholarship*, 33(1); 83–90.

Luker, K. and Kendrick, M. (1992) An exploratory study of the sources of influences on the clinical decisions of community nurses. *Journal of Advanced Nursing*, 17(4); 457–466.

Matteson, P. and Hawkins, J. (1990) Concept analysis of decision making. *Nursing Forum*, 25(2); 4–10.

McGrew, A. and Wilson, M. (1982) *Decision Making. Approaches and Analysis*. London: Taylor and Francis.

Miller, M. and Babcock, D. (1996) *Critical Thinking applied to Nursing*. St. Louis: Mosby.

Muir, N. (2000) Unpublished MSc thesis – *Clinical Decision Making by District Nurses*. London: Southbank University.

NMC (2006) *Consultation on a Framework for the Standard for Post Registration Nursing*. London: Nursing Midwifery Council.

Offredy, M. (1998) The application of decision making concepts by nurse practitioners in general practice. *Journal of Advanced Nursing*, 28(5); 988–1000.

Offredy, M. (2002) Decision making in primary care: Outcomes from a study using patient scenarios. *Journal of Advanced Nursing*, 40(5); 532–541.

O'Neill, E., Dluhy, M. and Chin, E. (2005) Modelling novice clinical reasoning for a computerized decision support system. *Journal of Advanced Nursing*, 49(1); 68–77.

Paniagua, H. (1997) Consultations: In practice. *Practice Nurse*, 8(8); 20–22.

Polanyi, M. (1983) *The Tacit Dimension*. Gloucester: Smith.

Pyles, S. and Stern, P. (1983) Discovery of nursing gestalt in critical care nursing: The importance of Gray Gorilla Syndrome. *The Journal of Nursing Scholarship*, 15(2); 51–57.

Rolf, G. (1998) Beyond expertise: Reflective and reflexive nursing practice. In Johns, C. and Freshwater, D. (Eds.) *Transforming Nursing through Reflective Practice*. Oxford: Blackwell Science.

Royal College of Nursing (2005) *An RCN Guide to the Nurse Practitioner Role, Competencies and Programme Approval*. London: Royal College of Nursing.

Rubenfeld, M. and Scheffer, B. (1995) *Critical Thinking in Nursing: An Interactive Approach*. Philadelphia: Lippincott.

Sackett, D., Rosenberg, W., Gray, J., Haynes, R. and Richardson, W. (1996) Evidence based medicine: What it is and what it isn't. *BMJ*, 312(7023); 71–72.

Sahler, O. and Carr, J. (2003) *The Behavioural Sciences and Health Care*. Germany: Hogrefe and Huber.

Thompson, C. (2001) Jan Forum: Clinical decision making in nursing: Theoretical perspective and their relevance to practice – A response to Jean Harbison. *Journal of Advanced Nursing*, 35(1); 134–137.

Thompson, C. (2002a) Human error, bias, decision making and judgement in nursing – The need for a systematic approach. In Thompson, C. and Dowding, D. (Eds.) *Clinical Decision Making and Judgement in Nursing*. Edinburgh: Churchill.

Thompson, C. (2002b) The value of research in clinical decision-making. *Nursing Times*, 98(42); 30–34.

Thompson, C. (2003) Clinical experience as evidence in evidence based practice. *Journal of Advanced Nursing*, 43(3); 230–237.

Thompson, C. and Dowding, D. (2001) Responding to uncertainty in nursing practice. *International Journal of Nursing Studies*, 38; 609–615.

Thompson, C., McCaughan, D., Cullum, N., Sheldon, T., Mulhall, A. and Thompson, D. (2001a) The accessibility of research-based knowledge for nursing in United Kingdom acute care settings. *Journal of Advanced Nursing*, 36(1); 11–22.

Thompson, C., McCaughan, D., Cullum, N., Sheldon, T., Mulhall, A. and Thompson, D. (2001b) Research information in nurses' clinical decision making: What is useful? *Journal of Advanced Nursing*, 36(3); 376–388.

Watson, S. (1994) An exploratory study into a methodology for the examination of decision making by nurses in the clinical area. *Journal of Advanced Nursing*, 20(1); 351–360.

White, S. and Stancombe, J. (2003) *Clinical Judgement in the Health and Welfare Professions: Extending the Evidence Base*. Maidenhead: Open University Press.

Health education and health promotion

6

Daryl Evans

Becoming a health-promoting nurse in general practice and walk-in centres: Introduction

The aim of this chapter is to encourage the development of a health-promoting culture in general practice (GP) and walk-in-centre (WiC) nursing. The promotion of health is an essential role for every nurse wherever they practice. The Nursing and Midwifery Council (NMC) Code of Conduct (2008:1) requires that nurses 'promote the health and wellbeing of those in your care, their families and carers, and the wider community'. It goes on to mention helping them to access relevant health information and supporting them to improve and maintain their health (NMC, 2008).

Nurses are part of the public health workforce, and when you look at the skill requirements for public health, it is easy to see the overlap. It was Acheson (1998) who defined public health practitioners as those who spend substantial time furthering health by working with community groups and individuals. He included community nurses.

The Public Health Skills and Career Framework (Skills for Health, 2008) sets out levels of public health practice aligned with suggested job expectations. A registered nurse is at level 5 and a specialist in community health nursing (health visitor, school nurse and occupational health nurse) at level 6. The 'Defined Area' of Health Improvement articulates the knowledge and skills required at level 5, which are a follows (a summary):

- work with communities to plan and deliver health improvement programmes;
- develop resources for specific audiences;
- communicate the health interests of the community to others;
- have knowledge of the wider determinants of health, principles of community development, theories of health promotion and approaches to improving health, including behaviour change;
- have an understanding of how health promotion can address inequalities.

Perhaps a more familiar document setting out levels of skills required is the National Health Service (NHS) Knowledge and Skills Framework (NHS, 2004). In this, health promotion is largely within Health and Wellbeing 1 (HWB1) and level 2 seems to be most often used to measure the skills of a registered nurse. There is a good match to the level 5 expectations mentioned above.

This chapter takes an approach to health promotion in nursing which recognises these competencies and skills and sets them in a framework, enabling a nurse to see the practical applications to the practice/centre workplace.

Learning Outcomes

- ▓ To examine the potential for health promotion within nursing practice
- ▓ To refocus actions on wider issues than immediate health education
- ▓ To consider a realistic framework for improving health promotion practice.

Background

The key to becoming a health-promoting nurse is not to make extra time to 'do' health promotion but to change to a way of practising that has promoting health embedded in the goals, methods and locations of everyday work. This makes health promotion an activity which surrounds the nurse–client encounter and reaches further to impact on others. It is about developing a culture of health promotion rather like a culture of safety or of hygiene, an integral part of the potential of nursing.

Creating a health-promoting culture for yourself and for the area in which you practice is a somewhat broader way of thinking than simply educating your clients about their illnesses. It incorporates the NMC notions of not only the client's immediate circle, but also the community in which your practice area is set. Your clients enter your practice area with not only an expectation of help with their problem of the moment, but also the trust that you will extend that help to their general and future well-being. Their visits can be opportunities to engage patients in gaining control over their own health and for families and carers to do the same for themselves. The practice area can become a community resource for health improvement.

To be a health-promoting nurse involves an element of personal learning, an awareness of current strategic plans, the management of individual patients and the creation of an environment of opportunity for them and the local community. The World Health Organisation (WHO) in its Ottawa Charter (1986) set out a way forward to a joined-up way of thinking of promoting health, with its call to address developing personal skills, strengthening community action, building healthy public policy, creating supportive environments and reorienting health services towards more prevention and the promotion of positive health. The Ottawa vision is a foundation for this framework for nursing (Figure 6.1).

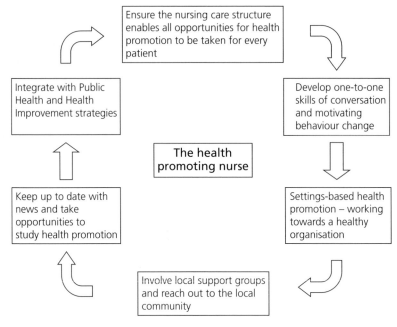

Figure 6.1   A framework for health promotion in nursing

Integrate with public health and health improvement strategies

Since 1998, the UK government has increasingly adopted the WHO (1986) guide-lines for improving health. Moving away from a predominantly victim-blaming philosophy, they have embraced partnership working, equity and community devel-opment, against a background of the wider socio-economic view of health.

Over the past 20 years or so, health promotion has become embedded in the function of community health services working in partnership with local govern-ment. Partnership is now seen as essential, involving organisations across sec-tors, for example, pharmacies, leisure centres, police, supermarkets, community groups, charities, youth services, schools, media and faith organisations. The pos-sible partnerships reflect the wide range of health determinants.

The WHO continues to base much of its work on equity in health care and on the wider determinants of health (WHO, 2003; CSDH, 2008). This way of think-ing acknowledges all aspects of living impact on health: income, housing, educa-tion, transport, leisure, employment and environment, for example (Dahlgren and Whitehead, 1991). The health of your patients is therefore not just about their age, gender, genetic makeup and medical history, but also about their lifestyles being limited by such wider determinants.

The government has focused on inequalities in health since they took office, com-missioning a report to suggest an action plan to reduce inequalities (Acheson, 1998). Previous governmental action had refused to acknowledge the widening gap in health chances between the well-off and the less well-off (Townsend et al., 1988).

Today addressing inequalities is essential to planning health improvement work, securing funding for projects, setting targets and attaining quality standards for practice. National and local organisations all focus their work towards lessening the gap.

Activity

Look up your local community health targets for inequalities. How is your practice/ centre contributing to those targets?
List some of the local issues such as...

- large number of low income families
- significant ethnic group

. . . and think of some ideas for what you could do as a nurse in your workplace to address these issues e.g., free offers; culturally sensitive approaches.

The current health improvement strategy – a white paper – was designed by the government in 2004. In England, this is *Choosing Health: Making Healthy Choices Easier* (DoH, 2004), a direct use of earlier WHO phraseology, demonstrating continued alignment with that organisation's stance. Targets in this strategy have been refocused away from an emphasis on specific disease prevention to enabling healthier lifestyle choices. There are:

Three underpinning principles: informed choice supported by the right environment for that choice; personalisation of services to meet the needs of deprived groups and communities, tailored to the realities of individual lives; and effective partnership.

Six overarching priorities
1. reducing the numbers of people who smoke;
2. reducing obesity and improving diet and nutrition;
3. increasing exercise;
4. encouraging and supporting sensible drinking;
5. improving sexual health;
6. improving mental health.

There are further documents giving more detailed plans for healthy eating and physical activity and updates on progress. Since 2004, some of the promises within the statute have been followed through, for example, the ban on smoking in enclosed public spaces. This manoeuvre is intended to empower people to make healthy choices through environmental control. Other policy decisions are in operation or under discussion, such as legislating for healthy school meals, controlling promotion of unhealthy lifestyles in the media, graphic warnings on tobacco and alcohol packaging, regulating the number of fast food outlets and making some areas alcohol-free.

Activity

Read the white paper Choosing Health (DoH, 2004).
  In what ways does your practice/centre meet these statutory principles and priorities?

As well as this white paper, there are national strategic plans related to specific topics. Some are governmental and some are in national partnership with charities and industry bodies, integrating partnership working through the national and local delivery. You will find such plans for sexual health, drugs, five-a-day (fruit and vegetables), at least five-a-week (physical activity), smoking, teenage pregnancy, suicide prevention and so on. As you can see, the list is long. Disease prevention strategies are more numerous than those devoted to lifestyle and behaviour change, but the National Institute for Clinical Excellence (NICE) has for a few years had a remit to review and advise on effective public health as well as treatments and drugs. They have guidelines on smoking cessation, physical activity and behaviour change, amongst other things – see their publications on http://www.nice.org.uk.

Ensure the nursing care structure enables all opportunities for health promotion to be taken for every patient

This is fundamentally concerned with reorienting nursing care to see the patient's visit as an opportunity for health promotion. Teaching the patients and their families about the diagnosis, treatment and follow-up care for the reason they attended is one big part of this, of course. Most nurses tend to do this very well; it is relevant to the moment, necessary for concordance and compliance, and usually relatively straightforward to deliver.

Taking opportunity for addressing other health issues to do with risk factors and the wider determinants of health while the patient is with you is more difficult. Time constraints need to be recognised, as consultations are short. Focused conversations controlled by the nurse can move the patient along a decision-making process. Having educational resources close to hand, ready to pull out and discuss with the patient cuts out going to find something. One effective action is to make sure the leaflets you are giving have space to personalise (or attach an extra fold of paper). Write or sketch the information or alter the leaflet as you speak or as the patient asks questions. Patients tend to learn more effectively when the information is contextualised to their circumstances.

One way to 'save' time is to set up or link with group sessions. Referring the patients to smoking cessation, weight reduction, exercise and chronic disease management group sessions means you have used a few minutes effectively and the learning will continue. Have the information at your fingertips.

Activity

Consider constructing a resource manual for each nurse area (desk, interview room etc) containing:

- All available leaflets
- Lists or cards with local addresses of support organisations
- Lists or cards of appropriate groups as above
- Instruction sheets or protocols for nurses on how to deliver health promotion for the main lifestyle issues and risk factors. Start with the common issues and build up a series; a set of teaching notes.

Reception staff also need resources nearby. They could hold a directory of local facilities such as patient support groups and smoking cessation, weight loss, etc. Patients could be offered a chance to look through this and take notes. Be sure to have some translations into other relevant languages as it will save everyone time trying to explain verbally.

A good patient record-keeping system is essential for patient care, but how well does it accommodate records of health promotion? Space is needed to keep records compatible with the practice/centre structure. If assessing, planning, implementing and evaluating are used in the paperwork, then the process can be applied to education needs as well as care needs. If integrated care pathway planning has been implemented, then this can include health education for the current problem as part of the paperwork. Opportunistic health promotion for wider health issues is by its nature unplanned before seeing the patient, but the paperwork may still allow a reminder to nurses to take action, and a space to record it.

Activity

Review your patient record system. Ensure it enables recording of:

1 Information given relevant to the reason for visit (tick box perhaps)
2 Broader, opportunistic, health advice and screening done
3 Suggested follow up actions, so that other nurses may continue.

Finally, it would be good to discuss as a practice/centre team the development of protocols for health promotion. It may seem very intrusive and uncertain to raise a broader lifestyle or health risk with patients, and without guidelines a nurse may feel unable to deal with more than the reason for the visit. Drawing up protocols for initiating health promotion with obese patients, smokers, alcohol drinkers at risk, those with high blood pressure or cholesterol, people who do not exercise, etc., could be a useful process of decision-making for the team as well as providing guides for future practice.

Develop one-to-one skills of conversation and motivating behaviour change

There are many suggested psychological theories and practical means of enabling health behaviour change in people. Health psychology is a large discipline and many researchers have tried to find the evidence for the most effective methods. NICE (2007) have produced a set of guidelines for organisations, training and research. Nurses are generally exposed to a few more commonly used models and methods in the health professional literature.

This chapter presents just two methods of behaviour change for your consideration. More detailed discussion of the whole background to influences on behaviour, such as beliefs, attitudes, values and judgement of risk to health, is not possible here, but you should consider these. A practical approach to trying the two methods and some suggestions for managing health conversations is shown.

Conversations can wander about all over the place, and as you probably already know patients can get you off the subject. Trying to focus on smoking can lead you at one point into the stress of organising a wedding and later into a catalogue of all the methods of quitting and why none of them seem to work for the patient. You must control the little time you have in order to achieve progress. Notice the emphasis on progress, not on achieving the end goal. In such a short interview, smoking cessation or achieving normal weight is not going to happen, and neither is the complete commitment to start giving up. All you can do is move the patient along the continuum of change a little more each time. If you are only going to see the patient once, then this means perhaps getting agreement to read a leaflet, or to stop using sugar in tea for a week and see how it goes. This plan needs to be communicated in the patient record especially if you or another nurse will see that patient again. At the next interview, another plan may move the patient further along towards permanent change.

Control the conversation.

1. Be bold in introducing the subject, for example, 'I want now to talk to you about your smoking/weight'. Do not ask any closed questions such as '*are you aware smoking is a problem?*' and '*do you have any difficulties with your weight?*' This will only allow the patient to deflect the focus by denial.
2. Ask the patient about their present behaviour, for example, 'how many do you/how long have you smoked?' 'What weight are you? How long have you been overweight?' Only ask one or two straightforward questions, and remain visibly and verbally non-judgemental. This will reassure the patient that you are not going to attack or accuse.
3. Then ask them to tell you what they have tried in the past or 'so far'. This will hopefully give you the chance to avoid suggesting a long list of possible methods of cessation and dieting – most of which will have been rejected already as ineffective. You may, with some people, have to interrupt firmly – 'let me stop you there, you've obviously really tried to do this, well done'.
4. Now, maintaining eye contact and waiting for an answer, ask them 'what do you think you need to do next?' Please resist the temptation to jump in with

multiple suggestions as in step 2; wait for the patient to make a suggestion. If needed, after a minute say 'you do need to make a plan'; keep eye contact.

5. Turn that suggestion into an achievable plan, one small step to be taken by a deadline and then rethink. If you do not approve of the suggestion, then be careful in making corrections or you will be back to step 1. Keep the patient positive.

6. Congratulate the patient for a hard decision well made.

Activity

Try this conversation structure with a patient. Tape-record it (with the patient's consent) if you feel strong enough! Does it work, did it save time?

Can you adapt it to suit your own style and can you see the adaptations which may be needed for some people of different cultures?

One method of behaviour change recommended in the literature is known as brief intervention. Popular with the medical profession, it too addresses the time factor. Usually described in the context of a health issue, for example, alcohol use, the structure is based on explaining health risks of the current behaviour, advising healthier behaviour and getting agreement for action. An example in detail related to alcohol is produced by WHO (Babor and Higgins-Biddle, 2001). The current Smokefree campaign from the NHS (2009) has the following structure to advise you:

- *ask* and record smoking status;
- *advise* patient of health benefits of quitting;
- *act* on patient's response and refer to NHS support.

Another popular structure for behaviour change management is the Stages of Change Model devised in 1983 (Prochaska and DiClemente, 2009). Their model purports to incorporate a range of theories (transtheoretical) of behaviour change and to suggest a series of stages patients may go through.

Precontemplation is the stage at which the patient has no intention to change behaviour and is unaware of their problems. Your intervention is likely to come as an unwelcome intrusion. What you can do is gain their interest and curiosity, perhaps at a health fair, through challenging with shock stories, or just being direct.

Contemplation is the stage in which a patient is aware that a problem exists and is seriously thinking about overcoming it but have yet to commit to action. Your actions could include directly asking for a plan of action, again arousing interest with success stories or showing more details of health risks.

Preparation is often when the patient is still tenuous about intent, but will be keen to seek information and advice. Now the patient is eager for information,

give appropriate responses to their multiple ideas, but continue to encourage a
decision.

Action is when your patient tries something, even a small step. Praise and reward
is needed now, 'keep it up, well done, give yourself a treat'.

Maintenance comes some time later and may last for the foreseeable future. The
patient gradually become secure and develops an 'expertise'. Continue the
praise and encourage the patient to set an example to and teach others.

Relapse may occur, so continue to encourage and do not let your patient see it as
failure.

Settings-based health promotion – working towards a healthy organisation

One of the most successful approaches to health promotion has been the WHO
settings-based programme. A setting is seen as any place where people live, work,
learn, play and so on, where there is a bordered area or organisation which can
work on health problems (WHO, 2009). The approach is an alternative to focusing primarily on a series of unconnected health issues for the same population and
instead takes a 'whole system' view of problems and planning. Within this plan,
a collection of relevant initiatives and projects may be undertaken. One of the
strengths of the approach is that projects need not be short term and transient,
as they often become when isolated from other projects, but can become more
embedded into the structure and agenda of the organisation itself.

Settings-based work began in 1986 with the creation of Healthy Cities (large urban
areas) of which there are now thousands across the world. On a smaller scale, the
UK names its local initiatives Healthy Neighbourhoods. Healthy Schools, Colleges,
Universities, Prisons and Health Promoting Hospitals are all found in this country
and information about them can be found at the Healthy Settings Development Unit
at the University of Central Lancashire (UCLAN, 2009). Health Promoting Hospitals
have had a more limited impact, largely due to lack of management commitment
and resources as well as constantly changing organisational structures. As an illustration of how a Health Promoting Hospital can work towards an agenda for smoking,
healthy eating, physical activity, sensible alcohol use, mental well-being and sexual
health, see some tips from the North East of England (Ubido et al., 2006).

Taking the 'whole system' approach into GPs and WiCs, it is possible see the
potential impact on patients, staff, visitors and the local community. People are
waiting, snacking, walking around, reading information, watching TV/video,
using computers, sitting and getting bored and/or anxious. The environment can
be enhanced to make use of opportunities for health promotion. Even when just
arriving, people can be soothed or cheered in some ways by a pleasant atmosphere and decor. It may be possible through negotiation to make travelling to the
practice/centre easier, and provision of cycle spaces for appropriate people, especially staff. Knowledge of and signposting to walkways in the grounds or nearby
would usefully and healthily occupy people who need to wait or take a break.

Staff health can be acknowledged through making a link with the local leisure centre for trial sessions and discounts.

A useful framework with which to formulate the creation of a 'healthy practice/centre' is that of Tannahill (Downie et al., 1996) who suggested that health promotion is comprised of health education, prevention services and health protection in three overlapping spheres. These are health education, prevention services and health protection.

Health education

Posters, notices and leaflets in ample supply and always up to date would seem to be an obvious starting point to making your practice/centre a place where people can learn about health. Information notice boards can be however ignored and become 'wallpaper', especially if they are boring in layout or colour, not easy to read or out of date and looking old. Real effort is needed to keep them interesting. A monthly change-over of new topics could be used. Specific, perhaps humorous, notices next to stairs and vending machines could make people think about healthier behaviour as they smile. Remember to get copyright permission. You could use joke cartoons and well-known characters to make your point.

Leaflets on a wide range of clinical conditions, investigations and treatments are available from various charity organisations which support patients and families. If you can get good supplies for free, then they can be given to every relevant patient; if they come with a charge, then they may be considered by managers to be an essential resource. As a professional, you will be able to obtain examples at least, or print from online sources.

Activity

Make a list (from the local directory of patient organisations and support services) of the relevant organisations for your patients.

Write to them all, or go online, and request examples of their literature. Make a considered choice of which to have available for your patients or to use as displays.

Plan how to use them. Audit your place of work; note the old leaflets, empty spaces and uninteresting displays. You may need leaflet dispensers, new notice boards, folders for reference etc.

Health education in written form is obviously of limited use. Many people are not by nature, ability or experience great readers of text. For some areas, resources need to be translated into relevant languages. This can be costly and may not solve the whole problem. Lengthy, wordy leaflets and notices may not suit your local needs. Perhaps you can raise the possibility of having a TV/DVD system which can show health advice alternating with service information and entertainment on a continuous loop. Look for some resources which put the point across visually; sometimes diagrams and representational images can get the message across with very few words. Models can help too.

Consider also tailoring material to your practice/centre. Many organisations now have relevant information on services available on their websites. It would be easy to include some pages of lifestyle advice and links to more comprehensive websites for further details. Have you thought of having a computer station accessible to patients, where they could look up your suggested online resources?

Prevention services

Clearly this overlaps with the functions you ordinarily perform for your patients when required. In addition, take opportunities to give information and offer services such as screening tests and smoking cessation to patients when they come for something else. Similarly this may be advertised to the local community and offered to staff. For example, offer screening for diabetes or blood pressure to all adults 'available at this practice/centre on request'. There are budget implications; perhaps ask a local pharmacy to come into partnership with you, seek sponsorship or charge a small fee. Of course, you could limit the time of this to one day a week or even to a one-month campaign in the year.

Campaigns based on an annual calendar can be useful for screening and raising awareness of risks. Breast cancer month, men's health week, no smoking day and mental health day could be interspersed with ideas of your own, perhaps for a significant ethnic or age group. The Department of Health and the relevant charities tend to hold information about these calendar events, but there is no one source of information.

Activity

Choose a calendar event for a future date (in good time to get set up). Try contacting your local health promotion/improvement unit, ask them to help you.

Collect resources and plan the day/week/month. One day could have several activities going on if you ask for volunteers and favours! Screening tests could be offered.

It is more difficult to sustain multiple activities over time, so a really interesting, colourful, multimedia display across the whole practice/centre for a period would work. Put up information about screening available for your chosen focus and advice on how to spot signs of e.g., diabetes, cancer or stroke.

Then plan to take it all away so as to keep the anticipation and improve the impact.

Health protection

This is the development of policies and the allocation of resources to health promotion. Some 'policies' are large and national, and some are locally operated. In a healthy setting, it is possible to raise awareness of the policies that protect us, for example:

- the local authority's ban on alcohol in public;
- food labelling regulations;
- school decisions to control children's eating;
- the local park notices encouraging walking, with exercise stations;
- laws which forbid the sale of tobacco to children.

Having local authority information available for browsers can be a good approach to partnership work in this way. Perhaps someone could be at one of your events.

As well as giving information in this way, as a healthy setting the practice/centre could itself have health policies. Consider banning snacks which are high in fat, salt and sugar – from vending machines, in front of children or in the staff room. Suggesting people use the stairs, making drinking water available (no fizzy drinks), and protecting time for staff breaks and possibly exercise and relaxation are all ideas for organisational policies.

Involve local support groups and reach out to the local community

Really this is an essential part of the settings-based approach to health promotion. The setting is more than the people inside the organisation. It reaches out to the local community and welcomes them into the organisation in order to impact upon their health and those inside the organisation – for mutual benefit.

Local support groups are of course resources for your patients who can contact them as individuals. Groups may also be at your health events in the practice/centre. Indeed if your place is convenient, the event could be opened to the wider public and advertised in local papers. Locally based specialist nurses sometimes arrange whole health fairs for their patient groups, for example, colorectal and diabetes patients. Local Age Concern or British Heart Foundation groups also like to have information stalls at events. Looking at this the other way around – have you thought of taking a stall to an event held perhaps at the local shopping mall? Tell people what your practice/centre can offer and give health advice as well.

Another way to tell people what you do and contribute to the dissemination of health education is to take space in the local free newspapers or get onto local radio. This can work well when timed for your health events. A website for your practice/centre is also useful – remember to advertise that you have one. As well as organisational information, weave in some health messages and make links to resources. You can get permission to use some of the health-related social marketing logos such as 5-a-Day and Drink Aware.

Returning to the subject of health fairs, there is a wide range of potential partners. An older persons' health fair may include police home safety, utilities advisors (safe gas and electricity use), fire safety, pensions and benefits, savings, leisure ideas, disability support and so on. The lifestyle topics include community dietician, low-cost supermarket, fitness opportunities, suitable shoe sales and foot care advice, drop-in medical advice, nurses giving health advice, etc. All this can be done in an atmosphere of a fun day out.

There are an increasing number of partnership referral schemes. Smoking cessation groups, weight loss groups and exercise on prescription at the local leisure centre address some of the lifestyle issues. For patients with chronic disease, patient education for arthritis and diabetes has been available for a few years. In addition, the Expert Patient Programme (EPP) is a system of courses run by volunteer lay trainers who have been patients themselves (EPP, 2009). The courses are attended by a mixture of patients with chronic disease. The government is committed to investment in these courses, which have already trained over 50,000 patients. All these referral examples contribute to health promotion as either secondary or tertiary prevention measures.

Activity

Find out how you refer patients to appropriate groups. Make a contact list for the practice/centre.

Ask to make a professional observation visit to a group; see what happens there.

Finally, you and the practice/centre are an integral part of the local community. Issues important to the community are also part of your professional role, the political part. Make sure you are aware of the health issues the community are lobbying for and objecting to. Do you enable them to use your premises to put up notices or hold meetings? Do you join in petitions and protests? Obviously there is no simple answer, but it may be a good question. Practice/centre managers and local community health managers may be wary, but may also recognise the need to support the community. It is a question for you to answer as a nurse, a public-sector employee and an individual.

Keep up to date with news and take opportunities to study

Public health-related news comes from research or from organisations who are stakeholders in some aspect of health. It is difficult to keep up with research findings without perhaps specifically searching databases for recent articles in journals, and not many nurses have time to do this on a regular basis. There are many government departments and other national organisations connected with health, and they may deal with more than one aspect of health, so nurses could find themselves trying to keep up with multiple topics.

One way to see what is new is to regularly read those broadsheet newspapers which tend to report research findings with a little more in-depth reporting than the sensationalising of the tabloid press. Responsible articles reporting new research, government decisions and position statements from legitimate organisations can give you something to follow up in your areas of interest. If the paper does not give the full reference, then a Google search can be useful if you put the right keywords in. Remember however to go to what seems to be a professional website source to find out more.

It is possible to sign up to e-mail or postal updates from some organisations. You do not want too many of these, but a select few may include the Department of Health, the NICE and one or two specifically relevant organisations such as Diabetes UK and the British Heart Foundation. Alternatively, it is relatively quick to check on their websites for news once a month. Organisations such as these are also good sources of resources for your clients and you can arrange to be kept informed of new materials this way.

Along similar lines, look out for new national campaigns. When you see some new example of social marketing (advertising techniques used to market health and other social benefits rather than products), look on the poster or leaflet or television advert for its source. Some recent examples are:

- *FAST* – a stroke awareness campaign, from the NHS, teaching people to recognise the signs of stroke and to act fast.
- *Drink Aware* – teaching about alcohol use, from the Drink Aware Trust. Their logo appears on all alcohol containers and advertisements originating in the UK.
- *Change 4 Life* – tackling childhood obesity, from the NHS.

Familiarise yourself with the campaign aims and rationale, think about what is good and not so good about it, and whether you would use the materials in your work. Send for or print some of the publications and perhaps discuss the campaign at a team meeting.

Spending any amount of time in these activities is a good use of development time and well worth recording in your portfolio as part of PREP, especially if you write up a short reflective account of your learning and how it will influence your practice. A more traditional approach to recording PREP is to attend study days and seminars. However, this can be a real problem. You need time to do this and also the money. However, there are some things where time can be organised differently and there are cheap or even free opportunities.

Most big nursing and public health conferences cost so much that you may not be given the chance to attend. There are however locally held seminars – usually by the Primary Care Trust/Local Health Board or by charity and other organisations which are sometimes free, and usually either based on the work they are doing such as launching a new plan or offering training in a method of helping people to take up healthy behaviours. Some offer the Foundation Certificate in Health Promotion. Look out for seminars by reading the professional press and checking websites relevant to your needs. Occasionally a leading manufacturer will organise a study day related to what they are selling as 'healthy', for example, a food product company organising training on helping people to eat a healthy diet.

Making good use of exhibitions can also be useful. The display stands and workshops offer chances to talk to other professionals and take something away for your portfolio. Nursing and Primary Care exhibitions are often free – for example, at RCN Congress – and often have exhibits from the Department of Health, the NICE, Public Health Observatories and the like. Go and find out what is new and collect further reading material; also talk to the stallholders about how they can help with your work. Commercial companies are usually present with their products.

The general advice regarding information and materials from brand name products would be to pick up the samples and the freebies but take them home for use by you and your family. Do not advertise their products to your clients, not even by using their pens with logos. However, some of the samples and publications could be useful for teaching in the workplace.

There are some learning packages and courses available by post or online. The NHS Smokefree campaign offers a free guide to giving brief advice to clients. The Department of Health has launched an Alcohol Identification and Brief Advice e-learning course at http://www.alcohollearningcentre.org.uk/eLearning/IBA/. Health Knowledge is developing e-learning modules for the public health competency areas at http://www.healthknowledge.org.uk/. Accessible from Canada, one online course in health promotion is available at http://www.ohprs.ca/hp101/main.htm.

Finally, remember to keep your professional portfolio up to date by recording the hours you spend on learning aspects of promoting health and reflecting on how this has influenced your practice.

Conclusion

Becoming a health-promoting nurse and creating a culture of health promotion in your place of work is going to be hard work, but will enhance your skills, your job satisfaction and your career. Success will depend on your determination, stamina and teamwork skills. Innovation and change take time and resources. Start with small plans, just like the patients' changing behaviour, and monitor the effects. Remember to seek recognition for your hard work. Make sure you have it acknowledged in your appraisal and incorporate it into your curriculum vitae.

As you make these changes, evaluate the effectiveness of your health promotion. Keep a note of the processes involved and the difficulties overcome. Measure the impact by auditing the number of patients given opportunities for health promotion in different topics. Ask some patients to give you their views on the changes. Ask some staff to give you feedback. Do make sure your managers receive this information; write a report or put a piece in the local press. Above all, enjoy the challenge.

References

Acheson, D. (1998) *Independent Enquiry into Inequalities in Health*. London: TSO.

Babor, T. and Higgins-Biddle, J. (2001) *Brief Intervention for Hazardous and Harmful Drinking: A Manual for Use in Primary Care*. Geneva: WHO. http://www.who.int/substance_abuse/publications/alcohol/en/index.html (accessed 31 March 2009).

CSDH (2008) *Closing the Gap in a Generation: Health Equity through Action on the Social Determinants of Health*. Final report of the Commission on Social Determinants of Health. Geneva: World Health Organization.

Dahlgren, G. and Whitehead, M. (1991) *Policies and Strategies to promote Social Equity*. London: Health Institute of Future Studies.

DoH (2004) *Choosing Health: Making Healthy Choices Easier*. London: Department of Health. http://www.dh.gov.uk/en/Publicationsandstatistics/Publications/PublicationsPolicyAndGuidance/DH_4094550 (accessed 31 March 2009).

Downie, R., Tannahill, C. and Tannahill, A. (1996) *Health Promotion Models and Values*. 2nd edn. Oxford: Oxford Medical.

Expert Patients Programme (2009) *Website Homepage*. http://www.expertpatients.co.uk/public/default.aspx?load=PublicHome (accessed 31 March 2009).

National Health Service (2004) *The NHS Knowledge and Skills Framework and the Development Review Process*. London: Department of Health.

National Health Service (2009) *Smokefree Campaign Website*. http://smokefree.nhs.uk/resources/campaigns/ (accessed 31 March 2009).

National Institute for Clinical Excellence (2007) *Behaviour Change at Population, Community and Individual Level*. http://www.nice.org.uk/Guidance/PH6 (accessed 31 March 2009).

NMC (2008) *The Code: Standards of Conduct, Performance and Ethics for Nurses and Midwives*. London: Nursing and Midwifery Council.

Prochaska, J.O. and DiClemente, C.C. (2009) *Prochange Website*. http://www.prochange.com/ttm (accessed 31 March 2009).

Skills for Health (2008) *Public Health Skills and Career Framework. Skills for Health/Public Health Resource Unit*. http://www.skillsforhealth.org.uk/page/career-frameworks/public-health-skills-and-career-framework (accessed 30 March 2009).

Townsend, P., Davidson, N. and Whitehead, M. (1988) *Inequalities in Health: The Black Report and the Health Divide*. London: Penguin.

Ubido, J., Winters, L., Ashton, M., Scott-Samuel, A., Atherton, J. and Johnstone, F. (2006) *Top Tips for Healthier Hospitals*. Liverpool Public Health Observatory and Cheshire and Merseyside Public Health Network. http://www.uclan.ac.uk/health/schools/sphcs/hospitals_health_services.php (accessed 31 March 2009).

University of Central Lancashire (2009) *Healthy Settings Development Unit – Web Pages*. http://www.uclan.ac.uk/health/schools/sphcs/healthy_settings_development_unit.php (accessed 31 March 2009).

WHO (1986) *The Ottawa Charter*. World Health Organisation. http://www.who.int/healthy_settings/about/en/ (accessed 31 March 2009).

WHO (2003) *Social Determinants of Health: The Solid Facts*. 2nd edn. World Health Organisation. http://www.who.dk/document/e81384.pdf (accessed 31 March 2009).

WHO (2009) *Healthy Settings – Web Pages*. World Health Organisation. http://www.who.int/healthy_settings/about/en/ (accessed 31 March 2009).

Domain 2
The Nurse–Patient Relationship

Working with individual patients and groups: creating and strengthening relationships

7

Karen Thompson

Introduction

The aim of this chapter is to address how practice nurses (PNs) and walk-in-centre (WiC) nurses can create and strengthen working relationships with patients and groups through good communication. Good communication is the bedrock of all nursing care. Nurses need to communicate with patients or clients and their families in an effective and meaningful way. All the current strategies for care make some mention of the client being involved in the decisions made about their care and treatment; good communication between nurse and client is where that involvement starts. Nurses in primary care, particularly in general practice (GP) or WiCs, need to use their interpersonal skills to quickly establish good communication channels with both individual clients and groups of clients. Good communication can enhance the caring aspect of nursing and it can be taught. For example, Ryden et al. (1991) found that nursing students who had undertaken a course on interpersonal relations demonstrated a level of helping skills akin to that of experienced psychotherapists.

Learning Outcomes

- To become aware of some basic theories of communication
- To understand the various aspects of verbal and non-verbal communication
- To understand how communication theory can inform practice
- To understand the nature of groups and the role of the group leader.

Background

Good communication begins with the nurse having a self-awareness of all the issues that may cause him or her to pre-judge a client, and biases and prejudices, beliefs and values that may influence the establishment of the nurse–patient relationship. To communicate well with other people, we need an understanding of ourselves as well as an understanding of those with whom we wish to communicate. We are conscious of the world around us which we all view and experience through our own particular frame of reference. We attribute meaning to experiences and actions through our own sense of self or identity and our individuality is expressed through the value we place on these experiences. Humans are social beings and encounters with other people and the social context in which these encounters take place also influence our sense of self. Experiences within this social medium can influence our views and perceptions of others and may lead to generalisations and stereotyping, socially derived expectations of the behaviour of a group of people. This can have a negative impact on the communication process if the nurse is unaware of underlying influences on his or her expectations of others.

Our own sense of self-esteem may influence our relationships with others. Self-esteem may be said to be a measure of self-worth, regarded in terms of the feelings we have about ourselves. It asks the question 'Do you like yourself'? It is important to recognise our own level of self-esteem and that of our patients. Low self-esteem often results in the setting of unrealistic goals, and a tendency to be overcritical and to undervalue oneself. High self-esteem, however, results in the feeling of possessing the necessary strengths to meet life's demands and regarding stressful events as challenges to be met (Niven, 2006).

Understanding ourselves will enable us to relate to other people, to those in our care, more effectively; therefore, it is necessary to identify important qualities or traits within ourselves. When others relate to us, they are relating to the people we are and their behaviour towards us is a response to our behaviour towards them. It means accepting that their behaviour says something about ourselves as well as something about them (Fontana, 1990).

Once we have achieved a level of self-understanding and awareness that will enable us to form good communication channels with our patients, how much of ourselves is it prudent to disclose? There is a belief, long held dear by some, that it is essential for nurses to maintain a professional distance from their patients, not get too involved. It is also argued, however, that judicious self-disclosure can foster a sense of empathy between patient and nurse for the benefit of the patient.

Luft and Ingham (1955) developed a model to demonstrate the four aspects of 'self' – the Johari Window (Figure 7.1). They state that in any given situation, one of the windows will take precedence over the others. In self-disclosure, the public self (open) window increases in size and the other three are diminished because self-disclosure brings information about ourselves into the open or public domain.

Self-disclosure, when used appropriately, has several functions.

The Public (Open) Self	The Blind Self
What we know about ourselves and what is known by others about us	*What is known by others but is unknown by us*
The Hidden Self	The Unknown Self
What is known by us but hidden from others	*What is unknown by us and unknown by others*

Figure 7.1   The jJohari window

- It can help develop a sense of empathy.
- It can encourage the patient to say what they want to say.
- It can emphasise the shared human experience of nurse and patient.

Self-disclosure can happen on three different levels, according to Niven (2006).

1. Sharing opinions – probably the easiest level to start with but it has the least affective value.
2. Sharing experiences – this can help provide the patient with a new perspective on their situation.
3. Sharing feelings – there are occasions when it is correct to share feelings and emotions and even to cry with patients.

Any decision to use self-disclosure must be made with due consideration of the benefit to the patient. The focus must remain at all times with the patient and his or her issues. Too much self-disclosure may make the patient feel burdened, not just with his or her problems but yours too! Self-disclosure which takes the focus away from the patient undervalues their feelings and experiences, perhaps suggesting that there are others with worse problems and they should just 'get on with it'. If there is any doubt about the benefits to the patient of self-disclosure, then it is probably best to leave it out.

   In seeking to gain a greater understanding of 'self' and how this influences interactions with patients, the ability to reflect is an invaluable professional tool. This can be achieved through regular personal reflection, perhaps maintaining a reflective diary, journal or log, and through regular supervision with a trusted colleague. Nurses in primary care settings spend a lot of their time working alone with patients. Clinical supervision can be essential in helping to keep practice in perspective through examining it with a 'reflective lens'.

Communication

Frameworks of communication

Finding a concise or succinct definition of communication is very difficult as it is a very broad concept encompassing many facets of how, as a society, we organise ourselves. As the context in which we communicate changes, so then our definition and understanding of communication also changes. Within nursing, as in other 'people-focused' professions, the word communication is usually taken to refer to interpersonal communication, that which is specific between two or more people.

Activity

Spend 2–3 minutes thinking of words and phrases that you associate with 'communication'. Try to formulate your own definition from these and write it down.

Crouch and Meurier (2005:129) define communication as:

a two way process in which information is transmitted and received. It also involves feedback between the recipient and the transmitter of information.

They go on to state that the process of communication has seven stages.

1. The sender encodes and formulates the message.
2. The sender states what the message is.
3. The sender sends the message.
4. The receiver receives and decodes the message.
5. The receiver establishes the meaning of the message.
6. The receiver feeds back to the sender.
7. The sender re-encodes and re-formulates the message.

Breaking down communication into a mechanistic process in this way suggests that it is cold and stark. Indeed, if communication involved merely the stating of certain words in a particular order, then this would be the case. Communication, however, involves much more than the exchange of words. Donnelly and Neville (2008) suggest that communication theories fall into four main frameworks.

- Mechanistic – favoured in radio and telephone communications where there is a lack of non-verbal cues; this incorporates a transmission model of communication.
- Psychological – this has far more emphasis on how we feel and our emotional responses to communication.
- Social constructionist – mainly concerned with how different realities are constructed from the same experiences.
- Systemic – looks at communication as part of a whole system and how, within that system, each constituent of the communication process is re-examined and re-worked.

All our senses may have a part to play in the relaying of a message – sight, hearing, taste, smell and touch – as well as our intellect, belief and values and understanding of cultural norms.

Models of communication

Shannon and Weaver (1949) produced one of the earliest and most basic models of communication. Their model is a transmission model and sits within the mechanistic framework. The model consists of five parts:

1. the source of information, for example, the nurse's mind;
2. the transmitter, for example, the nurse;
3. the channel, for example, the nurse's voice;
4. the receiver, for example, the patient's ears;
5. the destination, for example, the patient's mind.

The flow of the message is in one direction only and operates against a background of 'noise'. Noise can be taken to mean a variety of things which may impede the flow of the message. Noise can be physical – actual noise – and psychological such as strong emotion, anxiety and cultural barriers. It may be semantic (language or representation problems) or physiological – hearing or visual impairment, pain and discomfort (Donnelly and Neville, 2008). Noise can interrupt the communication at any stage; thus, if the message is not reaching its destination, then the solution lies in establishing the nature of the noise and employing strategies to eliminate or modify the noise. An example of psychological noise could be seen when a woman who has received an invitation for routine breast screening asks about the process of having a mammogram but does not seem very comfortable with the idea. The skilled PN or WiC nurse will discern that anxiety is present and is disrupting the flow of information. By allaying fears about the procedure and its possible outcomes, anxiety is lessened, the noise is modified or eliminated and the message is allowed to flow freely.

Activity

Make a list of all the things in your area of work that might constitute 'noise' and categorise them into physical, psychological, semantic and physiological.

Transmission models such as that of Shannon and Weaver's (1949) illustrate the flow of a message, but it is a linear, unidirectional flow. There is an assumption that the message is informative and needs only to flow from the giver to the receiver, that is, from nurse to patient. Nursing, particularly in primary care in the 21st century, is very dependent on the establishment of a relationship between the nurse and the patient. Rapport needs to be established quickly and a partnership for care fostered. Transaction models such as that of Wood (2004) allow for greater interaction between the communicators. Figure 7.2 illustrates the communication channels between two people using Wood's model.

Transactional models of communication are more complex than transmission models. There is still the concept of noise but this surrounds the communication

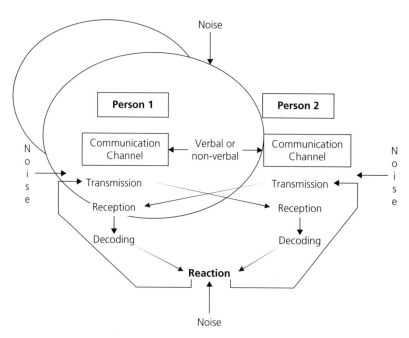

Figure 7.2   A representation of transactional communication

which is multidirectional and focuses on meaning and interpretation. Messages are being sent all the time, sometimes simultaneously. In the transactional model, multiple channels are used, including language, voice, tone, expression and posture. Non-verbal behaviours and the use of symbols in communicating play an important role in establishing the meaning of the message.

Non-verbal behaviours

As has been stated, communication depends on the message being sent, received and accurately interpreted. Non-verbal behaviours can affect the interpretation of the sent message, perhaps conveying a message different to that indicated by the use of words and language. Understanding something is a subjective experience with meaning constructed according to social contexts and behaviours that are culturally bound and age related.

In an average face-to-face encounter, 55% is communicated via body language, 38% by voice tonality and only 7% is communicated through the words used (Donnelly and Neville, 2008). Transactional models take into consideration multiple channels of communication and, therefore, perhaps are more accurate in depicting what happens in face-to-face communication than the transmission models which are more linear and unidirectional. For this reason, using a transactional model is a better basis for the creation of effective communication with patients and clients (Donnelly and Neville, 2008).

In choosing an effective way of communicating, consideration of the various channels of communication and how they may be interpreted is very important. These channels may include:

- words and word images;
- voice tonality;
- perception of role;
- facial expression;
- gaze;
- posture and body angle;
- presentation.

Remember that, in the transactional model, communication is multidirectional and also simultaneous – as the message is being sent, the sender is also receiving, decoding and interpreting messages at the same time. Memories, experiences and perceptions all influence the decoding and interpretation of messages. Normally, we do not consciously consider these factors in everyday life but when we are seeking to communicate in a helping capacity, we need to carefully consider all the factors which will impact on the effectiveness of our communication. Questions that need to be considered when planning a communication episode may include:

- How much time is available?
- How many people will be involved?
- What and how much information needs to be sent and received?
- What role will questions play in the episode?
- Which of the senses will be utilised in the episode?
- How will all the participants' needs be met?

Remember that many factors can influence the interpretation of a message. We communicate through the use of signs and symbols which are learned when we are young and these may be not just culturally specific, but also specific to our own close social group such as family and friends. For example, prolonged eye contact may be taken as a sign of a high level of interest in what one is saying or it may be interpreted as being threatening. Hand gestures which are acceptable in one culture may be offensive in another.

Facial expression

Most non-verbal communication is probably conveyed through facial expression. Rosenthal and DePaulo (1979) found that the most accurate channels for decoding information were: first, facial expression; second, the body (posture, proximity and body angle); and third, tone of voice. Ekman (2004) found that certain facial expressions were easier to decode than others, with happiness and surprise being the easiest and disgust or contempt being the hardest. Agreement across all cultures was found in the representation of happiness through smiling and sadness through frowning (Ekman and Freisen, 1975). The facial feedback hypothesis is referred to by McCanne and Anderson (1987) based on an experiment by Zuckerman et al. (1981) which concluded that positive and negative emotions increased with the use of facial expression and decreased with a lack of facial expression. Thus, greeting patients and clients with a smile could be seen to be beneficial as it encourages them to smile back and induces pleasant feelings. It is also worth remembering that a lack of facial expression in a client may indicate suppressed emotion, stress or tension. Ekman (2004) also states that true smiles can be distinguished from forced smiles through recognition of the contraction of the orbicularis oculi muscle which has the effect of narrowing the eyes and is almost impossible to achieve at will. The observant PN and WiC nurse will be able to detect nuances in facial expression that may indicate dissonance between overt behaviour and inner emotions.

Gaze

Closely linked to facial expression, gaze can be described as the fixing of one's eyes on another person. Mutual gaze or eye contact refers to two people focusing their eyes on each other and is generally thought to indicate friendliness and affection. Engaging in eye contact usually conveys the message that the person wishes to be friendly. Staring, on the other hand, can be taken as threatening – a prelude to attack, thus initiating feelings of uneasiness or discomfort in the person being stared at.

Lying to someone whilst maintaining eye contact is very difficult and if there is something uncomfortable to be said or uncertainty as to its reception, then eye contact is often broken. In the course of an interaction with a patient or client, the pattern of eye contact can provide the nurse with vital clues as to any hidden messages being conveyed.

A note of caution needs to be sounded, however, regarding the social and cultural differences in the use of gaze. Arabs, Latin Americans and Southern Europeans are more comfortable with direct focus, whereas Northern Europeans and Asians tend to avert their eyes and gaze less (Mayo and Le France, 1973). The use of eye contact or gaze should always be interpreted within the context of the culture and social norms of the patient or client.

Personal space and body posture

We all have a sense of our own 'space', an area surrounding us which, when invaded, produces feelings of unease or discomfort. An anthropologist, Edward Hall, came up with the notion of 'proxemics' and identified four main proximity zones.

1. Intimate (0–0.45 m) – accessible to spouses/partners and close family and friends.
2. Personal (0.45–1.2 m) – referred to as 'personal space'; invasion of this area causes anxiety, particularly if there is no means of escape.
3. Social (1.2–3.65 m) – day-to-day interaction with associates and strangers, and formal business purposes.
4. Public (3.65 to >7.6 m) – the distance kept from important or public figures (Niven, 2006).

These distances are average and there may be individual variations in how close others may get before the individual feels uncomfortable. Cultural differences may also affect perceptions of personal space. Conflict may arise where proximity may be seen as threatening or intrusive or distance may be perceived as cold and impersonal.

The very nature of nursing allows us the privilege of legitimately invading patients' or clients' personal – or even intimate – space and we need to recognise that this alone may cause feelings of unease or discomfort in both ourselves and those seeking our help. This can have a negative impact on the care episode. Careful use of other interpersonal behaviours such as appropriate language, voice tone, facial expression and gestures can help alleviate this. There is also a need to recognise that expressions of anxiety may simply be the result of close proximity and not necessarily indicators of deeper issues, although this may need to be explored with the client.

Body posture and orientation have also been shown to affect interactions between people. Posture can convey a wealth of non-verbal information about a person. An erect posture with the head held up, hand on hips and a direct gaze may portray a dominant character but a hunched posture and averted eyes may suggest submissiveness. Folded arms or clasped hands may be interpreted as inaccessible but open arms and hands, palms out, suggest openness and a willingness to interact. PNs and WiC nurses who are effective communicators take care to note their patient's or client's posture and to interpret the messages held therein. They are also conscious of their own posture, taking care to portray openness and friendliness rather than adopting a posture that may be seen as dominant or aggressive. Orientation of the body, the angle at which we position ourselves in relation to others, can increase or decrease the effectiveness of an interaction with patients and clients. Sitting at a 90° angle during a consultation has been found to produce a more meaningful interaction than sitting opposite, perhaps the other side of a desk (Niven, 2006).

Gesture and touch

It is very difficult to speak without gesticulating in some way. Try observing someone on the phone; they are likely to make gestures even though they know the person on the other end of the line is unable to see them! Gestures are a way of supplementing speech and language or sometimes replacing it altogether. Some gestures are universal such as a wave in greeting or farewell. Others are subject to social and cultural influences and may be variously interpreted.

Some gestures involve touch and can be used effectively to convey warmth, affection or friendship. The use of touch whilst communicating emotionally sensitive information, for example, breaking bad news, can indicate care and concern. Again, touching is subject to social and cultural influences. One example being that touch is used sparingly in the British culture, a handshake being regarded as a normal greeting, whereas Europeans and Americans are more likely to kiss and embrace on greeting one another. The use of touch in the therapeutic relationship must be judicious and within the social and cultural context of the patient or client in order to avoid offence. Generally to touch hands or upper limbs or to place an open palm on the shoulder is an acceptable way of conveying care and concern.

Therapeutic presence

This is probably the most difficult non-verbal behaviour to define. Words are a comfortable tool to use in patient or client interaction but there are times when silence or 'being with' is enough. Therapeutic presence is a category of presence suggested by McKivergin and Daubenmire (1994) along with physical presence and psychological presence. They talk of 'intuitive knowing' where the nurse just knows words are unnecessary. It is difficult, however, to discern when speech is needed and when it is not. Silence is not easy to tolerate and there is always a tendency to 'fill the gap'. The PN or WiC nurse who is self-aware and reflective is likely to accurately discern those occasions when all that is necessary to meet the patient's needs is to be with them.

Verbal or vocal behaviours

The use of language, tone of voice and the sequencing of interactions are fundamental factors in the transmission of a message but only account for 45% of communication and only 7% of the message is transmitted by the words used.

Voice and tonality

The tone of the voice can convey different meanings to the receiver of the message. Just think of how many ways in which you can say the word 'no'. The tone of voice can make the word mean a variety of shades of 'no' from the absolute and non-negotiable to the 'perhaps maybe' or 'I'm not sure'. It can be said with authority, playfulness or despair. All these messages conveyed use the same word but meaning is added by the tone of voice. Voice tone can be thought of in terms of:

■ volume – variations of volume can convey affection concern or threat;
■ resonance – a toneless voice may indicate low mood or feeling unwell;
■ pitch – may vary with volume and may indicate anger or excitement.

Activity

Think about a number of recent interactions with people. How did volume, pitch and resonance contribute to your understanding of the messages they were sending? How did you use your voice tone to convey the messages you wanted to send? Were any of them angry, upset, pleased or relieved? How did you respond to these emotions?

Self-awareness on the part of the nurse can enable the nurse to respond to patient's high levels of emotion in a calming and controlled way. It is how we behave professionally. We greet people in a calm and controlled manner which conveys calm, safety and a willingness to respond to the patient's needs. The self-aware PN or WiC nurse recognises his or her own potential responses to the patient's actions and interaction and is able to judge and measure responses in the most appropriate way.

Language

It has already been noted that tone of voice can alter or influence the words we use but what of the words themselves? Language may be a common factor in a communication episode but it has the capacity to create barriers. Words may be used in different contexts between different groups of people, for example, 'wicked' means bad or evil to one group of people but to another group it means something that was enjoyable or good.

Language is influenced by age, culture and social class. Add into that mixture education, professional language and jargon and the potential for poor communication is very real. It is easy to slip into the habit of assuming everyone knows our professional language and so can understand us when we use 'technical terms'. The balance between using an appropriate level of language and not 'talking down' to the patient is very fine and should be judged on an individual basis. It is worth listening carefully to the language used by the patient and taking that as your guide.

The use of questions

The majority of interaction with patients or clients will involve asking questions. Questions should elicit the information necessary for you to effectively assess the patient and plan interventions. Questions may be closed or open. Closed questions will elicit factual information but this will be limited to the scope of the question itself, whereas open questions allow the respondent to answer freely and fully.

During the course of a care episode, the PN or WiC nurse will probably need to use both open and closed questions. Niven (2006) suggests avoiding constant swapping between open and closed questions as this can cause confusion. Rather start with open questions to elicit broad responses and then gradually focus the questions more in order to provide some sort of sequence to the dialogue.

Fundamental to the effectiveness of using questions is the ability and willingness to hear the answers!

Listening attentively

Listening is active, not passive. It is not 'time out' from speaking or an interlude between episodes of talk. Active listening tells the patient that you are interested and that what they are saying is important. It indicates that you care. Niven (2006) suggests there are three ways in which active listening can be indicated.

■ Non-verbal signals: attention to body posture, engaging in appropriate eye contact, nodding the head and acknowledging comments with 'mms', 'uh-huhs' and suchlike.
■ Reflecting back: this involves repeating back key words and phrases which enables the speaker to hear the words they have used and gives the listener the opportunity to select what they think are significant words or phrases. There is a danger that this may sound like 'parroting' – repeating words without any real focus or meaning. Careful use of voice tone and body language can minimise the 'parroting' effect.
■ Paraphrasing: this involves identifying what someone has said and feeding it back to them in your own words. Like reflection, it enables the speaker to hear what they have said and offers the opportunity for expansion. It has the advantage over reflecting back in that there is little danger of 'parroting'.

Donnelly and Neville (2008) add 'summarising' to these skills, taking what has been said and making a précis or summary of it. This indicates to the speaker that you have been attentive to what they have been saying and offers them the opportunity to add or correct.

In a helping situation, listening to the patient is probably the most valuable thing you can do. It enables you to gather the information they are giving you, interpret it accurately and monitor their reactions. It has the effect of allowing them to feel valued and cared for.

Barriers to communication

Many barriers to effective communication may be encountered as you seek to help and support patients and clients. These may come under several broad headings:

■ language barriers;
■ social and cultural barriers;
■ limited understanding and receptiveness;
■ negative attitudes towards health professionals;
■ contradictory messages.

Dealing with patients or clients who speak a different language can be fraught with problems and independent interpreters are often thin on the ground. One option may be to use an English-speaking member of the patient's family but this should be approached with caution as family members may have their own agenda and may influence the patient to make decisions the family are comfortable with rather than what is best for the patient. Ewles and Simnet (1996) advocate learning some key words and phrases such as 'hello' and 'goodbye'. This may help break down cultural barriers and will indicate your care for the patient by attempting to make them feel at ease.

Physiological impairments such as hearing or speech difficulties may mean that the message transmission is blocked or distorted. Visual impairment may also play a part in distorting the visual cues of non-verbal communication. Awareness of the presence of such problems will prepare the nurse to adapt communication methods to overcome these barriers.

Language barriers often exist between people of different backgrounds, even if they seemingly speak the same language. Age, gender, social class, culture and accent can all give rise to differences in interpreting what is being said. Different beliefs and values also influence the flow of communication from patient to nurse and nurse to patient. In the primary care setting, good communication channels and trust in the relationship between nurse and patient need to be established very quickly. The nurse needs to have an acute sense of self-awareness of his or her values and beliefs when dealing with social and cultural differences and must take care to maintain a professional attitude at all times.

Patients may not be receptive to communication from the nurse and/or other health care professionals. The reasons for this may include:

- learning difficulties;
- confusion;
- tiredness or pain;
- stress and anxiety;
- being pre-occupied or distracted.

Previous experiences of health care interventions may colour the patient's perceptions, thus creating a barrier. A lack of trust may also be an issue.

It is not always possible to overcome all barriers to communication but careful attention to use of language, the fostering of self-awareness, the use of appropriate non-verbal behaviours and the offering of consistent and evidence-based advice should arm the PN and WiC nurse with strategies which will minimise barriers, if not overcome them.

Working with individual patients and clients

Modern nursing is a complex business with nurses performing tasks that were the traditional domain of the doctor (Lloyd et al., 2007). Nurses in primary care will

Table 7.1 Phases in the Therapeutic Relationship

Phase	Activity
Orientation	Nurse and client meet as strangers and orientate to each other, establishing rapport and working together to clarify and define the problem
Identification	Clarification of each other's perceptions and expectations
Exploitation	Client encouraged by nurse to assume active and responsible role in his/her care
Resolution	Nurse and client become independent of each other, original needs are met and therapeutic relationship is terminated

(From Lloyd et al. 2007).

routinely see a patient, and assess, diagnose and treat illness without reference to a medical practitioner. They will plan pathways of care for those with chronic illnesses, plan health promotion activities and educate patients. However, PNs and WiC nurses need to take care that they do not focus solely on the tasks and retain a patient-centred therapeutic relationship. Patients are no longer passive recipients of care but should be partners in their care processes. Nursing is concerned with relationships (Freshwater, 2003) and care delivery should always be within the context of a therapeutic relationship.

Primary care nursing offers a wide range of reasons why patients may have a one-to-one interaction with a nurse:

- a need for information;
- a need for health education;
- a need for assessment or re-assessment;
- a need for lifestyle counselling;
- monitoring of a chronic condition;
- the breaking of bad news.

In each of these, the patient should be regarded as a partner. According to Muetzel (1988), partnership, intimacy and reciprocity constitute three elements of a therapeutic relationship. Partnership is strongly represented in current health care practice and policies abound, inviting patients to participate in and make choices for their care. Peplau (1952) defined the therapeutic relationship in theoretical terms, speaking of four phases in the relationship as shown in Table 7.1.

Assessing needs and setting goals

When assessing patients, it may be helpful to think of the concept of need in three ways:

- normative;
- felt;
- expressed.

Normative need is said to occur when professional standards are set and activity is judged to fall short of those standards, for example, a diabetic nurse may judge that a certain level of understanding is desirable if a new diabetic is to manage his or her disorder and that a programme of education is needed to reach that level of understanding.

Felt need is said to occur when the client identifies what he or she wants, for example, the new diabetic may feel the need to understand more about diabetes and how he or she may be affected.

Expressed need is said to occur when the client says what he or she needs; thus, a felt need is converted into a request or demand, for example, the new diabetic asks for information about his or her condition.

It should be noted, however, that felt needs are not always converted into expressed needs and it is wrong for the nurse to assume that a lack of demand indicates a lack of need (Ewles and Simnet, 1996). Expressed needs may conflict with normative needs. The patient may not wish to have the level of information about diabetes that the nurse deems necessary and conversely, the nurse may feel the patient may be overloaded with too much information and stops short of the level of knowledge the patient feels he or she needs (Ewles and Simnet, 1996).

Goal setting

Once needs have been established, then goals and strategies can be negotiated. Goals may be short-, medium- or long-term but they must be acceptable to the patient. Long-term goals need to be broken down into manageable short-term goals – 'bite-sized chunks' – so that the patient does not feel overwhelmed by the size of the task. Using the acronym 'SMART' may be helpful in setting goals:

- Specific;
- Measurable;
- Achievable;
- Realistic;
- Time oriented.

Using counselling skills

Nursing and the establishment of caring or therapeutic relationships should not be confused with counselling, although many skills used in counselling can be used effectively in the nurse–patient relationship. PNs and WiC nurses must retain a good level of self-awareness, knowing their limitations and when it is appropriate to refer the patient on to other agencies.

PNs and WiC nurses are good communicators and will naturally use many skills and techniques in their interactions with patients that may be classed as 'counselling skills', but it is important to remember that counselling is a specific helping activity and should only be undertaken by those with the appropriate training and recognition. The British Association for Counselling and Psychotherapy (www. bacp.co.uk), Counselling and Psychotherapy in Scotland (www.cosca.org.uk) and the United Kingdom Register of Counsellors (www.ukrconline.org.uk) all provide information for professionals and the public about counselling.

Alongside all the communication techniques that have previously been mentioned, the works of Egan (1998) and Rogers (2002) are also worth a mention when considering the helping relationship. Rogers (2002) believes that helping relationships have three core conditions.

- Empathy – the ability of being able to see the world as the other person sees it.
- Congruence – the ability to be 'real', show your true self. To achieve this, it is necessary to be comfortable with whom you are and not pretend you are something you are not.
- Unconditional positive regard – setting aside your own attitudes and values in order to accept the person you are helping as they are and to be non-judgemental.

Rogers (2002) maintains that these conditions are necessary if an effective partnership is to be established.

Egan (1998) identifies three stages in the partnership.

- Exploration – encouraging the patient to tell their story, speak it out loud. The helper needs to create time and space for this and also to signal that they are listening actively.
- Understanding – supporting the patient in trying to understand and reflect on their story. What do they want to change or do differently? It is at this point that goals can be negotiated and set.
- Action – using the goals to effect the desired change. The helper will need to encourage and support the patient.

Throughout the interaction, attention should be paid to listening skills, body language and tone of voice – all the topics mentioned previously in this chapter.

Working with groups

Groups are formed for a variety of reasons. Some groups may appear to be a random collection of individuals, but do not be misled by appearance – all groups consist of members who have a sense of shared identity, defined membership criteria, a set of common objectives and their own particular ways of working (Ewles and Simnet, 1996). Group work can be a way of moving a patient from being a passive recipient to an active partner in their health care. Within the primary care arena, groups may exist for a variety of reasons and increasingly, experienced PNs and WiC nurses are finding themselves facilitating groups as part of their remit. Health promotion and health education are probably the likeliest areas to be chosen for group work but patients may also benefit from support groups where they can support and be supported by others experiencing similar health problems or patient action/participation groups where they can be partners in assessing and planning health care services in their area.

Leading a group

Group leadership can be very demanding and complex and specialist training in group leadership is available. There are, however, some basic considerations that can help the nurse in primary care who is involved with group work. Two major aspects to consider are:

- leadership style;
- responsibilities of the group leader.

Leadership style

There should be a clear agreement within the group who the leader is. Within this chapter, the consideration has been the nurse–patient relationship, so let us assume that, as a professional, the PN or WiC nurse will be the acknowledged group leader. Leadership styles depend largely on where the leaders see themselves on a continuum from authoritative to facilitative/participative.

Authoritarian leadership is directive or didactic. The leader relies on status and expertise to retain control. This style of leadership may enable weak or vulnerable members to feel secure but often group members become disempowered and unable to take decisive action. A facilitative or participative style allows a sharing of power between leader and group members. The leader needs not only to demonstrate empathy, tolerance and encouragement, but also the ability to confront difficulties with a problem-solving approach. The strength of this style is that members feel a sense of trust in their own abilities and judgements whilst at the same time appreciating other members' rights and opinions (Ewles and Simnet, 1996).

There is no right or wrong way to lead a group. Successful group leadership depends on several different factors:

- the leader's preferred style and personality;
- the specific circumstances of the group;
- the group's aims and objectives;
- the wider perspective of the group members – culture, age, gender and social class.

These factors need to be considered and the leadership style adapted to fit the purpose of the group.

Role and responsibilities of the leader

Before agreeing to run any group, it is advisable to find out what specific responsibilities you will have as you will need to manage your time accordingly. Will you be expected to organise the venue, for example, or refreshments, sending invitations and so on? Having said that, there are core responsibilities that go with the role of group leader:

- helping members to identify and clarify their needs and aims;
- helping to develop a relaxed and open atmosphere;
- offering expertise and professional knowledge;
- accepting and valuing all contributions and ensuring fairness in discussions.

It is also necessary to recognise that the group membership also has its responsibilities such as participating appropriately and acting within the boundaries set by the group.

Effective working with groups is more likely if the leader has some understanding of how groups behave and the different roles members may take. Tuckman's (1965) cycle of group behaviour is well acknowledged. He suggests all groups move through a number of stages before becoming effective:

- forming – getting to know each other and setting the agenda;
- storming – conflict stage;
- norming – conflicts are resolved and accepted practices are established;
- performing – group becomes effective and focuses on its task.

Belbin (1981) identified a mixture of eight roles that enabled a group to be fully effective:

- leader or chairperson – coordinates;
- shaper – action oriented;
- plant – creative source of ideas;
- monitor/evaluator – analyses and criticises;
- resource investigator – liaises with contacts and networks;
- team worker – supports and listens;
- company worker – organises and administers;
- finisher – ensures the task is completed.

Each person may play a variety of these roles but individual personality may influence the roles in which they are most comfortable. The effective leader may consciously adopt any of the roles if they are missing to maintain the effectiveness of the group.

Be aware of hidden agendas. Individuals often join groups for their own reasons, perhaps because they offer them the opportunity to air their own issues. The group leader needs to recognise and acknowledge these hidden agendas whilst valuing the individual. However, the leader may need to be assertive and not allow one person's issues to dominate the expense of the groups' aims and needs.

The meeting environment

As was stated earlier, the responsibilities of the leader in terms of organisational and practical issues need to be established at the outset. Practical issues that you may be expected to address may include:

- location;
- accessibility;
- facilities needed;
- space and seating arrangements;
- security.

Practical needs will vary according to the nature and remit of the group. An exercise class may need floor space and changing facilities. A Mums' and Toddlers' group may require security and baby changing facilities, whereas a health education group may require audio-visual equipment and comfortable seating.

Thought needs to be given to room layout and arrangement of seating as this can affect the way a group functions. A formal layout can promote an authoritative or didactic approach, whereas less formal arrangements may encourage a more participative or Socratic atmosphere (Figure 7.3).

Ground rules

Different assumptions and expectations of the group and how it will run could give rise to conflict among the group members. Encouraging the group to consider and set ground rules early on in the group's life will possibly prevent this or at least limit the damage! Ground rules may cover such issues as:

- confidentiality;
- good listening skills;
- respect for each other's viewpoints;
- acceptable behaviours, for example, use of mobile phones;
- expected attendance patterns.

There needs to be a sense of ownership of any ground rules by the whole group. Consensus needs to be achieved for both the rules themselves and the use of any sanctions when the rules are broken.

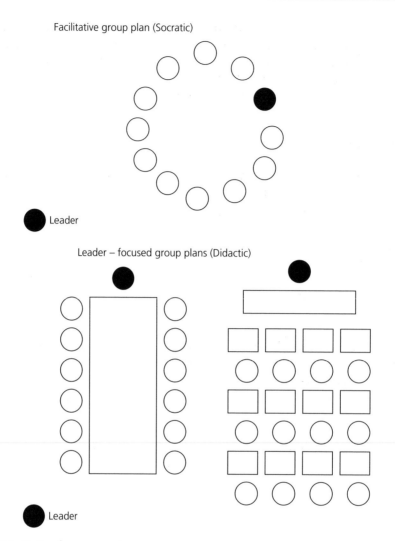

Figure 7.3   Seating for group work

Planning meetings

Group meetings require some planning – they will not just happen! The plans and the work required before the meeting will depend on the nature and remit of the group. Consider the following:

■ Does the group need to follow a set programme, for example, smoking cessation?
■ Are there particular activities that must be included, for example, 'weigh-in' or exercise session?
■ How much time is allowed for each activity?

Initial meetings of any group need to be well planned so that people get to know each other and become comfortable within the group. Ice breakers that involve movement around the room and talking to each other to find out something can be fun and get people chatting.

Working with groups can be difficult, as has been said, but a good starting point is to consider your strengths as a communicator. Underpin your practice with sound theory and maintain honesty, integrity and professionalism at all times.

Conclusion

In this chapter, the concept of communication within GP and WiC nursing has been explored with reference to relevant literature. Various communication skills have been discussed, both verbal and non-verbal, and these have led to a consideration of the establishment of effective relationships with both individuals and groups. Underpinning this is a recognition that the integrity of the nurse–patient relationship depends on the nurse's self-awareness, professionalism and ability to be a reflective practitioner.

References

Belbin, M. (1981) *Management Teams*. London: Heinmann.

Crouch, A. and Meurier, C. (2005) *Vital Notes for Nurses: Health Assessment*. Oxford: Blackwell Publishing.

Donnelly, E. and Neville, L. (2008) *Communication and Interpersonal Skills*. Exeter: Reflect Press.

Egan, G. (1998) *The Skilled Helper*. Chichester: Wiley.

Ekman, P. (2004) *Emotions Revealed: Understanding Faces and Feelings*. London: Orion.

Ekman, P. and Friesen, W. (1975) *Unmasking the Face*. New Jersey: Prentice Hall.

Ewles, L. and Simnet, I. (1996) *Promoting Health: A Practical Guide*. 3rd edn. London: Bailliere Tindall.

Fontana, D. (1990) *Social Skills at Work*. Leicester/London: BPS Books/ Routledge.

Freshwater, D. (2003) *Counselling/skills for Nurse Midwives and Health Visitors*. Maidenhead: Open University Press.

Lloyd, H., Hancock, H. and Campbell, S. (2007) *Vital Notes for Nurses: Principles of Care*. Oxford: Blackwell Publishing Ltd.

Luft, J. and Ingham, H. (1955) *The Johari Window: A Graphic Model for Interpersonal Relationships*. California: University of California, West Training Laboratory in Group Development.

Mayo, C. and Le France, M. (1973) *Gaze Direction in Interracial Dyadic Communication*. Paper presented at the Eastern Psychology Association Conference, Washington, DC.

McCanne, T. and Anderson, J. (1987) Emotional responding following experimental manipulation of facial electromyographic activity. *Journal of Personality and Social Psychology*, 52; 759–768.

McKivergin, M. and Daubenmire, J. (1994) The essence of therapeutic presence. *Journal of Holistic Nursing*, 12(1); 65–81.

Muetzel, P. (1988) Therapeutic nursing. In Pearson, A. (Ed.) *Primary Nursing in the Burford and Oxford Development Units*. London: Chapman and Hall.

Niven, N. (2006) *The Psychology of Nursing Care*. 2nd edn. Basingstoke: Palgrave MacMillan.

Peplau, H. (1952) *Interpersonal Relations in Nursing*. London: MacMillan.

Rogers, C. (2002) *Client Centred Therapy*. London: Constable.

Rosenthal, R. and DePaulo, B. (1979) Sex differences in eavesdropping on non-verbal cues. *Journal of Personality and Social Psychology*, 37; 273–285.

Ryden, M., McCarthy, P., Lewis, M. and Sherman, C. (1991) A behavioural comparison of the helping styles of nursing students, psychotherapists, crisis intervenors and untrained individuals. *Archives of Psychiatric Nursing*, 5; 185–188.

Shannon, C. and Weaver, W. (1949) *The Mathematical Theory of Communication*. Illinois: Urbana University of Illinois Press.

Tuckman, B. (1965) Developmental sequence in small groups. *Psychological Bulletin*, 63; 384–399.

Wood, J. (2004) *Communication Theories in Action: An Introduction*. New York: Belmont Wadsworth/Thomson Learning.

Zuckerman, M., Klorman, R., Larrance, D. and Spiegel, N. (1981) Facial, autonomic and subjective components of emotion: The facial feedback hypothesis versus the externaliser – internaliser distinction. *Journal of Personality and Social Psychology*, 211; 929–944.

Confidentiality, privacy and dignity: ethical, legal and cultural issues 8

Nicola L. Whiteing

Introduction

The aim of this chapter is to consider cultural issues, patient consultations, ethical issues and legal issues within the context of confidentiality, privacy and dignity in practice nursing (PN) and walk-in-centre (WiC) nursing. This will be achieved by framing both PN and WiC nursing within the context of advanced practice. Advanced practice nurses (APNs) are accustomed to addressing the multiple dimensions of health and illness with responsibilities and duties that lie outside of the nurse–patient relationship. Changes in health care delivery systems and financing have created conflicts of interest for those who must be both a provider of care and a gatekeeper for services (Anderson and Pope-Kish, 2001). Therefore, it is imperative that the APN keeps the concept of caring central to his/her care and his/her nurse–patient relationships.

Research has shown that APNs have a positive impact on patient care, particularly in terms of patient choice, accessibility and quality of care (Carnwell and Daly, 2003). Indeed, Horrocks et al. (2002) found nurse practitioners were as effective as GPs in dealing with common presentations and scored higher in terms of patient satisfaction. Perhaps some of this can be put down to the effects of a good nurse–patient relationship.

There are times, however, when the APN finds himself/herself faced with dilemmas which may mean that his/her approach to the nurse–patient relationship needs to be altered. In this chapter, some of the issues that may arise when dealing with patients in a variety of primary care settings are explored. Throughout this chapter, the reader will find activities and a case study to consider in relation to some of the topics raised. In addition, individual competencies from within this domain will appear in brackets where relevant. Relevant competencies associated with the nurse–patient relationship are cited numerically (e.g. C1 or C7) next to the competency discussed.

Learning Outcomes

■ To consider some of the dilemmas that an APN working within the primary care setting may come across in relation to Domain 2
■ To explore the importance of cultural awareness and competence in providing effective health care
■ To consider when the APN's relationship with the patient may need to alter due to ethical or legal issues
■ To explore issues surrounding record keeping and confidentiality, considering relationships with patients and their families.

Background

As advanced nursing practice becomes more complex and demanding, nurses must reflect more on the professional ethical and legal implications of their work (Humphris and Masterson, 1998). Greater legal and professional accountability has been highlighted with advanced practice (Peysner, 1996) and as a greater level of responsibility is assumed with ever increasingly complex patient health needs (Jones and Davies, 1999), the APN must define, assume and document a greater level of accountability.

With increased autonomy and subsequent accountability, the role of the nurse–patient relationship may, at times, need to take on a different dimension. Traditionally, nurses acted as patient advocate in the very 'doctor-biased' doctor–patient relationship (Porter, 1991). As the APN takes on a more active and autonomous role in managing patients' health problems and the GP slips into the background, the APN may find himself/herself facing legal, ethical, professional and cultural dilemmas which alters his/her approach to the relationship with the patient.

As the boundaries between medicine and nursing become increasingly blurred, APNs must not forget that one of the main advantages of care delivery by a nurse is that of the ability to work with the patient as a partner (Crumbie, 1999) (C1). As the role of the nurse changes to accommodate the many roles formerly undertaken by a doctor, there is a risk that patients will perceive the APN in a different way and may be less willing to enter into the relationship. The APN must therefore consider the importance of the nurse–patient relationship and how this may be enhanced in order that effective health care is delivered.

The relationship that is established between patient and nurse becomes the vehicle through which patients participate in their care (C3). By meeting the competencies within this domain, the APN provides the opportunity for the patient to incorporate feelings of self-efficacy and empowerment in relation to choices that are made in both the short term and the long term in relation to their care (Cox, 2001) (C7). Indeed, Green-Hernandez (1997) wrote that without the patient being actively involved in the participation of their health care, the successful implementation of any health care plans made may be consider-ably lessened.

The APN's relationship with a patient must be formed as a partnership with the patient getting involved or being allowed to become involved in the decision-making process regarding the delivery of care (C1, 7). Within the primary care setting, this partnership is likely to be formed on a one-to-one relationship between the nurse and patient; however, it may be that more complex partnerships need to be formed involving the patient's family, other members of the health care team and the local health authority (C1). This can have a direct impact on the nurse–patient relationship with wider issues around maintaining confidentiality and pro-fessional, ethical and legal issues.

Activity

Consider how you form a partnership with a patient.
  What are the key components of establishing a therapeutic relationship with the patient?
  Describe how you form an effective partnership with patients, carers and the multi-disciplinary health care team.

The following section will focus on aspects of culture, privacy and dignity, confi-dentiality and some legal and ethical issues in relation to Domain 2.

Domain of practice area with specific competencies

Table 8.1 outlines the 10 competencies that contribute to Domain 2.

Cultural issues

Culture is an important part of who we are and how we interact with the world, providing learned ways of thinking and feeling that affect the development of our attitudes, values and beliefs (McGee, 2003). Nursing is a patient-centred caring profession, however; providing care to an ever-changing multicultural and mul-tilingual population whilst still maintaining patient-specific personal delivery can be a challenge to the APN. A culturally competent system of health care recog-nises and integrates the importance of culture on multiple levels, including policy making, administration and practice.

The way in which individuals view health and illness has its base in their culture. What is defined as a health problem or illness, when and where to seek health

Table 8.1   The 10 Competencies of Domain 2

1. Creates a climate of mutual trust and establishes partnerships with patients, carers and families
2. Validates and checks findings with patients
3. Creates a relationship with patients that acknowledges their strengths and knowledge, enabling them to address their needs
4. Communicates a sense of 'being there' for the patient, carers and families and provides comfort and emotional support
5. Evaluates the impact of life transitions on the health/illness status of patients, and the impact of health/illness on patients' lives (individuals, families, carers and communities)
6. Applies principles of empowerment in promoting behaviour change
7. Develops and maintains the patients' control over decision-making, assesses the patients' commitment to the jointly determined plan of care and fosters personal responsibility for health
8. Maintains confidentiality, whilst recording data, plans and results in a manner that preserves the dignity and privacy of the patient
9. Monitors and reflects on own emotional response to interaction with patients, carers and families and uses this knowledge to further therapeutic interaction
10. Considers the patients' needs when bringing closure to the nurse–patient relationship and provides for a safe transition to another care provider or independence

(RCN 2008:14).

care and preventative services, what is expected from treatment and the way in which the sick role is enacted are all part of one's culture (Gerber et al., 2001). The use of herbal remedies and other 'alternative' healing methods are becoming increasingly popular and easily accessible in the UK. A thorough patient assessment should include a respectful discussion of such methods. Patients may be reluctant to discuss such alternative methods if they think they are going to be met with a negative attitude by the APN; thus, attention may need to be paid to establishing a therapeutic relationship with the patient prior to tackling such issues (C3).

Without an understanding of the many diverse beliefs, health care providers, who practice from a traditional Western medicine framework, will be confused about the meaning of these beliefs and practices for their patients (Gerber et al., 2001) and this will ultimately impact on the success of the nurse–patient relationship. If the APN is not knowledgeable about the health beliefs and practices of other cultures, misdiagnosis or ineffective treatment may occur (Paniagua, 1994) with potentially disastrous consequences and ineffective utilisation of health care resources.

A large component of the primary care APN is the ability to carry out an assessment of the patient and formulate an effective treatment plan. APNs need to develop an awareness of the biological variations in individuals of different racial and ethnic groups, such as the diversity of individual response to drug therapy, variations in laboratory results and clinical significance, disease risk and the pathophysiology of disease entities (Meiner, 2001). What at first seems to be a simple assessment of pain can become increasingly complex when issues such as cultural responses to the expression of and management of pain are considered. McGee (2003) wrote that not taking into account the patients' cultural variations devalues their experiences and beliefs and can contribute to the perpetuation of health inequalities.

Activity

Consider a patient that you have recently seen in which there were cultural differences.

- How thoroughly do you feel that cultural issues were addressed throughout your assessment?
- How could the assessment have been improved?
- What potential negative implications could the lack of focus on cultural aspects within your assessment have meant for your patient?

McGee (2003) writes of numerous studies that have been undertaken in the UK demonstrating that people of ethnic minorities suffer health inequalities. Suggestions put forward as to why this occurs include: inappropriate services and stereotypical assumptions (Ahmad, 2000), poor communication and a lack of knowledge amongst health professionals (McGee, 2003). Cultural competence is therefore important for all health professionals and it has been given a high political agenda through various documents such as the National Service Framework for older adults (DoH, 2001) which states that the needs of local members of minority ethnic groups must be taken into account. APNs working in the community have the opportunity to make services more readily accessible, sensitive and responsive to local needs (McGee, 2003), thus contributing to the competencies within this domain (C5, 6, 7).

Actively incorporating culture into care is regarded as a dimension of the moral work of nursing in helping people to make sense of their illness or disability in ways that are meaningful to them and in doing so helping them to accept and enjoy their life (Mendyka, 2000). A large part of this lies in health promotion activities. Readers should consider Domain 1 (Chapter 6) alongside the points outlined in this chapter.

Being comfortable with cultural diversity can be difficult and due to the power that culture has, it may take the APN a lot of effort to learn to be comfortable with people who do things differently. It is important to remember that people of varying cultures not only are of varying ethnicity, but also have differing sexual preferences, live in different regions, are of varying gender type or are of different ages (Clark, 1999).

APNs have a responsibility in fulfilling the competencies of the domain 'nurse–patient relationship' to learn about the different cultures that dominate in their practice area. Not all of this can be learnt from books and the importance for the APN to engage in dialogue with patients from such cultures to learn about their health beliefs and practices cannot be over-emphasised. In working towards achievement of competencies affected by culture within this domain, the APN should strive to work with a range of different cultural groups represented within the locality and have the chance to check and validate information with other members of the patient's culture (McGee, 2003) as simple intuitive interpretation is not enough (Paniagua, 1994) (C1, 2, 10). In doing so, issues around confidentiality must be considered; all too frequently, inappropriate people are being called upon to assist in translation, due to time constraints and lack of forward planning (C8). It may not be appropriate for the nurse to be including family members or reception staff, for example, in discussions regarding the patient's assessment as meanings may be distorted and transmitted information incomplete (Bickley and Szilagyi, 2007). Translators and cultural liaison nurses may be available and should be utilised where possible.

It is neither necessary, nor possible to know everything about the large variety of different cultures to provide effective health care (Meiner, 2001). However, APNs do need to continually gain an awareness of their own beliefs, stereotypes and prejudices prior to being able to build a completely effective nurse–patient relationship and so provide effective health care. Stereotyping or stigmatising may interfere with care (Morrisey, 1996) and therefore the ability to see each patient without being influenced by personal biases and judgements is a goal for all APNs to work towards in seeking to understand, respect and adapt to cultural differences (Meiner, 2001) (C9). The APN must demonstrate respect for people as unique individuals (Clark, 1999) so that a climate of mutual trust and established partnerships with patients, carers and families are created (C1). It may be that once the APN reflects on his/her own views and beliefs and considers the patient's needs, a decision is made to hand over the care of a patient and in doing so there is a closure to the nurse–patient relationship, ensuring provision for a safe transition to another care provider (C9, 10). However this may not always be possible, and therefore the APN must seek additional support in managing the patient's episode of care. In addition, the APN should remember that they cannot pick and choose which patients he/she will or will not care for (Callaghan, 2006).

Whilst it is important to learn of other cultures and how they may impact on health care practices, it is also important for the APN to recognise his/her own unique cultural attributes. Nursing and medicine has its own professional culture and there will also be organisational cultures present (McGee, 2003). Each of these individual cultures may present the APN with a difficult and challenging task in understanding the patient's views and problems and the subsequent effect

---

Activity

What cultural backgrounds comprise the patients within your practice or WiC setting?
   What barriers do you face within your practice or WiC setting in terms of working with patients from cultural backgrounds other than your own?
   How do you overcome these barriers?

of this on building effective relationships with patients should be recognised. In addition, for the ANP working as a district nurse, PN or community matron, it is likely that they will have the opportunity to build relationships with patients over many visits. However, for the ANP working in a WiC, for example, managing just one episode of care, they will have to build a therapeutic relationship with the patient much more quickly taking into consideration cultural issues.

Patient consultations

No matter whether the primary care ANP is working as a PN, district nurse, within a WiC or as a health visitor, a fundamental element of the role is to carry out an advanced health assessment taking a health history, obtaining physical data through a systematic assessment and ordering and interpreting the appropriate diagnostic tests (RCN, 2008). Taking the history alone may well take you into some sensitive areas but to obtain a holistic picture of the patient's health status, the APN must obtain truthful information in such a way that the therapeutic relationship between nurse and patient can be established and maintained (Clark, 1999) (C1). For treatment to be culturally competent, this assessment must have a cultural dimension in which the APN takes into account the individual's beliefs, values and practices (Barkauskas et al., 2002). This cannot be done by simply looking at a patient and their surname. An assessment tool can be useful in aiding the APN in taking his/her history. There are a number of assessment tools that have been designed to ensure a culturally competent assessment (Kleinman et al., 1978; Rooda, 1992; Campinha-Bacote, 1994; Leininger, 1995). The APN is advised to seek these out as it is beyond the scope of this chapter to discuss them here.

One important aspect of the consultation worth highlighting here, however, is that of the APN's non-verbal communication and the impact that this can have on obtaining a successful history. The APN should pay close attention to eye contact, facial expression, posture, head position and movement such as shaking or nodding, interpersonal distance and placement of the arms and legs such as crossed, neutral or open (Bickley and Szilagyi, 2007). Being aware of such non-verbal communication is the first step to building up a good rapport (C1) with the

---

Activity

Consider how you have taken a patient's history in the past. What are the strengths and weaknesses of your history taking?

How might you go about improving your history-taking skills?

What services, policies and procedures do you have in place within your organisation to help you carry out a culturally competent assessment of your patient's?

How do these services, policies and procedures contribute to/hinder the relationships that you build up with your patients/clients?

patient and obtaining as much information from them as possible. Be aware of the cultural variations with non-verbal communication. For example, the crossing of legs in some cultures is seen as a mark of disrespect by the nurse.

Ethical issues

When considering ethics in advanced practice, the fundamental element is the nurse–patient relationship and the responsibility it entails, making decisions within an implicit agreement between patient and nurse (Gray et al., 2001). A number of complex ethical decisions need to be made by the APN when considering the involvement of the patient with the health care process. Veath and Fry (1995) suggest that nurses face ethical issues in a unique manner because of the special relationship that they have with not only the patient, but also families and other members of the health care team. This relationship in which collaboration is achieved must be one built on trust (C1) in which confidentiality and privacy is central. Many models have been put forward to help the APN in ethical decision-making and issues of autonomy, freedom, objectivity, privacy, paternalism, beneficence, non-maleficence and justice should be considered as each will help to inform decisions about the level of involvement a patient should have in the nurse–patient relationship (Husted and Husted, 1995; Crumbie, 1999; Anderson and Pope-Kish, 2001) (C7). By focusing on such issues, the APN will respect each individual patient as a human being and provide full and appropriate information, allowing them to become fully informed, thus helping them to include themselves in the decision-making process (C1, 3, 6, 7) and making ethical dilemmas easier to manage.

It is important to remain sensitive to the patient's wishes (Elwyn et al., 1999; Levinson et al., 2005). Some patients will want to become actively involved in the maintenance of their health with little input from the APN on some or all decisions and others may be passive in their involvement, relying on the APN to make all decisions and carry out all aspects of care (Brearley, 1990; Elwyn et al., 2000; Whitney, 2003). For the APN working in many primary care settings, he/she is able to build and develop the nurse–patient relationship over time, encouraging patients to become actively involved in their care (C7).

The APN makes many decisions every day, some unconsciously and some with more thought; however, even with small decisions, a decision-making process is used (refer Chapter 5). It is when faced with more significant decisions that the APN may find it difficult to maintain the nurse–patient relationship that has been previously built in quite the same way. Indeed, it may seem that the best choice might well be the one chosen from several equally unsatisfactory options and this is when the APN becomes faced with an ethical dilemma.

The case study given in Box 8.1 outlines a scenario in which an APN is torn between what he/she feels his/her role is ethically as an APN and what he/she feels is right for working within the domain of nurse–patient relationship. Read the case study and complete the questions at the end of the activity before continuing

---

Box 8.1   Case Study

Mr Baker came to see you in your practice complaining of a change in bowel habit, PR bleeding, weight loss and lethargy. Following your examination and subsequent referral to the local hospital, he has recently been diagnosed with bowel cancer. Mr Baker has come to see you for a routine follow-up appointment for his hypertension and tells you of his diagnosis and the options that he has been given. Mr Baker tells you that he can either do nothing or that the consultant has recommended surgery±chemotherapy afterwards. None of the options guarantee a cure and all involve a level of discomfort and so Mr Baker tells you that he has decided that he will do nothing and wait and see if the symptoms get any worse before doing anything further. He also has concerns regarding surgery as he has been told that there may be the need for a stoma.

  Although this is not your area of practice, you are aware of the importance of making a decision regarding further intervention rather than 'waiting' for worsening of symptoms. You have a good relationship with Mr Baker that has been built up over many years; he has just retired at the age of 61 years and lives independently with his wife. Based on your relationship with Mr Baker, you feel that he should seek treatment of some sort immediately and that delaying this could lead to further spread of the cancer.

- What are the ethical dilemmas that you are faced with in this scenario (you may need to consult an ethics text)?
- Should you try to change Mr Baker's mind? And if so, how will you go about this?
- If you decide not to try and change Mr Baker's mind, based on your own feelings, would you consider doing anything else regarding the matter?
- Three months later, Mr Baker comes back to you and tells you that he has now decided that he wants to have the surgery but is afraid to contact the hospital due to refusal of treatment previously. What are your actions?
- Discuss your thoughts with other health professionals within your practice area.

---

to read the text. This case study will be used as the basis for discussion of some of the ethical issues for working within this domain.

In the case study illustrated in Box 8.1, Mr Baker has the right and duty to make his decision regarding his care and, in accordance with the principle of autonomy, there is an expectation that the APN is required to respect, accept and even support such decisions, even when the decision does not agree with what the APN would have wanted (C7). This can be difficult to do, particularly when a patient's choice is something that the APN knows will ultimately cause him harm. The APN may, however, have a role in helping Mr Baker examine the options with as much information as possible made available to him in understandable terms. This may be difficult as the primary care APN may not have the expertise in this area to consult on this and may need to ask Mr Baker's consent to seek a further appointment with a specialist nurse or the GP. The APN could direct specific questions beyond his/her scope of practice to the appropriate provider to ensure that the patient has an additional perspective (C10); furthermore, there may be the option of asking a patient who has had similar experiences to meet Mr Baker (Anderson and Pope-Kish, 2001).

There is the potential for conflict within the nurse–patient relationship in this case study; the patient obviously feels that he has a good relationship based on mutual trust and respect with the APN to even bring up the subject for discussion (C1). However, the APN knows that for any chance of success in eliminating the cancer, Mr Baker must undergo treatment for which he is refusing. This potential conflict between respect for the patients' autonomy and the APN's interest in doing good (beneficence) can be a dilemma for the APN.

Mr Baker's decision not to have treatment requires support by the APN and any signs of disapproval on the APN's part should not become apparent (C3, 7). The APN must show acceptance and respect for the decision, whatever it is, even if it does not conform to the APN's belief or to the decision that he or other patients would have made (Wheeler, 2000). Whilst the APN may feel that he/she is supporting the patients' decisions and accepting the decision, he/she should also remember that non-verbal cues given by the APN can also have a powerful effect (Gray et al., 2001).

The APN can enable decision-making by providing Mr Baker with relevant information and impartial guidance and an understanding that he can contact the APN for further advice in the future (C4). In this way, the APN is acting as the patient's advocate. In this case, this presupposes that the patient is willing to have the information provided, that the APN either knows or has access to the information needed by the patient and that the APN has the capacity to frame the information in words understandable to him and any other significant people involved in his decision-making process. A plan of care should be formulated with the patient in which he is empowered to take responsibility for his health and symptom management (C7).

Baldwin (2003) delineated three main attributes of patient advocacy:

- maintaining a therapeutic nurse–patient relationship in which to secure a patient's freedom and self-determination;
- promoting and protecting the patient's rights to be involved in decision-making and informed consent;
- acting as an intermediary between patient and their families and between them and health care providers.

In considering the case study given in Box 8.1, it can be seen that the APN is able to fulfil each of these attributes through supporting Mr Baker in his decision and through acting as an intermediary between the patient and the hospital staff both in obtaining further information and in organising later treatment. This willingness to share power with the patient helps build mutual trust (C1) and enables the APN to consider the unique details of his illness within the context of his life (C5) and continue to build upon the already established therapeutic nurse–patient relationship. This is important as it is not only the ideal outcome of removing the cancer that should be considered, but also the patient's quality of life. Quality of life is subjective, reflecting the patient's personal views (Anderson and Pope-Kish, 2001) and may be considered more important than a cure at that present time.

Activity

What ethical issues to you face in your daily practice?

Within your practice or WiC setting, are there established guidelines indicating the type of information you can share with patients?

Legal issues

Primary care APNs are personally and professionally accountable for their practice and as such must ensure that they have the competence to undertake and perform advanced practice activities to the same reasonable standard as the person that would have normally undertaken and been entrusted with those activities (e.g. a GP) (Whiteing, 2008). Difficulties will arise when APNs are poorly prepared for their roles with insufficient knowledge and skill to perform the functions of the advanced nursing role (Jones and Davies, 1999). Indeed, in law, being inexperienced is no defence and APNs, at whatever level of their development, will be judged by the same standards as more experienced colleagues unless they have sought the advice of someone more experienced than themselves (Furlong and Glover, 1998; Jones and Davies, 1999; Tingle, 2002; Callaghan, 2006). In working alongside other members of the health care team, procedures and protocols can be adapted to reflect the APN's legal accountability and aid protection against claims of clinical negligence (Tingle, 2002).

It is important that APNs are honest with patients (C1) in discussing when they feel that they are working outside their scope of practice so that they can seek help and advice from more experienced members of the team. This may involve discussing confidential information with others and it is important that the APN gains the patient's consent and full awareness in doing so in order that the patient's privacy and dignity are preserved (C8). Whilst the nurse–patient relationship is one built on confidentiality, it is paramount that the APN does not compromise the care delivered by not seeking help from others when out of their scope of practice (C10).

Indeed, without explaining to the patient that he/she is a nurse, the APN may invalidate the patient's consent if the patient assumed by the very nature of the task being performed that the APN is a doctor. It may be that the patient does not give consent for anyone other than a doctor to perform the task and therefore the APN must explain his/her status to the patient (Dowling et al., 1996).

Confidentiality

Competency 8 of the nurse–patient relationship domain addresses the issues of recording and keeping records of the patients care episode(s). This includes how the record is made, where it is stored and who has sight of it. The APN should be aware of both the Nursing and Midwifery Council (NMC) guidelines (2005) and also the National Heath Service (NHS) confidentiality code of practice (DoH, 2003). Good record keeping promotes good-quality patient care, safeguards the APN in case of legal or disciplinary action and empowers the APN to practice to the highest standard of care (Callaghan, 2006). Confidentiality and the maintenance of clear, comprehensive health care records is part of the professional responsibilities of all health care professionals and a fundamental role of the nurse (Dimond, 2003; Whiteing, 2008); however, due to the unique nature of the relationship between the APN and the patient in primary care, the APN will often have access to a considerable quantity of confidential information, which may continue over a significant period of time (Pennels, 2008). In addition, the APN will often have built up a relationship with the patient's family (C4) and it can be challenging to maintain this relationship and confidence, knowing exactly which information the patient wishes to remain entirely confidential and which he/she is happy to share with those around him/her. The APN requires good communication skills in order that he/she can explain to the relatives or next of kin that their request for information regarding the patient will only be disclosed with consent from the patient. Confidentiality is an important consideration in record keeping, as in any other area of professional practice (Dimond, 2004). As such, confidentiality must remain the priority of the APN and it may be that he/she can make reference to a document which will answer questions that the relative may have without actually showing them the relevant record/document.

This can be made more difficult depending on what types of records are used, particularly if care is being provided in the patient's own home and the APN must consider the professional and ethical issues of record keeping in this environment where greater protection of confidentiality is required. Patients should be able to access their records in order that they can participate in their own health care. Patient participation in record keeping should become the norm. Records should therefore be written in a manner that the patient is able to understand and contain only information that the patient agrees to. Records of consultations should form part of the summary and closure of the nurse–patient relationship (Thome, 2008) (C10).

In the past, patients would receive treatment from one GP. Today owing to the number of specialists involved in care and the extended scope of nurses and physiotherapists, patients are likely to be treated by a team of health care professionals. This delivers great benefits to the patient regarding quality of treatment; however, it also means that the many different professionals also need to be able to communicate effectively between themselves (Thome, 2008). It is commonly agreed that relevant information regarding the patient is shared amongst health care professionals on a need-to-know basis (DoH, 2003); however, it should not be assumed that the patient is aware of this. Therefore, the APN must inform the patient that their information will be shared with their consent.

Good record keeping does take practice, especially when the APN is required as part of his/her advanced role to be documenting histories and physical examinations that do not traditionally form part of the nurse's documentation. The APN must review his/her findings and the future treatment decisions with the patient where possible when recording them in the notes (Thome, 2008) (C2). This process can be difficult at first, trying to document at the same time as maintaining communication with the patient displaying interest in what the patient is saying and trying to utilise effective listening skills. In sharing the content with the patient, the APN is able to validate his/her findings (C2), establish partnerships (C1) and develop and maintain the patient's control over decision-making (C7).

Following the death of a patient, the APN may still continue to have a therapeutic relationship with the family who may wish to discuss the care and treatment of the deceased (C1, 4). As the legal duty of confidentiality extends into death, the APN's professional and ethical duty of confidentiality to the patient continues (C10) and the APN and the employing organisation must ensure appropriate measures are in place to hold patient records, only releasing them where relevant (DoH, 2003; Pennels, 2008).

Another difficult situation in which the APN will need to rely on good communication skills is if the patient is unable to consent to disclosure of information, for example, if they have dementia. The APN must balance the rights of the patient with the expectations of the relatives (Pennels, 2008).

Activity

Look at Table 8.1.
  What competencies do you already feel that you meet in relation to Domain 2 and more specifically in relation to the topics covered in this chapter? What evidence do you have for your portfolio to demonstrate this?

Key points in relation to the competencies for Domain 2

- A climate of mutual trust and partnership must be established with the patient and their families through appropriate communication skills, cultural awareness and emotional support.
- The APN can help patients participate in decision-making by providing relevant information and impartial guidance.
- The APN must take a step back from the nurse–patient relationship at times to examine his/her ethical and professional obligations to the patient.
- Accurate and consistent records should be kept by the APN and stored according to the organisation's storage and retrieval policies.
- The APN must be aware of his/her responsibilities under the NMC (2005) guidelines for records and record keeping and the DoH (2003) confidentiality code of practice, regarding the confidentiality of records.
- The APN should reflect on situations that have challenged the nurse–patient relationship in order that further learning and development can take place.

- The APN has a responsibility to learn about the different patient cultures within his/her locality and his/her professional and organisational cultures, and to have an awareness of his/her own biases and stereotypical assumptions.
- The APN cannot pick and choose which patients he/she sees based on cultural or ethical challenges; however, the APN must seek help from other members of the health care team if it is felt to be in the patient's best interest or beyond the APN's scope of practice.

Conclusion

This chapter has examined the nurse–patient relationship in relation to issues of confidentiality, culture, ethics and law, privacy and dignity and record keeping. It has been noted that:

- APNs have a unique relationship with their patients and it is through this relationship that the APN can become the vehicle through which patients participate in their care.
- Through the APN, patients can become empowered to make the decisions upon which they can provide a change in health behaviours, take personal responsibility for their health and work in partnership with health care providers.
- As the boundaries between nursing and medicine become blurred, APNs should consider how their relationship with the patient and their families may need to alter.

This chapter has considered just a few situations in which APNs may feel challenged in maintaining the therapeutic nurse–patient relationship whilst addressing the many professional, ethical, legal and cultural dilemmas they may face. It is only by working through such situations and reflecting on practice that APNs will be able to strive towards excellent provision of care within an effective nurse–patient relationship.

References

Ahmad, W. (2000) *Ethnicity, Disability and Chronic Illness*. Buckingham: Open University Press.

Anderson, M. and Pope-Kish, C. (2001) Decision making for ethical practice. In Robinson, D. and Pope-Kish, C. (Eds.) *Core Concepts in Advanced Practice Nursing*, pp. 224–236. St. Louis: Mosby.

Baldwin, M. (2003) Patient advocacy: A concept analysis. *Nursing Standard*, 17(21); 33–39.

Barkauskas, V., Baumann, L. and Darling-Fisher, C. (2002) *Health & Physical Assessment*. 3rd edn. St. Louis: Mosby.

Bickley, L. and Szilagyi, P. (2007) *Bates' Guide to Physical Examination and History Taking*. 9th edn. Philadelphia: Lippincott.

Brearley, S. (1990) *Patient Participation: The Literature*. London: Scutari Press.

Callaghan, C. (2006) The professional and legal framework for the nurse practitioner. In Walsh, M. (Ed.) *Nurse Practitioners Clinical Skills and Professional Issues*. 2nd edn., pp. 356–368. Edinburgh: Elsevier.

Campinha-Bacote, J. (1994) Cultural competence in psychiatric mental health nursing: A conceptual model. *Nursing Clinics of North America*, 29(1); 1–9.

Carnwell, R. and Daly, W. (2003) Advanced nurse practitioners in primary care settings: An exploration of the developing roles. *Journal of Clinical Nursing*, 12; 630–642.

Clark, C. (1999) Taking a history. In Walsh, M., Crumbie, A. and Reveley, S. (Eds.) *Nurse Practitioners Clinical Skills and Professional Issues*, pp. 12–23. Oxford: Butterworth-Heinemann.

Cox, C. (2001) Alteration in comfort: Caring for the patient using complementary therapies. In Cox, C.L. and Reyes-Hughes, A. (Eds.) *Clinical Effectiveness in Practice*, pp. 123–144. Hampshire: Palgrave.

Crumbie, A. (1999) The patient as partner in care. In Walsh, M., Crumbie, A. and Reveley, S. (Eds.) *Nurse Practitioners Clinical Skills and Professional Issues*, pp. 239–248. Oxford: Butterworth-Heinemann.

Dimond, B. (2003) Legal and ethical issues in advanced practice. In McGee, P. and Castledine, G. (Eds.) *Advanced Nursing Practice*, pp. 184–199. Oxford: Blackwell.

Dimond, B. (2004) *Legal Aspects of Nursing*. Essex: Pearson Education.

DoH (2001) *Modern Standards and Services Models. National Service Framework: Older People*. London: Department of Health.

DoH (2003) *Confidentiality – NHS Code of Practice*. London: Department of Health.

Dowling, S., Martin, R., Skidmore, P., Doyal, L., Cameron, A. and Lloyd, S. (1996) Nurses taking on junior doctors' work: A confusion of accountability. *British Medical Journal*, 312(7040); 1211–1214.

Elwyn, G., Edwards, A. and Kinnersly, P. (1999) Shared decision-making in primary care: The neglected second half of the consultation. *British Journal of General Practice*, 49(443); 471–482.

Elwyn, G., Edwards, A., Kinnersley, R. and Grol, K. (2000) Shared decision-making and the concept of equipoise: The competencies of involving patients in health care choices. *British Journal of General Practice*, 50(460); 892–899.

Furlong, S. and Glover, D. (1998) Legal accountability in changing practice. *Nursing Times*, 94(39); 61–62.

Gerber, D., Luggen, A. and Wishnia, G. (2001) Basic concepts in cultural diversity. In Robinson, D. and Pope-Kish, C. (Eds.) *Core Concepts in Advanced Practice Nursing*, pp. 457–466. St. Louis: Mosby.

Gray, P., Anderson, M. and Pope-Kish, C. (2001) Foundations for ethical practice. In Robinson, D. and Pope-Kish, C. (Eds.) *Core Concepts in Advanced Practice Nursing*, pp. 205–223. St. Louis: Mosby.

Green-Hernandez, C. (1997) Application of caring theory in primary care: A challenge for advanced practice. *Nursing Administration Quarterly*, 21(4); 77–82.

Horrocks, S., Anderson, A. and Salisbury, C. (2002) Systematic review of whether nurse practitioners working in primary care can provide equivalent care to doctors. *British Medical Journal*, 324(7341); 819–823.

Humphris, D. and Masterson, A. (1998) Practising at a higher level. *Professional Nurse*, 14(1); 10–13.

Husted, G. and Husted, J. (1995) *Ethical Decision Making in Nursing*. 2nd edn. St. Louis: Mosby.

Jones, S. and Davies, K. (1999) The extended role of the nurse: The United Kingdom perspective. *International Journal of Nursing Practice*, 5(4); 184–188.

Kleinman, A., Eisenburg, L. and Good, B. (1978) Culture, illness and care. *Annals of Internal Medicine*, 88(2); 251–258.

Leininger, M. (1995) *Transcultural Nursing: Concepts, Theories and Practices*. 2nd edn. New York: McGraw-Hill.

Levinson, W., Kao, A., Kuby, A. and Thisted, R. (2005) Not all patients want to participate in decision-making: A national study of public preferences. *Journal of General Medicine*, 20(6); 531–535.

McGee, P. (2003) Cultural competence and advanced practice. In McGee, P. and Castledine, G. (Eds.) *Advanced Nursing Practice*. 2nd edn., pp. 129–143. Oxford: Blackwell Publishing.

Meiner, S. (2001) Racial/ethnic group issues and health care. In Robinson, D. and Pope-Kish, C. (Eds.) *Core Concepts in Advanced Practice Nursing*, pp. 513–523. St. Louis: Mosby.

Mendyka, B. (2000) Exploring culture in nursing: A theory-driven practice. *Holistic Nursing Practice*, 15(1); 32–41.

Morrisey, M. (1996) Attitudes of practitioners to lesbian, gay and bisexual clients. *British Journal of Nursing*, 5(16); 980–982.

NMC (2005) *Guidelines for Records and Record Keeping*. London: Nursing and Midwifery Council.

Paniagua, F. (1994) *Assessing and treating Culturally Diverse Clients: A Practical Guide*. California: Sage.

Pennels, C. (2008) The legal and regulatory implications of advanced nursing practice. In Hinchliff, S. and Rogers, R. (Eds.) *Competencies for Advanced Nursing Practice*, pp. 21–49. London: Edward Arnold.

Peysner, J. (1996) Physicians assistant: Legal implications of the extended role. *British Journal of Nursing*, 5(10); 592.

Porter, S. (1991) The poverty of professionalization: A critical analysis of strategies for the occupational advancement of nursing. *Journal of Advanced Nursing*, 17(6); 720–726.

RCN (2008) *Advanced Nurse Practitioners: An RCN Guide to the Advanced Nurse Practitioner Role, Competencies and Programme Accreditation*. London: Royal College of Nursing.

Rooda, L. (1992) The development of a conceptual model for multicultural nursing. *Journal of Holistic Nursing*, 10(4); 337–347.

Thome, R. (2008) Domain 1: The nurse–patient relationship. In Hinchliff, S. and Rogers, R. (Eds.) *Competencies for Advanced Nursing Practice*, pp. 50–70. London: Edward Arnold.

Tingle, J. (2002) The legal implications of extending nurses' roles. *Practice Nursing*, 13(4); 148, 150, 152.

Veath, R. and Fry, S. (1995) *Case Studies in Nursing Ethics*. Boston: Jones & Bartlett.

Wheeler, P. (2000) Is advocacy at the heart of professional practice? *Nursing Standard*, 14(36); 39–41.

Whiteing, N. (2008) Domain 6: Monitoring and ensuring the quality of advanced health care practice. In Hinchliff, S. and Rogers, R. (Eds.) *Competencies for Advanced Nursing Practice*, pp. 192–219. London: Edward Arnold.

Whitney, S. (2003) A new model of decisions: Exploring the limits of shared decision-making. *Medical Decision Making*, 23(4); 275–280.

Domain 3

Education Function

Anticipatory guidance: National Service Frameworks

9

Victoria Lack

Introduction

The aim of this chapter is to examine how nurses working in general practice and walk-in centres (WiCs) can implement anticipatory guidance as described by the Royal College of Nursing (RCN) in the education domain for advanced practice. The National Service Framework (NSF) for diabetes mellitus will be used to illustrate the practice of anticipatory guidance in primary care.

Learning Outcomes

- To assess the need for practice nurses (PNs) and WiC nurses to provide anticipatory guidance
- To illustrate the knowledge necessary to achieve the anticipatory guidance role of nurses with reference to the NSF standards
- To give examples of how the necessary knowledge can be achieved or accessed.

Background

Anticipatory guidance is defined by 'Bright Futures', the national health promotion initiative in the USA for maternal and child health, as 'information that helps families prepare for expected physical and behavioural changes during their child's or teen's current and approaching stage of development' (Bright Futures, 2008:1). It is a term that is widely used in the USA to describe, as the definition implies, information and advice given by health workers to carers of children in order for them to be able to anticipate and prepare for normal changes during childhood and adolescence. The term anticipatory guidance is used in the RCN third domain of advanced practice (2008) and implies a wider definition of guidance given throughout the life span. In this chapter, the broader understanding of the term will be used which is to include information given to all age groups, throughout life. Anticipatory guidance is only a part of one of the competencies described by the RCN in the education domain of practice. In this chapter, reference will be made to the 14 competencies within the domain.

Domain 3: The education function

Domain 3: the education function of advanced PNs as described by the RCN and validated by the Nursing and Midwifery Council (NMC) is set out as follows:

Dimension – timing:
1. Assesses the ongoing and changing needs of patients, carers and families for education based on the following:
   a. needs for anticipatory guidance associated with growth and the developmental stage,
   b. care management that requires specific information or skills,
   c. the patients' understanding of their health condition;
2. assesses the patient's motivation for learning and maintenance of health-related activities using principles of change and stages of behaviour change;
3. creates an environment in which effective learning can take place.

Eliciting:
4. Elicits information about the patient's interpretation of health conditions as a part of the routine health assessment;
5. elicits information about the patient's perceived barriers, supports and modifiers to learning when preparing for patient's education;
6. elicits the patient's learning style to facilitate an appropriate teaching approach;
7. elicits information about cultural influences that may affect the patient's learning experience.

Enabling:
8. Enables patients by displaying a sensitivity to the effort and emotions associated with learning about how to care for one's health condition;
9. enables patients in learning specific information or skills by designing a learning plan that is comprised of sequential, cumulative steps, and that acknowledges relapse and the need for practice, reinforcement, support and re-teaching when necessary;
10. enables patients to use community resources when needed.

Providing:
11. Communicates health advice and instruction appropriately, using an evidence-based rationale.

Negotiating:
12. Negotiates a jointly determined plan of care, based on continual assessment of the patient's readiness and motivation, re-setting goals and optimal outcomes;
13. monitors the patient's behaviours and specific outcomes as a guide to evaluating the effectiveness and need to change or maintain educational strategies.
Coaching:
14. Coaches the patient by reminding, supporting and encouraging, using empathy (RCN, 2008).

The third domain of practice: the education function is relevant to all nurses, although not all nurses may achieve all the competencies within it. This domain of practice reflects the view that advanced PNs, at least, should be able to provide education to patients, carers and families which is accurate, appropriate, timely and sensitive to the individual's needs, in an atmosphere which is conducive to learning. It is expected that most nurses, working in general practice or WiCs, would be able to identify with the competencies to a greater or lesser extent.

Activity

After reading the domain of practice, think of examples from your practice in which you provide anticipatory guidance.

Practice nursing, as practiced today, has largely developed in response to changes in the health care system, notably the GP contract (DoH, 1993) which encouraged general practitioners (GPs) to take on more preventive work with cash incentives for chronic disease management clinics and which also relocated much of routine chronic disease management into primary health care. The New GMS Contract (DoH, 2003) formalised health education in general practice, by making health education activities necessary for achieving 'QoF' points. It is normal for PNs to take much of the responsibility for attaining the QoF targets; therefore, PNs should be equipped for an educational role within the practice. For example, the QoF for diabetes has 17 indicators for ongoing management of the condition (DoH, 2003; Table 9.1).

Many of these, if not all, involve the patient knowing what to expect and being able to manage and plan for their condition: they rely on the patient having received anticipatory guidance in its broader sense. For example, consider the targets DM 6–11. These rely on the patient knowing to expect that they will have their blood taken, feet checked, blood pressure recorded and eyes checked. This information giving is not only to achieve income for the practice, but is also good sense in terms of diabetes management.

The focus and context of WiC nursing is different from that of the PN. The role of WiCs includes provision of information surrounding minor health conditions and health promotion (Salisbury et al., 2002). Nurses working in WiCs are therefore

Table 9.1   QoF Points attainable for the Management of Diabetes Mellitus (DoH, 2003). Reproduced under the terms of the Click-Use Licence

All minimum thresholds are 25% indicator	Points	Maximum threshold (%)
Ongoing management		
DM 2. The percentage of patients with diabetes whose notes record BMI in the previous 15 months	3	90
DM 3. The percentage of the nGNf patients with diabetes in whom there is a record of smoking status in the previous 15 months except those who have never smoked where smoking status should be recorded once	3	90
DM 4. The percentage of patients with diabetes who smoke and whose notes contain a record that smoking cessation advice has been offered in the past 15 months	5	90
DM 5. The percentage of diabetic patients who have a record of HbA1c or equivalent in the previous 15 months	3	90
DM 6. The percentage of patients with diabetes in whom the last HbA1C is 7.4 or less (or equivalent test/reference range depending on local laboratory) in past 15 months	16	50
DM 7. The percentage of patients with diabetes in whom the last HbA1C is 10 or less (or equivalent test/reference range depending on local laboratory) in past 15 months	11	85
DM 8. The percentage of patients with diabetes who have a record of retinal screening in the previous 15 months	5	90
DM 9. The percentage of patients with diabetes with a record of presence or absence of peripheral pulses in the previous 15 months	3	90
DM 10. The percentage of patients with diabetes with a record of neuropathy testing in the previous 15 months	3	90
DM 11. The percentage of patients with diabetes who have a record of the blood pressure in the past 15 months	3	90
DM 12. The percentage of patients with diabetes in whom the last blood pressure is 145/85 or less	17	55
DM 13. The percentage of patients with diabetes who have a record of micro-albuminuria testing in the previous 15 months (exception reporting for patients with proteinuria)	3	90
DM 14. The percentage of patients with diabetes who have a record of serum creatinine testing in the previous 15 months	3	90
DM 15. The percentage of patients with diabetes with proteinuria or micro-albuminuria who are treated with ACE inhibitors (or A2 antagonists)	3	70
DM 16. The percentage of patients with diabetes who have a record of total cholesterol in the previous 15 months	3	90
DM 17. The percentage of patients with diabetes whose last measured total cholesterol within previous 15 months is 5 or less	6	60
DM 18. The percentage of patients with diabetes who have had influenza immunisation in the preceding 1 September to 31 March	3	85

fundamental to provision of this role. However, Abbott et al. (2008) say that WiCs may not be the best place for health education, if this is to be more than simply passing on information, due perhaps to a lack of time per consultation to be able to provide such detailed information.

It seems evident that general practice is an ideal setting for anticipatory guidance to be provided by PNs. There are many opportunities during preventive consultations: childhood immunisation clinics, cervical cytology, family planning clinics, chronic disease management clinics and new patient health checks, for example. Time may be limited to 15 or 20min per consultation, but the PN usually has the advantage of previous notes, and the opportunity to ask the patient to return for follow-up. Anticipatory guidance in a WiC is more difficult, as time needs to be spent developing a rapport, discussing previous history and assessing the readiness of the patient to engage in discussion. However, it is a key function of the WiC and one which should not be overlooked. One advantage of the WiC is that there are usually no appointment times, so time can be spent with the presenting patient as needed. However, this depends to an extent on the discretion of the WiC management. It is possible to spend an hour with patients presenting at aWiC with extremely complex needs, knowing that the WiC nurse could send a patient away very quickly if the patient presenting is not strictly in WiC criteria (consulting for 'minor' and urgent injury or illness). Recently in a WiC, one such patient had human immunodeficiency virus (HIV) and kidney failure and was consulting because she had been menstruating for several weeks without pause. The patient did not have a GP, and as a 'non-documented migrant' was unlikely to find it easy to obtain one. The nurse conducting the consultation felt it was correct to try to give as much information and practical help as possible regarding the issue of registering with a GP (which was seen to be the most important issue at that moment). The patient needed to be 'guided' through the NHS system, and told what to expect (and also what not to expect). The patient's per vagina bleeding was also dealt with. The WiC management at this particular centre instituted a system of 20min 'slots' for patients in order to keep the queue down and minimise the risk of 'breaching' the 24h Accident and Emergency (A&E) target. However, the nurse had the opportunity to override that as she had in effect no booked patients. This example is illustrated to make the point that it may actually be easier to give guidance in a WiC than in general practice, when time factors are considered.

Education and anticipatory guidance are accepted as being an essential part of nursing. WiC nurses and PNs are therefore expected to practice such guidance throughout their consultations. The NSF for diabetes will now be discussed to illustrate how nurses working in these two environments can use the NSFs to facilitate and/or provide anticipatory guidance for their patients. The example of the NSF for diabetes can then be extrapolated to the other NSFs.

The NSFs

Following the Labour party's victory in the 1997 general elections, the Department of Health quickly issued a White Paper which described the proposed direction of the NHS over the life of the Labour government. *The NHS, Modern Dependable* (DoH, 1997) discussed quality and uniformity in the NHS. The old internal market of the conservative era was to be disbanded and there was to be a new emphasis on standards and clinical excellence and an end to regional variations in practice and outcomes. The way to achieve this was termed clinical governance. Clinical governance was and is a key feature of Labour's NHS policy and aims to 'produce within every health organisation a structure and system to assure and improve the quality of clinical services' (Vincent, 2001:62). Put more simply, it is about the 'patients/carers receiving the right care at the right time, from the right person, in a safe environment' (McSherry and Pearce, 2002:18).

Clinical governance has three overlapping elements which are:

- development of national standards and guidelines to improve and standardise care;
- NSFs (mental health, elderly, CHD and diabetes);
- National Institute for Clinical Excellence (DoH, 1998).

NSFs were first described in the White Paper *A First Class Service: Quality in the New NHS* (DoH, 1998). NSFs are long-term strategies for improving specific areas of care. They set national standards which identified specific interventions to be completed within agreed time scales (DoH, 2008). The two main roles of NSFs are to set clear requirements for care and to offer strategies and support to health care organisations to achieve these requirements or standards (NHS Direct, 2008).

There are currently 10 NSFs covering key chronic diseases, such as diabetes, age groups (children and older people) or areas of care (mental health). They are 'care blueprints' to tackle unacceptable variations in care across the country. The National Institute for Health and Clinical Excellence (NICE) was developed at the same time to advise health workers on best practice according to the best available evidence. Coupled to both the NSFs and NICE was the concept of lifelong learning, to enable and assure that health workers have the opportunity to remain up to date in their chosen fields. Indeed, the concept of lifelong learning and providing the most contemporary evidence-based practice is an essential requirement of all nurses, midwives and community public health specialist nurses (which includes PNs and WiC nurses) as is evident from *The Code Standards of Conduct, Performance and Ethics for Nurses and Midwives* (NMC, 2008).

A First Class Service: Quality in the New NHS (DoH, 1998) continues to have far-reaching implications for all health workers. WiC nurses and PNs have significant roles to play in assuring quality in the NHS, and a high standard of anticipatory guidance is met throughout the 10 NSFs. First of all, it is important that nurses are familiar at least with the broad outline of each NSF. The standards are clearly stated in the executive summary of each NSF and it is important that nurses – along with all health workers – have a grasp of at least the background assumptions and summary of the standards. Second, it is essential that both groups of nurses are experts in their own field of practice, and know where to refer or direct patients to when the issue is outside of their sphere of knowledge.

How does anticipatory guidance relate to the NSFs?

As discussed in the section 'Introduction', the NSFs are 'care blueprints' to help achieve a high standard of clinical care across the NHS. A large part of the NSFs is concerned with the provision of anticipatory guidance to patients, carers and families. In order for this guidance to be effective, it needs to be accurate, appropriate, timely and sensitive to an individual's needs, in an atmosphere which is conducive to learning. In this chapter, the NSF for diabetes illustrates how the NSF requires nurses to be able to provide anticipatory guidance regarding the prevention and management of Type II diabetes.

Standard 1 of the NSF for diabetes states the following:

> The NHS will develop, implement and monitor strategies to reduce the risk of developing Type II diabetes in the population as a whole and to reduce the inequalities in the risk of developing Type II diabetes.

The key interventions are described as follows: the overall prevalence of Type II diabetes in the population can be reduced by preventing and reducing the prevalence of people being overweight, obesity and the prevalence of central obesity in the general population, particularly in sub-groups of the population at increased risk of developing diabetes, such as people from minority ethnic communities, by promoting a balanced diet and physical activity. Individuals at increased risk of developing Type II diabetes can reduce their risk if they are supported to change their lifestyle by eating a balanced diet, losing weight and increasing their physical activity levels (DoH, 2001). The NSF then continues with a discussion of these interventions and approaches to the interventions in more detail.

Nurses working at an advanced practice level should be able to implement an anticipatory guidance function relating to the prevention of Type II diabetes in the practice or WiC population that they are managing, as well as work towards reducing inequalities in risk between different sub-groups of that population. In order to carry out effectively the education function in relation to this one standard in one NSF, the nurse must be knowledgeable in many areas. The nurse will also need to have knowledge of health promotion theory in order to be able to assess the patient's readiness to learn and make positive changes in their lifestyle. Anticipatory guidance as related to the NSF is clearly an advanced practice role, but one which is essential for PNs and WiC nurses to adopt if they are to provide a high quality of care in the NHS.

Standard 1 requires knowledge of the local population, along with particular risk factors for diabetes. It also requires knowledge of primary and secondary prevention strategies associated with diabetes mellitus (DoH, 2001). Diabetes UK presents the main risk factors for Type II diabetes on the organisation's website (Box 9.1).

Besides the risk factors associated with the onset of Type II diabetes mellitus, there are other associated risk factors as shown in Box 9.2.

Box 9.1   Risk Factors for Type II Diabetes

Ethnic background

- The prevalence of diabetes is around 2.4% in Caucasians.
- In some Black and minority ethnic (BAME) groups, it can be as much as three to five times higher for Type II diabetes compared to their Caucasian equivalents.
- Type II diabetes also tends to develop around five years sooner in people from Black and minority ethnic groups.
- In the South Asian population, it is around 10 years earlier and at lower levels of obesity (Diabetes UK, 2008).

Box 9.2   Other Associated Risk Factors associated with Type II Diabetes

Other risk factors

1   White people >40 years and BAME people >25 years with one or more of the following risk factors:
   - first degree FH DM;
   - BMI 25 or above and a sedentary lifestyle;
   - waist measurement 94 cm or above (White and Black men);
   - waist measurement 94 cm or above (Asian men);
   - waist measurement 80 cm or above (White, Black and Asian women);
   - people who have IHD, cerebrovascular disease, PVD and treated hypertension;
   - PMH of gestational diabetes;
   - PCOS with a BMI 30 or above;
   - known IGT;
   - severe mental health problems;
   - hypertriglyceridemia not due to alcohol or renal disease (Diabetes UK, 2008).

Knowledge of preventive strategies

Primary preventive strategies for prevention of Type II diabetes are varied. The NSF for diabetes advocates the promotion of healthy diet and exercise to prevent obesity and particularly central obesity, especially among those at higher risk. The White Paper *Our Health, Our Care, Our Say* (DoH, 2006a) recommends multiagency action to reduce the numbers of people who are physically inactive or who are overweight. According to the government paper *Turning the Corner: Improving Diabetes Care* (DoH, 2006b), action must be taken in childhood to have the greatest impact. Most PNs and WiC nurses will not be directly involved in such programmes, but there is no reason why they should not be, especially if they work in areas where the population is at higher than average risk of diabetes. They may also support others such as school nurses, dieticians, etc., in the implementation of such programmes. Preventive programmes, especially when targeted towards higher risk groups, can work in practice.

There are many local initiatives in which WiC nurses and, perhaps more likely, PNs will be involved. For example, the *Do Activity Stay Healthy Scheme* (DASH) is run by Somerset PCT to tackle the growing problem of obesity in school children. The programme is run as a school-based club where children aged five to nine years are encouraged to exercise and eat healthily through 'fun' activities. The anticipatory guidance to the children and families here is to discuss with the participants why it is important to eat well and exercise well and the consequences of not having a healthy lifestyle in later life (DoH, 2006b).

Secondary prevention of diabetes involves screening for diabetes. At present, there is no nationally agreed strategy for screening (Diabetes UK, 2008) although many local initiatives are running. In addition, there is no definitely agreed protocol for screening for Type II diabetes, or agreement about how to interpret the results. Fasting venous blood samples are the usual method although capillary glucose measurement may be sufficient. Glucose tolerance tests can be used in cases where the diagnosis is in doubt (Patient UK, 2008). A large, UK-based study used the classification given in Box 9.3 to decide on the need and direction of further intervention (Greaves et al., 2008).

Box 9.3   A Simple and Pragmatic System for detecting New Cases of Type II diabetes and Impaired Fasting Glycaemia in Primary Care

- Fasting plasma glucose of <6.1 mmol/l: unlikely to have impaired glucose metabolism and should be re-enlisted for further screening at a later date (probably in a further three years or so);
- fasting plasma glucose of 6.1–6.9 mmol/l defined as having IGT ('pre-diabetes');
- two results >7 mmol/l defined as having probable frank diabetes;
- fasting or random plasma glucose, on one reading, of >11.1 mmol/l is diagnostic of diabetes (Greaves et al., 2008).

It is essential that if nurses are to administer screening tests, then they are able to manage the results in collaboration with the patient. They need to be able to give guidance pre- and post-testing to ensure the patient is not made unduly anxious, or indeed given false reassurances. For example, if a client is found to have impaired glucose tolerance (IGT), then the nurse must be confident in explaining this to the individual, and also what is to be expected and what should be done by the patient about the condition. In short, the nurse must be competent in anticipatory guidance in this area. In a WiC setting, the patient may not return to the WiC for the results, but the nurse must be prepared for this eventuality and ensure the patient is followed up by someone also competent in giving results and identifying a future plan of action.

Follow-up for Type II diabetes is hopefully reasonably well established within most general practices, but follow-up for IGT is less well managed. Patients with increased risk of Type II diabetes have a 50% risk of progression to Type II diabetes within 10 years, and double the risk of cardiovascular disease (Tuomilehto et al., 2001). Lifestyle intervention can reduce the risk of progression to diabetes, and may have an impact on cardiovascular disease (Wylie et al., 2002). The Joint British Societies (JBS) recommends the following for patients with IGT: apparently healthy individuals with a CVD risk >20% over 10 years who have IGT should receive appropriate lifestyle and risk factor intervention, including the use of cardiovascular protective drug therapies, to achieve the risk factor targets including glycaemic control (British Cardiac Society; British Hypertension Society; Diabetes UK; HEART UK; Primary Care Cardiovascular Society; Stroke Association, 2005; JBS, 2005). Nurses may not be responsible for the provision of drug therapies such as the aforementioned, but they should be able to advise the patient on the anticipatory guidance surrounding their condition.

Pre-requisites for giving anticipatory guidance

PNs and WiC nurses should be able to guide and support all individuals with risk factors for diabetes, IGT and overt diabetes, or at the least know where and how to refer them in order that they receive such support elsewhere. For this, nurses need to have the knowledge (or resources to find the knowledge) at their fingertips. They must also have the ability to give guidance in a way that the patient will respond to. Although the RCN (2008) competencies state that nurses in advanced practice should be competent in anticipatory guidance, it is hard to find discussion on how this can be achieved. First of all, it is apparent, from the above discussion, that nurses need to know their subject, their resources and their methods of referral, but discussion regarding actual implementation of anticipatory guidance, the how, when and where, is more difficult to find. However, by examination of the educational domain of practice, it is possible to deconstruct what is necessary for nurses to implement effective anticipatory guidance. The domain areas of timing, eliciting, enabling, providing, negotiating and coaching give an idea of what pre-requisites are needed in order to facilitate effective anticipatory guidance. The nurse needs to ensure that the time is right for the patient: the health education concept of being ready to change is very important here. The nurse also needs to gain information from the patient about what the patient already knows, what they need to know and how much the patient wants to know at this time. The nurse needs to then enable the patient to learn by provision of a conducive atmosphere, culturally appropriate information and appropriate back-up resources to leave with the patient. Finally, the nurse needs to provide the patient with the information, negotiate a plan of action and coach the patient to retain and implement the information (see Box 9.4).

Box 9.4   Example from a Walk-in-Centre

The prevalence of diabetes in the population can be reduced by increasing the activity levels and by promoting a healthy diet in the population, especially among groups at higher risk.

The nurse needs therefore to know which groups are at higher risk (as above) and which groups are at higher risk in the practice population (or catchment area) due to different ethnic backgrounds.

PNs especially may be involved in primary prevention on a more public health level. They may be involved or manage community assessments and implementation of preventive strategies at a community level. All PNs and WiC nurses however will be involved in secondary prevention on a one-to-one basis or in small groups, to patients at higher risk.

A Pakistani man of age 42 years arrives at the WiC with complaints of headaches. On history and examination, serious causes of the headache are excluded. However, on history taking, it is found that the man has a family history of Type II diabetes in both parents, he eats a diet which is high in processed foods and he does little exercise. He is overweight, but not obese. According to the NSF for diabetes mellitus, it is not enough to assess and treat the above man for the complaint for which he has come in. It may not be the time in the consultation to raise the possibility of diabetes mellitus, but it is the nurse who must realise the patient is at high risk, and assess whether, and if, to discuss the potential risk to the patient, or refer him back to his general practice for follow-up. However, in this particular case, the patient had already considered the possibility (not surprisingly given that his parents had diabetes) and was worried that he may have the condition himself. He had not, however, discussed the concern with anyone else. Having raised the possibility of a chronic illness with a patient, the nurse must of course be competent to carry on the consultation and make a positive action plan with the patient. In this case, the man was dispatched with request forms for fasting blood sugar, written advice regarding diet, exercise and weight, and advised to make a follow-up appointment with his PN for the results and further advice and investigations as needed.

Having raised the possibility of a serious disease, it is essential, as the above example shows, that the nurse is able to continue the consultation and give the patient something meaningful to take away with them. Preventive strategies on health diet and physical exercise are difficult to give when time is limited, especially when the patient may not be known to the nurse and may not be able or willing to return for follow-up. The nurse needs to know what is possible in the consultation, where to find relevant written information and where to refer to for follow-up.

Activity

Think of an encounter with a patient you have cared for with Type II diabetes. What information have you given to them? How did you assess what information to give them? Use the domain of practice headings of timing, eliciting, etc., to help organise your answer.

Nurses of course are not able to have all knowledge for all conditions. It is therefore essential that nurses work according to the needs of their populations and the role which they are fulfilling. For example, a WiC nurse may be less concerned with prevention of Type II diabetes in her day-to-day role than a PN working in an area with a high population of BAME groups. However, the WiC nurse should be able to recognise 'high-risk' patient for diabetes coming through the door and assess whether to give advice immediately, refer to a colleague, or merely recommend that the patient makes an appointment to see their PN or GP for a general health review. The NSFs and the advanced practice domains suggest that in order to provide quality care, it is not enough to treat the presenting problem, but anticipatory guidance should be given (or recommended to be given) for perhaps the more serious problem which has yet to manifest itself.

Activity

Think of a real-life situation where you have considered a patient to be at high risk of Type II diabetes, or other chronic condition. What did you do about it? Was there any knowledge that you were lacking in order to be able to carry out the consultation effectively? How would you do things differently if the situation arose again?

Anticipatory guidance for patients with a long-term condition

Standard 4 of the NSF for diabetes considers patients already living with Type II diabetes (DoH, 2001). The standard is:

> To maximise the quality of life of all people with diabetes and to reduce their risk of developing the long-term complications of diabetes.

It is immediately evident that this standard applies equally to WiC nurses and PNs and that nurses will need to be competent in the education domain of practice. Consider the patient who has an appointment in the general practice for a routine review of his diabetes, shown in Box 9.5.

Box 9.5   Case Study

Mr Paterson is 78 years old and lives with his wife. He has Type II diabetes, hypertension and heart failure. He has had his left leg amputated four years ago. He lives in an adapted ground-floor flat. He can push himself round in a wheelchair inside. He is breathless on transferring bed/chair and is sometimes wheezy. He has orthopnoea and nocturnal cough. His wife is the main carer, but cannot lift him.

Past Medical History

1987: Type II diabetes;
1988: hypertension;
1996: left heart failure;
2003: peripheral vascular disease and peripheral neuropathy;
2003: left below knee amputation for ascending infection.

Social History

Lives with wife in an adapted ground-floor flat. Has no children but has a niece who lives close by and visits nearly every day. Smokes for only three to four days now (previously a lot more). Alcohol on family occasions. He goes to a day centre three days a week which he enjoys.

Medication History

No known allergies;
aspirin 75 mg OD;
bendrofluazide 2.5 mg OD;
enalapril maleate 20 mg OD;
atenolol 50 mg OD;
digoxin 125 mcg OD;
metformin 500 mg TDS;
gliclazide 80 mg OD;
atorvastatin 10 mg OD;
Co-dydramol 10/500 2 PRN;
diazepam 5 mg nocte.

Services received

Daily carer for personal hygiene;
DN monitors diabetes;
day centre three times per week.
BP lying 110/65 mmHg; standing 120/70 mmHg

- P 84 bpm and slightly irregular;
- random BSL 14 mmol (post-breakfast);
- heart – apex beat displaced to left; RRR, S3 heard;
- chest – equal expansion, wheezes and crackles bilat bases.

Looking at the history of this complex patient, it is difficult to know where to start as he has multiple pathologies and is significantly impaired in mobility. However, going back to the education domains, it becomes easier perhaps to ascertain needs and priorities. First, the need for anticipatory guidance: Mr P has already suffered some of the long-term effects of diabetes mellitus including amputation of his left leg, and probably needs no reminder of the risk to his remaining leg. However, this does not reduce his risk of further macro- or micro-vascular risk and/or damage to his kidneys or peripheral nervous system. Mr P may not want to hear this, or this may not be his priority. He also needs ongoing care management. He already has a large input from the community health services and social services. Questions should be considered as to:

- Is this the right sort of input?
- Is it sufficient?
- Does it help Mrs P, as the main carer, to maintain a reasonable quality of life?
- What is Mr P's understanding of his condition?
- Mr P has lived with his chronic illnesses for a long time, but does he understand what is happening physiologically even at a basic level?
- Does he know why he takes the numerous medications that he takes?
- Does he want to know?
- Does he actively try to take care of his health?
- Does he want to stop smoking altogether?
- Does he want to listen to you here today?

The PN needs to be able to assess all of the above, a process which is often helped as the patient and nurse will hopefully have developed a rapport over previous consultations. The nurse in the WiC may have different priorities and a different agenda: her role is less concerned with management of long-term conditions, but with dealing with immediate problems. Quality care will not be provided in WiCs, if longer term guidance is ignored. The WiC nurse can refer and/or recommend that the patient self-refers for further educational needs. There is a dilemma as to how to strike the balance between the two.

Conclusion

Anticipatory guidance is an advanced skill, requiring considerable clinical knowledge, knowledge of health promotion theory, effective use of resources and good team working. The NSFs, among other components, are central to the concept of quality in the NHS and necessitate the use of health education and anticipatory guidance for their effective implementation. It is the role of primary care nurses in the 21st century to be a part of the implementation of quality standards. This requires nurses to extend their consultations beyond the immediately apparent, to discuss and guide patients through the issues with which they present and to work as a part of the wider team to ensure patients have access to all the information and guidance they need.

References

Abbott, S., Bickerton, J., Daly, M. and Procter, S. (2008) Evidence based primary health care and local research: A necessary but problematic partnership. *Primary Health Care Research and Development*, 9; 191–198.

Bright Futures at Georgetown University (2008) *Glossary*. http://www.brightfutures. org/healthcheck/resources/glossary.html (accessed 20 June 2008).

British Cardiac Society; British Hypertension Society; Diabetes UK; HEART UK; Primary Care Cardiovascular Society; Stroke Association (2005) JBS 2: Joint British Societies' guidelines on prevention of cardiovascular disease in clinical practice. *Heart*, 91(Suppl. 5); 1–52.

Diabetes UK (2008) *Causes and Risk Factors*. http://www.diabetes.org.uk/Guide-to-diabetes/What_is_diabetes/Causes_and_Risk_Factors/ (accessed 20 June 2008).

DoH (1993) *The GP Contract*. London: Department of Health.

DoH (1997) *The New NHS: Modern, Dependable*. London: Department of Health.

DoH (1998) *A First Class Service: Quality in the New NHS*. London: Department of Health.

DoH (2001) *National Service Framework for Diabetes*. London: Department of Health.

DoH (2003) *The New General Medical Services Contract*. London: Department of Health.

DoH (2006a) *Our Health, Our Care, Our Say: A New Direction for Community Services*. London: Department of Health.

DoH (2006b) *Turning the Corner: Improving Diabetes Care*. London: Department of Health.

DoH (2008) *National Service Frameworks*. http://www.dh.gov.uk/en/Healthcare/ NationalServiceFrameworks/index.htm (accessed 20 June 2008).

Greaves, C., Stead, J., Hattersley, A., Ewings, P., Brown, P. and Evans, P. (2008). A simple pragmatic system for detecting new cases of type 2 diabetes and impaired fasting glycaemia in primary care. *Family Practice*, 21(1); 57–62.

JBS (2005) http://www.hmr.nhs.uk/userfiles/documents/Joint%20British%20Society %20Guidelines%20full%20doc.pdf (accessed 4 March 2009).

McSherry, R. and Pearce, P. (2002) *Clinical Governance; A Guide to the Implementation for Health Care Professionals*. Oxford: Blackwell Science Ltd.

NHS Direct (2008) *What are National Service Frameworks?* http://www.nhsdi-rect.nhs.uk/articles/article.aspx?ArticleId=1080 (accessed 20 June 2008).

NMC (2008) *The Code Standards of Conduct, Performance and Ethics for Nurses and Midwives*. London: Nursing and Midwifery Council.

Patient UK (2008) *Screening for Diabetes*. http://www.patient.co.uk/showdoc/ 40024556 (accessed 22 June 2008).

RCN (2008) *Advanced Nurse Practitioners. An RCN Guide to the Advanced Nurse Practitioner Role, Competencies and Programme Accreditation*. London: Royal College of Nursing.

Salisbury, C., Chalder, M., Manku-Scott, T., Nicholas, R., Deave, T., Noble, S., Pope, C., Moore, L., Coasr, J., Anderson, E., Weiss, M., Grant, C. and Sharp, D. (2002) *The National Evaluation of NHS Walk in Centres: Final Report*. Bristol: Bristol University.

Tuomilehto, J., Lindstrom, J., Eriksson, J., Valle, T., Hamalainen, H., Illanne-Parikka, P., Keinanen-Kiukaanniemi, S., Laakso, M., Louheranta, A., Rastas, M.,

Salminen, V. and Uusitupa, M. (2001) Prevention of Type 2 diabetes mellitus by changes in lifestyle amongst subjects with impaired glucose tolerance. *The New England Journal of Medicine*, 344(18); 1343–1350.

Vincent, C. (2001) *Clinical Risk Management: Enhancing Patient Safety*. 2nd edn. London: BMJ Publishing Group.

Wylie, G., Hungin, A. and Neely, J. (2002) Impaired glucose tolerance: Qualitative and quantitative study of general practitioners' knowledge and perceptions. *British Medical Journal Online*, 324(1190); 403–404, http://www.bmj.com/cgi/content/full/324/7347/1190 (accessed 22 June 2008).

The creation of an environment for effective learning 10

Marie C. Hill

Introduction

The aim of this chapter is to explore the factors that influence and motivate adult learning. Adult learning theories will be explored and suggestions made on how a practitioner can facilitate an effective learning environment for adult learners. Reference will be made to Domain 3: The Education Function (RCN, 2008). The emphasis in this chapter will be on how a practitioner needs to be able to create an effective learning environment starting with their own development in order to enable them to become effective and competent to educate, motivate and mentor their clients.

Examples will be provided in this chapter focusing on how some primary care nurses (e.g. practice nurses (PNs) and walk-in-centre (WiC) nurses) may create an effective learning environment for their clients.

Learning Outcomes

- To explore adult learning theories
- To examine factors that can motivate adult learners
- To emphasise the importance of adhering to Domain 3: The Education Function to promote client learning
- To provide examples from primary care nurses on factors that create and promote an effective learning environment to enable them to empower and facilitate their patients to understand their illness.

Background

The Shorter Oxford English Dictionary (1973) defines learning as the action of being able to learn (i.e. to obtain knowledge of a subject or skill by study, experience or teaching). A survey of adults exploring the question 'what is learning' revealed a number of categories emerging, namely that learning was:

- a quantitative increase in knowledge;
- memorising;
- acquisition of facts;
- the abstraction of meaning;
- the interpretation process aimed at understanding reality;
- developing as a person (Brockbank and McGill, 2007).

Indeed, learning is an integral part for the professional development of today's PN and WiC nurse in terms of preparing them for their respective roles within the changing primary care setting. The need to maintain contemporary skills and knowledge for all registered nurses, midwives and community public health nurses (which includes PNs and WiC nurses) is explicit in the Nursing and Midwifery Council's (NMC, 2008) *The Code: Standards of Conduct, Performance and Ethics for Nurses and Midwives*. These state:

> You must have the knowledge and skills for safe and effective practice when working without direct supervision.
> You must recognise and work within the limits of your competence.
> You must keep your knowledge and skills up to date throughout your working life.
> You must take part in appropriate learning and practice activities that maintain and develop your competence and performance. (2008:7)

However, as Rogers (2001) points out, learning does not always occur with teaching, in which she focused on the adult learner, which has implications and challenges for those involved in providing education and training. As PNs and WiC nurses fall into the adult category, it is important that educationalists understand the various factors that can influence and motivate adult learning, including adult learning theory and the educational implications that these theories have on the learner. Likewise, the PNs and WiC nurses must be aware of these theories and drivers when educating, coaching and mentoring their clients, so that their teaching will ultimately promote learning for their clients.

Adult learning theories

There are a number of different theories on learning. This section will examine some of these, namely the constructivist, experiential learning and humanistic theories.

The constructivist theory views learning as continuous building on previous structures as new information and learning is assimilated (Fry et al., 1999). There is an assumption with this theory that learning is taking place because new information is introduced to the student. Matheson (2008:40) explores constructivist theory further by stating that 'meaning and understanding are built up in a process that depends on the specific knowledge foundations and cognitive operations of each individual and the learning activities they engage in'. The influences to constructivist theory can be linked to the philosophical approach to knowledge (epistemology). Two different strands of epistemology can be traced to the Greek philosophers, Plato and Aristotle. Plato is associated with rationalism. This strand of epistemology states that our minds contain innate knowledge or ideal forms of knowledge. On the other hand, Aristotle argued that the senses were the ultimate origin of knowledge.

Immanuel Kant (known as the father of modern constructivism) explored and synthesised these two strands and concluded that there was commonality between these epistemological strands. There have been other significant constructivist thinkers who have contributed to understanding the nature of education such as Dewey, Piaget, Vygotsky, Kelly and Ausubel, to name but a few. The implications for teaching, taking the constructivist approach, are manifold and include that a teacher:

- find out a student's prior knowledge;
- activate their prior knowledge, for example, the teacher could summarise previous learning or she/he could elicit the students' prior learning through questioning and discussion;
- build on existing knowledge;
- challenge existing knowledge and create cognitive dissonance.

In Festinger's *Theory of Cognitive Dissonance*, he argued that knowledge and beliefs about oneself (i.e. cognitions) could be either consonant or dissonant. It was indicated that:

> The presence of dissonance gives rise to pressures to reduce or eliminate the dissonance. The strength of the pressures to reduce the dissonance is a function of the magnitude of the dissonance. (Festinger, 1957:18)

Therefore, a student who has new information that challenges and even refutes their existing knowledge will be forced to make a decision on what information they agree with in order to negate their feelings of cognitive dissonance. Cognitive dissonance can be negated through activities such as:

- using group work (i.e. the integration of group work activities to aid learning and comprehension);
- promoting the concept that the learner is proactive in their approach to learning. The student will take responsibility for their own learning (Matheson, 2008).

The second learning theory – experiential learning or learning by experience – is a model usually attributed to Kolb (Cowan, 1998) and is based on the notion that ideas are not fixed but are formed and reformed through experience. Kolb was influenced by the ideas of Carl Jung and Carl Rogers. Unlike constructivist theory, experiential learning theory provides a mechanism for how learning takes place (Matheson, 2008). This process of learning is perceived to be continuous, is represented by a cyclical process, and implies that we all bring to learning situations our own learning experiences. This is an important area to remember, as adult learners will bring with them a plethora of both work and life experiences, that will have and continue to have an impact on their behaviour.

The Kolb learning cycle has four identified abilities which are listed as follows:

- Concrete experience: This is the origin of the Kolb cyclical process. It implies that learners are fully and freely involved in new experiences and, therefore, actively seek these new experiences, without the implication of coercion.
- Reflective observation: It is necessary for learners to take time to reflect on their experiences.
- Abstract conceptualisation: This implies (having received feedback) that learners will be able to process their new ideas into sound logical theories.
- Active experimentation: The theories are now used to make decisions. In this part of the cycle, the individual tests out the new learning.

The Kolb learning cycle would seem to assume that there is homogeneity amongst learners and even learning. Homogeneity amongst learners has been a criticism of the cycle in assuming that one learning theory embraces all the activities involved in human learning (Brockbank and McGill, 2007). Kolb used his framework to develop his Learning Styles Inventory (LSI) (Matheson, 2008). Perhaps the best known categorisation of learning styles is that of Honey and Mumford (1982) with each of the four styles linked to particular preferences to their learning, which is displayed in Table 10.1.

Activists respond most positively to learning situations offering challenge, to include new experiences and problems in their learning. Reflectors respond most positively to structured learning activities where they are provided with time to observe, reflect and think, and allowed to work in a detailed manner. Theorists respond well to logical, rational structure and clear aims, where they are given time for methodical exploration and opportunities to question. Finally, pragmatists respond most positively to practically based, immediately relevant learning activities, which allow scope for practice and incorporate theory (Fry et al., 1999). Many other learning style models have been proposed. One such model examines how information is received and processed by the senses, making use

Table 10.1　Learning Styles (Fry et al., 1999)

Learning style	Preferences
Activists	Respond to new experiences and problems, excitement and freedom in their learning
Reflectors	Respond to structured learning activities, allowed to work in a detailed manner
Theorists	Respond to a logical and rational structure
Pragmatists	Respond to practically based, immediately relevant learning activities

of sight, hearing and touch (Daines et al., 2006). The three groups respond and process information differently.

Given the diversity of adult learners' backgrounds (e.g. in terms of academic ability and achievement), it is important for those involved in nurse education to be aware that their student group may comprise these different learning styles. Likewise, a practitioner needs to recognise that their clients' academic background will influence their ability to integrate and internalise learning. This has led some writers to argue that it is more important to be aware of the learning style of the learner rather than the subject matter (Grow, 1991). Others such as Fry et al. (1999:31) have commented, 'An awareness of learning styles is important for the teaching; planning a course module, as a variety of strategies to promote learning should be considered'. Of course, it may not be possible for nurse academics to be aware of their students' learning styles prior to the start of their programme of study. Certainly, this will be the case with the majority of educational interactions that occur between a practitioner and a client within a consultation, particularly if this may be the first and only time that a practitioner meets a client, for example, a WiC practitioner teaching a client about the impact a diet high in saturated fats will have on their lipid levels. In this example, the consultation time will be limited to approximately 15 mins and it will not be possible for a practitioner to determine a client's preferred learning style.

However, the validity of Kolb's LSI has been questioned recently, as the inventory was compiled based on student self-reporting through responses to a questionnaire (Brockbank and McGill, 2007). A critical review by Coffield et al. (2004), who examined several different models of learning styles, identified a number of serious design weaknesses including low reliability and poor validity (Daines et al., 2006). However, even Kolb recognised that the use of learning styles did not fit the complete range of explaining how individuals learn or have preferential learning styles. Kolb (1984:63) indicated that 'Psychological categorizations of people such as those depicted by psychological types can too easily become stereotypes that tend to trivialize human complexity and thus end up denying human individuality rather than characterizing it'. Indeed, Daines et al. (2006) have postulated that since one of the main aims of any educator is to enhance individual learning, an effective teacher should be using a variety of teaching methods and styles to promote learning.

Reflecting back to the first part of this section on adult learning, what are the teaching implications for a practitioner taking a constructivist approach to their teaching? A number of practical suggestions have been made such as:

- A variety of teaching experiences, such as problem solving and asking questions.
- Reflection. This is a key element of experiential learning.
- Providing feedback. Reflection will be strengthened by the provision of constructive formative feedback.
- Mental models, practical skills and attitudes. Students should be able to model their experiences onto the experiences of others in the literature.
- Hypothesis testing and planning. It is imperative that students test out their knowledge. This can be achieved by discussion and interaction with facilitators and other students.

▪ Logbooks and portfolios. The completion of either will enhance the learning of students through keeping a written account of their learning experiences using reflection on action. Furthermore, the completed data can provoke and promote discussion with their facilitator and/or clinical assessor.

The possibilities for implementing a constructivist approach to teaching students will vary considerably between a nurse academic (i.e. based in a higher education institution) and a PN or WiC nurse in primary care. It is proposed that the opportunities for a nurse academic to teach students would be greater due to the volume of student numbers they encounter. The opportunities for PNs and WiC nurses on the other hand may be significantly reduced due to the small number of student placements (or in some cases there may be no student placements) to which they are exposed. However, the opportunities for PNs and WiC nurses to have one-to-one and group teaching, coaching and mentoring consultations with their clients must not be underestimated.

Activity

Consider constructivist and experiential learning styles. Which learning style is your preference from the lists provided? If none of these meets your own learning style, list your preferences for learning.

  How best do you learn? Reflect on the most recent example where you had a positive learning experience.

  Why was this effective? What were the factors that made the learning effective for you? List these.

Finally, adult learning theory has been influenced by humanistic psychology (Quinn and Hughes, 2007). The development of humanistic psychology occurred in the USA and was a reaction to the behaviourist school, as having reduced human qualities to 'mere physical entities' (Curzon, 2004:111). Two of the principal exponents of the humanistic approach were Abraham Maslow and Carl Rogers, who developed a humanistic or person-centred approach to the individual. This has been found to be a useful framework for dealing with individual learners (Matheson, 2008). Maslow, in a study on human motivation, developed his *Hierarchy of Needs*. He emphasised the concept of self-actualisation (i.e. the best we can possibly be) but in order to achieve the experience a number of basic needs must initially be fulfilled (Matheson, 2008). Maslow's model is presented as a pyramid and starting at the base of the pyramid are the human being's fundamental physiological needs (i.e. for thirst and hunger) followed by safety needs, belonging needs, need for self-esteem and finally, at the apex of the pyramid, self-actualisation. This step-by-step approach may seem to indicate that once these basic needs are met (e.g. physiological to self-esteem needs), an individual will self-actualise. However, Maslow reported that self-actualisation was rare and that few experienced such an event, although he did rate that individuals may experience occasional moments of peak experiences (Curzon, 2004).

Nevertheless, Curzon (2004) argues that Maslow's *Hierarchy of Needs* has significance for the classroom setting, as students' basic needs must be achieved before effective teaching can occur. However, one could argue that the achievement of the fundamental physiological and safety needs of an individual is beyond the remit of educationalists and that this is the responsibility of governments to ensure that their populations have access to these fundamental needs.

The other exponent of the humanistic school was Rogers (Curzon, 2004). Carl Rogers advocated a student-centred approach to education. This approach placed emphasis on feeling and thinking, recognition of the student's personal values, interpersonal communication and the development of positive self-concepts (Curzon, 2004). This humanistic or person-centred approach has been found to be a useful framework for dealing with individual learners and their educational environment (Matheson, 2008).

According to this approach, the role of the teacher is one of assistance and facilitation, rather than being the imparter of information. Therefore, great emphasis is placed on the role of the facilitator and the qualities that are required such as genuineness, trust, acceptance and having empathy. However, a criticism of this approach has been the lack of empirical evidence to support its claims and assumptions regarding human behaviour (Quinn and Hughes, 2007). There are a number of different implications for teaching using a humanistic approach, namely that the educationalist and/or practitioner needs to:

- Respect their students'/learners'/clients' learning needs.
- Start with the student's/client's own knowledge and understanding of a topic, when initiating learning.
- Pay attention to the learning environment to ensure that this is conducive for learning. One example could be to ensure that the room temperature is neither too hot nor too cold.
- See learning as a relationship between the facilitator and the student/client.
- Provide constructive feedback.
- Ensure that the student/client has sufficient time for self-directed learning. In the clinical setting, a PN may suggest another appointment for a client to ensure at the next consultation that they have understood and applied the initial learning (e.g. inhaler technique).
- Be optimistic that the student/client will achieve their learning outcomes (Matheson, 2008).

Activity

Consider the humanistic theory of learning. Is there a way that this type of learning theory could be employed in your practice? If so, how would go about employing it? Are there any barriers to using this method? If 'yes', what are these and is there a way you could overcome these?

Adult learning

There has been considerable work into the field of andragogy (i.e. the art and science of helping adults learn). Knowles (1984) is associated with the term andragogy, and from his work spanning over 30 years Knowles considered andragogy to have five basic principles:

- As a person matures, they become more self-directed.
- Adults have accumulated experiences, which can be a rich resource for learning.
- Adults become ready to learn when they experience a need to know something.
- Adults tend to be less subject-centred than children; they are increasingly problem-centred.
- For adults, the most potent motivators are internal (Fry et al., 1999).

There has been support for the use of andragogy in nurse education (Richardson, 1988; Burnard, 1991). With the change in nurse education from the traditional/vocational training to a more professional academically structured education, there has been a move to support nurses to become more self-directed learners (Milligan, 1997). Certainly, this would support the first principle of andragogy (i.e. being self-directed learners) as well as one of the principles of humanism that views adult learners as being able to plan and manage their own learning (Quinn and Hughes, 2007).

It is further argued that life experiences appear consistent with much of modern-day nursing (Milligan, 1997). This is relevant to Knowles' (1984) second principle. Knowles' third principle relates to the readiness and willingness of the student to learn. The fourth principle relates to adult learning being more problem-centred and Knowles' final principle is that the most fundamental motivator for learners is internally driven.

The study of motivation has been central to Maslow's identification of his *Hierarchy of Needs*, as mentioned previously. What other factors can motivate adults to learn? Box 10.1 demonstrates these can be multifactorial.

Some of the factors listed in Box 10.1 will resonate with the reader, others will not. The following activity provides an opportunity to reflect on motivation and adult learning. You may wish initially to consider your own motivation for learning and second to consider your client's motivation for learning (reflect on either a recent client or a group of clients) when you were involved in an educational initiative.

Activity

What motivates you to learn? List the factors.

Are there any barriers that you feel affect your ability to learn? If the answer is yes, what can you do to overcome these barriers?

Box 10.1   Factors that motivate Adults to Learn (Daines et al., 2006:16)

- Vocational or professional development:
    i.   to access some further learning opportunity;
    ii. to obtain a qualification;
    iii. to fulfil vocational requirements;
    iv. to broaden vocational horizons and possibilities.
- An aspiration of further learning or creativity:
    i.   to develop a new/existing interest, idea or skill;
    ii. to create something;
    iii. to satisfy curiosity;
    iv. to engage in the process of learning.
- A personal development goal:
    i.   to discover 'if I can/if I still can';
    ii. to enhance confidence in the subject;
    iii. to enhance self-esteem;
    iv. to gain the approval of others.
- A social need:
    i.   to meet like-minded others;
    ii. to make social contact;
    iii. to gain social self-confidence.

Domain 3: The Education Function

The third domain of practice is divided into six distinct sections and focuses on the importance of the health professional's role as educator, motivator and mentor to enable clients to understand their illness and to empower them to take more control over their illness or long-term condition. Domain 3 consists of the sections and competencies shown in Box 10.2.

Box 10.2   Sections and Competencies in Domain 4 (RCN, 2008:15)

Timing

- Assess the ongoing changing needs of patients, their carers and families for education based on the following:
    i.   needs for anticipatory guidance associated with growth and the development stage;
    ii. care management that requires specific information or skills;
    iii. the patient's understanding of their health condition.

- Assess the patient's motivation for learning and maintenance of health-related activities using principles of change and stages of behaviour change.
- Create an environment in which effective learning can take place.

(Continued)

Eliciting

- Elicits information about the patient's interpretation of health conditions as a part of the routine health assessment;
- elicits information about the patient's perceived barriers, supports and modifiers to learning when preparing for patient's education;
- elicits the patient's learning style to facilitate an appropriate teaching approach;
- elicits information about cultural experiences that may affect the patient's learning experience;
- enables patients, by displaying sensitivity to the effort and emotions associated with learning about how to care for one's health condition.

Enabling

- Enables patients in learning-specific information or skills by designing a learning plan that is comprised of sequential, cumulative steps, and that acknowledges relapse and the need for practice, reinforcement, support and re-teaching when necessary;
- enables patients to use community resources when necessary;
- communicates health advice and instruction appropriately using an evidence-based rationale.

Providing

- Negotiates a jointly determined plan of care, based on continual assessment of the patient's readiness and motivation, re-setting goals and optimal outcome.

Negotiating

- Monitors the patient's behaviours and specific outcomes as a guide to evaluating the effectiveness and need to change or maintain educational strategies.

Coaching

- Coaches the patient by reminding, supporting and encouraging, using empathy.

This domain clearly outlines the expected role of the practitioner as an educator and motivator. However, this is assuming that the practitioner has the requisite training and skills to undertake this role. Consider, for example, the changing role of the PN in meeting the increasing clinical outcomes of the new General Medical Services Contract or the WiC nurse adapting to the role of providing more acute care than was originally planned when their WiC opened (e.g. diagnostics and non-medical prescribing). Certainly, the developmental needs of PNs and WiC nurses will differ. Chapter 15 sets out the diverse role and responsibilities of a PN, which are significantly focused on preventive health care whilst WiC nurses are dealing with acute care. Regardless of the type of care in relation to Domain 3, the following activities provide an opportunity to examine how you can address these problem-solving cases. The first activity deals with practice nursing and the second with a WiC scenario.

Activity (relating to Practice Nursing)

You are working in a general practice with approximately 10,000 patients. You have been employed there for the past 4 years. The area that the practice serves is one of the most deprived in the country.

There are three other PNs and two nurse practitioners (NPs) in the practice. Besides you, only one NP works full time. You are finding it increasingly difficult to keep up to date with the volume of work that is generated from the Quality and Outcome Framework and the focus on chronic disease prevention and management. Although you have a specialty in the management of patients with diabetes mellitus (Types I and II), you are beginning to see patients with other chronic conditions that you need to refer to senior colleagues in the practice. You feel that a lack of knowledge on your part is undermining your position in the practice, particularly as you are the senior PN and the expectation from senior colleagues (e.g. NPs and general practitioners (GPs)) is that you should be knowledgeable about other chronic conditions.

You have read the RCN document – *Advanced Nurse Practitioners: An RCN Guide to the Advanced Nurse Practitioner Role, Competencies and Programme Accreditation.* Although you are not employed as a NP, your pay scale is linked to the achievement of these domains of practice, some of which you are not meeting in your current role as a senior PN.

Furthermore, you are considering applying for an increase in your pay scale.

You are aware that you need to come up with a solution and are going to develop a plan of action to address the gap in your knowledge.

The main issues you know you need to action are:

1   identifying specifically the areas in Domain 3 that you must achieve;
2   planning how you are going to achieve these.

How would you address the above issues?

Activity (relating to WiC Nursing)

You are working in an increasingly busy WiC, located in one of the city's train stations. When the WiC was initially opened (i.e. 2 years ago), the aim was to provide treatment for minor ailments (e.g. sprains, bruises and general health advice). Positive local press and national TV coverage in the last year have marketed the WiC location and services. However, the workload has noticeably increased beyond the remit of the original aim. Conditions seen more regularly now are clients with asthma exacerbations, other long-term conditions, chest pain and only last week a cardiac arrest! You have considered (along with your other colleagues) that you are a product of your own success, particularly since the recent media interest on the positive impact the WiC has had on reducing patient numbers to the local accident and emergency department.

The workforce is comprised of 15 registered nurses (with a varied skill mix of acute and PN experience). Although the majority of the care that is provided is acute, you are aware of the need for the majority of the team to be competent in meeting the RCN domains and competencies. You feel that Domain 3: The Education Function is viewed as being the remit of other primary care nurses such as PNs and NPs. However, the

(Continued)

majority of the WiC nurses are employed as advanced NPs with the assumption that they are competent in all seven domains of practice.

You have been asked by the WiC lead to devise a plan on how to ensure that all senior staff function competently in this domain.

How would you address this? Provide a time scale for planning and implementation.

Creating a learning environment

This chapter so far has examined some of the adult learning theories, the implications these theories have for education and some of the motives attributed to adult learning. These can have ramifications for individuals, some more so than others in how they learn. However, caution must be exercised by the reader not to extrapolate these theories and motives to the general population. Populations are not homogenous, in terms of gender, socio-economic status, demography and ethnicity. These influences must not be underestimated on not only how practitioners learn, but also, fundamentally, how they educate, motivate and mentor their clients. Concerning learning and ultimately promoting a learning environment, there is no 'one size fits all' to this approach.

What can a practitioner do to create a learning environment? This could be related to one-to-one teaching or a group learning/health promotion activity. Certainly, Domain 3 provides a template for the practitioner to enable them to assist and promote client learning, whilst acknowledging the significant role of the client's carers and family. Promoting an effective learning environment therefore will need, on some occasions, to be tailored to meet more than just the client. Bearing in mind the intended target audience, the practitioner must consider issues such as the environment in which the teaching will occur. Does this allow good practitioner/client communication and discussion that is uninterrupted? What time is allocated for client teaching? Is this time sufficient?

Consideration may have to be given as to when the teaching takes place, particularly for clients that work. Do the opening hours in the setting in which you work ensure that a client can access a practitioner before or after their working hours so that they can engage in learning? Box 10.3 delineates the factors required to create a learning environment.

Communication skills are paramount to promoting an effective practitioner/client relationship and ultimately an effective learning environment.

Activity

Consider the verbal and non-verbal skills that you utilise in your client consultations. Reflect on your most recent teaching experience with a client or group of clients. What verbal and non-verbal skills were successful in this consultation? How do you know they were successful?

Finally, reflect on your communication skills. Identify your strengths and your areas for improvement. How are you planning to develop and improve on areas for development?

Key to any consultation is knowing, understanding and respecting your audience. Who is going to be the recipient of your teaching and coaching? Consider what theory of education you subscribe to. Now critically appraise the implications for teaching in this identified theory. Other areas to consider are the willingness of the client to learn and the motives listed for adult learning in this chapter. How can you ascertain these?

Box 10.3   Factors to create a Learning Environment

The practitioner must have:

- good communication skills;
- empathy and understanding;
- an environment that is private with uninterrupted consultation time and welcoming;
- an environment that promotes access at times convenient for clients;
- leaflets about various health/illness conditions that are language specific.

The following examples give an insight into the preferred learning styles of a PN and a WiC nurse including their own motives for learning and how they create an effective learning environment for their clients:

A PN perspective:

It is clear to me that there is no particular environment or type of education that suits me best. It depends on what I am learning. However, for me, the attitude of the person teaching me can make or break my interest in a subject, whether or not I need to understand it as part of my sphere of practice.

Health education and promotion are two of the most important aspects of healthcare. It is therefore very important to try and ensure that health professionals create an environment that enables patients to understand their conditions and encourages them to take control of and improve their health.

Practice nurses are in the perfect situation to provide health education and promotion. This might involve providing advice about a number of areas such as weight-loss, smoking cessation or sexual health. It is common to see patients on a regular basis and this enables nurses to build relationships with them, creating a supportive environment which helps patients make positive decisions and changes about their health. A good relationship with your patients is therefore, central to providing an effective educational environment. Health professionals need to make it clear that they are there to help and support their patients. They can do this by displaying posters and leaflets about issues, as well as advertising the clinics that are available. They must also not feel awkward about bringing up what might be seen to be an uncomfortable subject – such as sexual health or obesity. Placing a piece about our obesity clinic in the surgery's newsletter seemed to encourage a number of people to use this service. However, it is also important to remember that patients, like health professionals, are individuals. If we are to make a positive contribution to their health we must tailor our approach according to the person. Some people might find group sessions more helpful as they can seek support from their peers – people who really understand them. Others prefer the one-to-one approach which also can offer more flexibility for them as they are in control of making the appointment at a convenient time. If we are to be truly effective we need to support both approaches. There are both quantitative and qualitative ways in which nurses can assess the effectiveness of their learning environments. If a patient is trying to lose weight you can see if your programme is helping them by measuring his/ her weight. However, you can also talk to your patients about their expectations and wishes, as well as asking for feedback during and after the appointment or programme. If you are approachable and supportive you can hope to receive an honest response, thereby enabling you to find out if the advice you are giving your patients is relevant. If health professionals make it clear that they are there to support change through posters and leaflets and approaching subjects with their patients they can start to support an effective learning environment. I believe that only by tailoring your approach to the patient and assessing what motivates them, can you really hope to achieve their – and therefore your – goals. (Rebecca Cosgrave, PN)

WiC perspective:

I am suited to any type of education that consciously updates professional knowledge and improves professional competency throughout my working life. Classroom based learning gives me the opportunity to impact, generate and assimilate ideas with a wider group.

The nature of my work as a NP currently places more emphasis on work place learning as this offers a hands on approach to the acquisition of skills which is critical in skills and competency development. However, I feel it is important that the theoretical underpinning to work place learning is obtained away from the clinical area.

Overall, I have utilised different types of learning such as: group based learning, learning on the job, experiential learning, competency based learning, distance and e-learning to fulfil my educational and professional development needs.

The main motivating factor that encourages me to learn is the ability to make a significant difference in patient care based on my knowledge and skills acquired through learning. My ability to utilise the knowledge and skills acquired to create a positive patient learning experience spurs me on to develop even more skills and knowledge through learning. Other factors that influence my desire to learn are the potential reward of career advancement with concomitant opportunities to influence the way learning and training is delivered to advance nursing practice.

Creating an effective learning environment for my clients in my current role is vital as most presentations seen in the clinic could be managed at home if patients' had the right information and education about their conditions. Although time constraints are an issue in my role, having the right environment and adequate information means that time spent with a client can make a huge difference to their health. Some of the factors used in creating an effective learning environment for my clients include:

- using a language appropriate to the client's or relative's understanding;
- demonstrating confidence and knowledge on the subject under discussion.

The nature of my work is such that clients' are not monitored for effectiveness of a specific learning outcome but usually a quick recap of issues discussed can determine whether patients' have learnt from the experience. (Daniel Apau, RGN, MSc (Advanced Nursing Practice), Clinical Lead and Nurse Practitioner, Newham Walk-in Centre)

Conclusion

This chapter has explored some of the main adult learning theories and the implications these theories have for education. The adult learner, whether a student within a higher education institution or a client within the primary care setting, will bring with them some form of learning and/or preconceived ideas that may affect their learning potential. This, of course, could lead to a positive or negative learning experience. Therefore, it is essential that the academic or practitioner involved in the education process ascertain the individual's current knowledge level to build on or supplant this knowledge.

The ultimate aim of any teaching experience is for learning to occur. Domain 3: The Education Function provides a framework which practitioners can utilise to ensure that learning meets both an individual and/or groups needs. However, it would be erroneous and naive to suggest that the education process is so straightforward. Populations are not homogeneous and, therefore, educationists must be mindful that individuals and/or groups will have diverse learning needs. Therefore, it is essential to find out the motives these adult learners bring to the learning environment. It is only with an understanding of these motives and an eclectic range of teaching preferences that teaching, mentoring and coaching can lead to effective learning.

References

Brockbank, A. and McGill, I. (2007) *Facilitating Reflective Learning in Higher Education*. 2nd edn. Maidenhead: SRHE/Open University Press.

Burnard, P. (1991) *Learning Human Skills*. 2nd edn. Guildford: Butterworth-Heinemann.

Coffield, F., Moseley, D., Hall, E. and Ecclestone, K. (2004) *Learning Styles and Pedagogy – In Post 16 Learning: A Systematic and Critical Review.* London: Learning and Skills Research Centre, Institute of Education.

Cowan, J. (1998) *On becoming an Innovative University Teacher.* Buckingham: SRHE/Open University Press.

Curzon, L. (2004) *Teaching in Further Education. An Outline of Principles and Practice.* 6th edn. London: Continuum.

Daines, J., Daines, C. and Graham, B. (2006) *Adult Learning Adult Teaching.* 4th edn. Cardiff: Welsh Academic Press.

Festinger, L. (1957) *A Theory of Cognitive Dissonance.* Stanford: Stanford University Press.

Fry, H., Ketteridge, S. and Marshall, S. (1999) *A Handbook for Teaching and Learning in Higher Education.* Glasgow: Kogan Page.

Grow, G. (1991) Teaching learners to be self directed. *Adult Education Quarterly,* 41; 125–149.

Honey, P. and Mumford, A. (1982) *The Manual of Learning Styles.* Maidenhead: Peter Honey.

Knowles, M. (1984) *Andragogy in Action.* San Francisco: Jossey-Bass.

Kolb, D. (1984) *Experiential Learning.* Englewood Cliffs, NJ: Prentice Hall.

Matheson, D. (2008) *An Introduction to the Study of Education.* 3rd edn. London: Routledge.

Milligan, F. (1997) In defence of andragogy. Part 2: An educational process consistent with modern nursing's aims. *Nurse Education Today,* 17(8); 487–493.

NMC (2008) *The Code: Standards of Conduct, Performance and Ethics for Nurses and Midwives.* London: Nursing and Midwifery Council.

Quinn, F. and Hughes, S. (2007) *Quinn's Principles and Practices of Nurse Education.* Cheltenham: Nelson Thornes.

RCN (2008) *Advanced Nurse Practitioners: An RCN Guide to the Advanced Nurse Practitioner Role, Competencies and Programme Accreditation.* London: Royal College of Nursing.

Richardson, M. (1988) Innovating andragogy in a basic nursing course: An evaluation of the self-directed independent study contract with basic nursing students. *Nurse Education Today,* 8; 315–324.

Rogers, J. (2001) *Adult Learners.* 4th edn. Buckingham: Open University Press.

The Shorter Oxford English Dictionary (1973) *On Historical Principles.* 3rd edn. Oxford: Clarendon Press.

Domain 4

The Professional Role

Clinical supervision: reflective practice; learning through experience

11

Christopher Johns

Introduction

The aim of this chapter is to share the experience of an e-mail dialogue based on a walk-in-centre (WiC) nurse's reflection on a patient she worked with within the WiC clinic. In this dialogue, Chris (the clinical supervisor) guides the nurse (named in this chapter as 'Mary') to reflect on an experience. Mary quickly adapts to this learning milieu, gaining insight about herself and her practice, suggesting the value of guided reflection for WiC practitioners. The nature of guided reflection and the insights Mary gained through reflection are considered. Reflection is then framed within a reflective model for clinical practice and the way it can help to address the clinical governance agenda (NHS, 2006).

Learning Outcomes

- To understand the nature of guided reflection
- To discover how to frame reflection within a reflective model for clinical practice
- To consider how reflective dialogue can be used as a mechanism for monitoring and developing clinical effectiveness.

Background

This chapter begins with a reflective dialogue and then depicts the evolving sequence of guided reflection.

Reflective dialogue

Dear Mary,

I would like you to write a description of a recent experience. The experience can be about anything about your practice, perhaps something that's been bothering you or something mundane that happened on your last shift. Just write continuously – do not think too much about what you are writing – just let it flow for as long as it takes – then take a step from the description and move into reflection. Try using the model for structured reflection [MSR] to guide you [I've attached it] (Box 11.1).

    The first MSR cue is 'what is significant about this experience'? This may seem to be obvious at first glance but as you begin to reflect, other issues may emerge as significant. Each cue has depth, so be patient, try not to hurry. I won't say anymore about the cues now, just let you play with them and see where it leads you. The last cue guides you to draw insights from the reflection. Insights are changed perspectives that lead you to see and respond to the world differently. They may be quite subtle and often come to us in a flash . . . or in other words they are intuited rather than reasoned. Try and hold these insights in your mind when you return to practice to see whether they influence the way you approach new clinical situations. When you have done this please e-mail me your reflection and then I will commence a reflective dialogue with you. It will be great to do this with you.

Best wishes, Chris

Mary responds:

Dear Chris,

Toward the end of a shift a few weeks ago, my Nurse in Charge asked me to see a difficult patient who came back for follow-up as she was not happy with the result of the consultation from the previous day. She is a 30 year old female who came to the WiC the previous day with a few days history [hx] of abdominal pain. After a thorough consultation, one of my colleagues advised her that she needed to go to A&E for further investigation. An A&E triage nurse told her that her problem was not of an emergency nature and that she should see her GP. She came back to the WiC the next day and informed us that A&E turned her away and her symptoms persisted. She was very unhappy and wanted to be seen again at our WiC. When I heard the above brief history of this case, my first reaction was: 'Oh, I hate seeing difficult patients'.

    I had no choice but to take the courage to see this patient. I started the consultation as usual, keeping in mind that she was a very unhappy patient who continued to have abdominal pain. The patient answered all my questions with a slight attitude that some might call an aggressive manner. Well, I appreciated that she had reason to be upset, but this kind of attitude never makes the consultation easy. My prime aim was to rule out the most serious medical conditions based on her symptoms and history. I admit, in her case, my other aim was to see her leave the consultation room satisfied and without complaints.

    Well, the patient's main complaint was abdominal pain with no urinary symptoms. The record of yesterday's consultation stated that the urine dipstick was negative and HCG was also negative. On examination, her abdomen was soft and did not suggest any acute surgical problems and all her vital signs were normal. But she insisted that her abdomen was painful; of a constant dull nature. The only red flag was that she had not had a normal bowel movement for three days, which I was so happy to tease out as it enabled me to conclude that her abdominal pain was due to constipation!

I started to end the consultation by summarising my findings and helping the patient to make sense of them. But the patient was still not happy and did not agree with my diagnosis! 'It is normal for me not to have my bowels opened for 3 days', she said. I thought to myself, 'Indeed what a difficult patient. I think she is making this up just to be difficult. But my value system dictates that I must listen to my patient. But what am I going to do now'?

We are a bit stuck; I thought I made a correct diagnosis, but the patient does not agree. I am happy with my diagnosis at this point, but my patient is not. I have to listen to the patient even though I think she may be being difficult. I was compelled to start from square one and disregarded all the test results from yesterday and proceeded to perform a urine dipstick test.

I have never been so excited with my findings: The urine dipstick was positive with prot, leuk, blood and nitr, HCG was negative! I now had a diagnosis based on lab results, history and symptoms. When I asked the patient again if she had any urinary symptoms i.e., frequency, urgency or burring sensation, she remembered that she has been going to the toilet more frequently but with no burning or urgency! I could now put everything together and make the correct diagnosis of simple UTI (but not with typical symptoms). What a relief!

This time, when I explained to the patient about my findings and plan of treatment, the patient agreed, and her attitude changed! I prescribed a treatment of antibiotics and advised that she needed to follow up with her GP if she was no better in 3–5 days. She thanked me for listening to her carefully.

This had been a very long consultation, but it was a good one. The patient was satisfied and so was I. One the one hand, I am humbled by my assessment and consultation skills. But on the other, I am proud that I overcame my own limitations and learned from this experience.

In some ways, I feel good about this experience as I believe I did my best to make a diagnosis and provide the best care I could. I feel that I communicated with my patient in a professional and therapeutic manner. In another way however, I feel sorry for the patient. The patient had been kicked around the system and I wouldn't have wanted to be in her situation, travelling from one WiC to an A&E and then back to the WiC; never mind the waiting and travelling time involved. I also feel guilty for thinking that all the initiatives that the NHS have made in an effort to increase patient access have not been as effective as expected. Perhaps what I am trying to say is that at the end of the day, the patient did receive help: but at what cost, to the patient or the practitioner?
Regards, Mary

Dear Mary,

Many thanks for the text. Before you do anything else – pause a moment and read your story again. List some words that capture what seems significant about this experience . . . for example

> *'my response to difficult patients'*
> *'difficulty of abdominal examinations'*
> *'professional manner'*

I guess most patients are not 'difficult' – so where does the idea of 'difficult' come from? Is there literature that informs you – or is it embodied in you in some way in response to being told that this patient was 'difficult'?

You say 'my value system' – what are your values as a WiC practitioner? Do you have a vision for your practice? If not – write one. What might it say?

From your experience I suspect it might say 'Listen to people carefully with respect and an open mind'?

Where do your values come from? Is there any literature that informs you?

Is there any contradiction between your values and the way this woman was treated and responded to? If so – what is it?

Consider the MSR cue 'Did I act for the best'? What ethical principles are relevant within this situation? Were there any other factors that influenced the way you saw and responded to this woman besides the difficult label? Think deeply about this . . . for example – did you adopt a medical manner because of the nature of the WiC? Maybe you were having a bad day etc.

Use the attached influences grid as check-list [Table 2].

Say more about your feelings. You mentioned exasperation with her and excitement . . . guilt.

What might you do differently given the situation again? – use your imagination/literature/be creative and playful with this question/generate different options and consider their potential consequences.

At the end of your text you ask yourself – 'at what cost'? Can you say more about this?

NOW – consider what insights you have gained – remember insights change us; the way we see and respond to the world. Has this experience changed your practice? For example, have you seen any more 'difficult' people since this event?

Be patient dwelling with these questions.
Many thanks, Chris.

Mary responds:

Dear Chris,

Regarding Ms. A, reflecting on my reaction to difficult patient, as I have become more experienced as a nurse in the WiC setting, I have learnt that there are many factors that contribute to a patient being considered or labelled 'difficult'. My experience with a 'difficult' patient is almost always, at first, uncomfortable and off-putting, but often ended satisfactorily thanks to a thoughtful consultation process. Although I suppose that most patients are not 'difficult', and the difficulty arises from conflicting expectations and misunderstanding of behaviours. Take Ms. A for example, Ms. A expected someone to tell her what was wrong with her, and until she was given an explanation of why her abdomen was hurting she remained unhappy and she kept coming back. It was not until after I put aside the 'difficult' label and started to really listen to her complaints that I was able to think and act more clearly and work-out a preliminary diagnosis. This has been a good consultation and it is one of those that involved a lot of emotional labour. I felt quite drained after this consultation as I felt her pain and her frustration and at the same time a sense of inadequacy with my clinical skills and an urge to upgrade myself so that I will be more at ease in similar situations. This kind of consultation is taxing but rewarding. And it is never easy. I do enjoy the pleasure as well as the pain that are part of this kind of experience and this is one of the attractions of working in a WiC environment.

Reflecting on the challenge of abdominal examination, there are at least 30–40 conditions that can present as abdominal pain, and it takes years of practice for a practitioner to become competent and confident in assessing and diagnosing patients with abdominal pain. Furthermore, nurses are not traditionally trained to assess and diagnose; these are advanced skills that require non-traditional training. The WiC environment, in addition, provides very limited diagnostic facilities. As a result, the WiC practitioner is compelled to refer patients to the next level of care and this sometimes contributes to patient anxiety, frustration and the concomitant dissatisfaction.

I have contradicting views on WiC services. Sometimes I think it does a fine job in increasing patient access, but often I wonder at what cost. To make my point clearer, I shall take a look at the cost to the health care system and society in Ms. A's case taking into account that she had immediate access to the health care system, no less three times within 24 hours! Ms. A needed to budget between one and four hours to be seen by a WiC nurse in her first visit, this includes the process of completing a registration form and then administration staff manually registering the patient onto the computer system and followed by a consultation. Ms. A is then referred to A&E and the above process is repeated and when she is seen within 4 hours only to be told that her problem cannot be dealt with at A&E and she should see her GP. At this point, a very unhappy patient, Ms. A again takes time off work and returns to the WiC and goes through the same process of registration and is again seen by a nurse and luckily this time a preliminary diagnosis could be established. The whole process cost Ms. A at least a total of 8 hours and in relation to the health care system there were 2 WiC administration staff, 2 WiC nurses, 1 A&E administrative staff and 1 A&E triage nurse.

The alternative is that the patient sees her GP/Nurse Practitioner directly in which case it only involves one GP/Nurse Practitioner where there is already a pre-established relationship between the patient and the surgery which can make a difference in patient care and patient satisfaction. A significant reduction of time required for both the patient and the health care system would occur should the patient be able to access her GP. Whenever I come across this kind of situation, I lament the unintended consequence of increasing patient access through the creation of WiCs. However, the NHS could save substantial sums by strengthening the existing General Practice system to effectively increase patient access and patient satisfaction.

My value system as a health care professional stems from my personal beliefs, educational background, personal and professional experiences. The unique setting of WiC requires the WiC practitioner to be a good clinician, a good educator, a good health promoter, a good counsellor, a good psychotherapist, a good social worker etc. These are advanced skills and in order for an individual practitioner to practice at this level they must possess high level critical thinking and problem solving skills. The way I treated Ms. A reflects my beliefs in patient empowerment and part of this is being open and honest with the patient about the scope of WiC practice and sharing with the patient of clinical findings. Most patients are honest when giving the history of their illness; even though I may get frustrated when my diagnostic reasoning is not leading me to a conclusion and I begin thinking that patient has an agenda or is making things up. However, I am bound by my professional code of conduct to not let personal judgment affect my consultation. Instead I forced myself to listen perceptively to Ms. A.

As an autonomous WiC practitioner, I am bound by local (trust or WiC) policy and the general WiC scope of practice, but the skills one can exercise in a WiC setting are boundless. I often compare a WiC nurse to a GP doctor. On some level, the WiC nurse functions as a GP doctor, but sometimes more than a GP doctor. The fact that WiC nurses are nurses rather than doctors is a double-edged sword. On the one hand some patients seem to be more comfortable with the fact that they are consulting a nurse about their health and they are comfortable asking all sorts of questions and nurses are good at making sense of things *for the patients. On the other hand, some patients possess a certain degree of mistrust of nurses' diagnostic abilities since traditionally nurses are not meant to diagnose and treat patients autonomously. Establishing trust and a therapeutic relationship in a short consultation is yet another challenging, but rewarding, aspect of WiC practice.*

In the situation under discussion, I acted for the best in terms of ethics, as I believe the patient has a reason to be dissatisfied and therefore it is ethical to listen to her complaints perceptively and show genuine concern about her problem. I did, at one point, feel at my wit's end, but I would have been comfortable to either make the decision to do an A&E referral or to advise her to self observe and to follow up with her GP after an appropriate length of time. This takes experience and confidence in one's own clinical judgment as the main goal of WiC practice is to treat patients when necessary or, when treatment is not applicable, to provide advice and a safety net.

Given the same situation again, the only thing I would do differently is to conduct a structured consultation and not to allow any previous assessment or lab findings to interfere with this approach, simply due to the fact that previous findings can change! This experience also confirmed that most patients are not difficult and that a successful WiC encounter resides in the art of consultation complimented by solid clinical skills. As a WiC nurse I am acutely aware that there is so much to learn and there is so much I don't know and striving to provide a safety net is not enough in the long run. My mixed feelings are that I am proud when I am able to come to a diagnosis, but I also feel inadequate in many clinical situations. Working in a WiC setting motivates me to be a life long learner.

Note:

1. *This reflection does not distinguish Nurse, Nurse Practitioner and Advanced Nurse Practitioner. They all perform the same tasks, diagnose and treat patients autonomously in the WiC*
2. *A list of glossary of abbreviations used are given below. I realise that perhaps I shouldn't have used any abbreviations.*

Glossary:
  abdo: abdomen
  abx: antibiotics
  A&E: accident and emergency
  HCG: Human chorionic gonadotropin
  hx: history
  leuk: leukocytes
  nitr: nitrite
  prot: protein
  Rx: prescription
  UTI: urinary tract infection
  WiC: walk-in-centre
Regards, Mary

Dear Mary,

Many thanks for this. You may want to follow up the literature on unpopular patients and emotional labour. How would you summarise any learning/insight gained from this reflection? Or put another way – how might this reflection begin to change your practice? Have you had any similar experiences – where you might have applied any learning, however subtle?
Best wishes, Chris

Mary responds:

Dear Chris,

The main lesson to be learned when dealing with the so-called difficult patient is that in most cases these difficult patients simply feel that the health care professional dealing with their concern is not taking sufficient time to understand the problem. In most circumstances, difficult patients are difficult for a very good reason. Getting to the root of this reason can lead to the practitioner learning something new.

The second lesson is that the results of tests that have been given during previous consultations should not always be taken at face value. This can be due not only to the possibility of mistakes having been made in the previous tests, but also the fact that test results can quite naturally change over time. This aspect of medical testing does not form part of the standard nursing curriculum, and therefore is something that nurses working in a diagnostic role, such as in a WiC, must learn in the course of everyday practice or through CPD.

I am constantly reminded, therefore, of the limitations of my training with respect to diagnosis of patients presenting for treatment. However, I feel that my basic approach to the problem is sound, and simply requires a little more patience when dealing with a so-called difficult patient. After all, I have been practicing nursing for quite a long time, and consider that I have the experience necessary to deal with most situations. Even though I have not had any similar experiences since, the lessons learned can be applied to many different cases. When practicing nursing in the context of a WiC, one is constantly reminded that each patient is unique. Keeping to the sound fundamentals of practice, and always giving each patient the care and attention that they deserve will always serve to provide the highest probability for success in each case. I look forward to hearing from you, when I return to London on September 1 from voluntary work in remote South Africa.
Regards, Mary

Deeper reflection

Mary draws her insights. Her values have been confronted and clarified. She is more aware of ethics. Her frustration has been worked through positively. She has reflected on abdominal examination – acknowledging the risk of jumping to an early diagnosis without careful differentiation. She has voiced her concerns about WiC practice and use of time. She has reflected on her relationship with the patient, recognising that sometimes, under pressure, she can miss seeing the person with a focus on the presenting symptom. Mary can conclude that she has learnt through the reflective experience. Is the fact that she has become mindful or aware of herself in relation to her practice. Reflection is a wake-up call to pay attention, especially when we are experienced and think we have the knowledge. Our knowing is always tentative simply because every situation is a unique human – human encounter. We are sure that other WiC practitioners reading this text can relate to many of these issues.

Reflection

Reflection on experience creates the opportunity for practitioners to access and learn through their everyday lived experiences of practice. The intention of reflection on experience is to help the practitioner appreciate the *creative tension* between an understanding of the situation and what can be termed as desirable practice (Senge, 1990). An understanding of the situation always involves a critique of self in context of the situation. The text reveals the way a guide (Chris) might help the practitioner (Mary) tease out contradiction between her vision of desirable WiC practice and the way she actually practices – this is the learning opportunity through reflection, the reason why Chris challenges Mary to identify her values as a WiC practitioner and to make a clear statement about her vision of WiC practice. This is more vital given the risk of slipping into a medical model frame of mind. A vision gives purpose and direction to clinical practice (Johns, 2004).

Activity

Pause for a moment and consider what your own vision might say?

Through understanding *creative tension*, Mary can explore other, more effective ways of responding that are planted like seeds in her mind to germinate in future situations. In doing so, it enables the subtleties and nuances of everyday practice to emerge, especially those of areas of practice that Schön (1983, 1987) alludes to as the 'swampy lowlands'. The swampy lowlands is a metaphor for those complex and indeterminate areas of practice that characterise much of nursing practice grounded in human–human situations of suffering. Such situations have no easy answers to the dilemmas they pose.

In the process of reflection, Chris first invited Mary to write a description. Then he asked her to stand back from the description to reflect on it using the Model for Structured Reflection (Box 11.1), moving from significance towards gaining insights using the reflective cues to guide her. It is like going from the surface of the experience into its depths where meaning and insights are revealed.

Chris guides Mary to go over old ground, going deeper, spinning out something new with each turn. He draws her attention to any relevant literature, for example, on: difficult patients (James, 1989), emotional labour (Ramos, 1992) and therapeutic relationships (Johnson and Webb, 1995; Bolton, 2000). Taking therapeutic relationships as an example, Ramos notes two impasses to therapeutic relationships within the nurse. The first is an emotional impasse, where the nurse struggles with her own emotional response to the patient. The second is control, where the nurse struggles to let go of her need to control the therapeutic environment. Both impasses are very evident within Mary's reflection. Ms. A's frustration is viewed as a threat by Mary, confirming the label applied to her by another nurse. In response, Mary feels anxious and projects this anxiety into Ms. A reinforcing the difficult label. It is only when Mary realises through the diagnostic testing that Ms. A's complaint is valid can she let go of her anxiety and accept Ms. A for who she is. This is important learning, for otherwise patients like Ms. A will continue to be seen as difficult, whereas the truth is it is the practitioner who is difficult – who projects this into the patient to deal with her anxiety. Such understanding seems so obvious when looking objectively. In practice, it is profoundly difficult as practitioners get wrapped up in emotional labour.

Box 11.1   The Model for Structured Reflection (Edition 15ᵃ) (Johns, 2006)

Reflective cue

- Bring the mind home.
- Focus on a description of an experience that seems significant in some way.
- Note any wider organisational, professional or social factors that impact on your experience.
- What particular issues seem significant to pay attention to?
- How do I interpret the way people were feeling and why they felt that way?
- How was I feeling and what made me feel that way?
- What was I trying to achieve and did I respond effectively?
- What were the consequences of my actions on the patient, others and myself?
- What factors influence the way I was/am feeling, thinking and responding to this situation?
- What knowledge did or might have informed me?
- To what extent did I act for the best and in tune with my values?
- How does this situation connect with previous experiences?
- How might I reframe the situation and respond more effectively given this situation again?
- What would be the consequences of alternative actions for the patient, others and myself?
- What factors might constrain me responding in new ways?
- How do I *now* feel about this experience?
- Am I more able to support myself and others better as a consequence?
- What insights do I gain through reflection?
- Am I more able to realise desirable practice?

Activity

Reflect on a time when you were wrapped up in emotional labour. How did you deal with this?

As such, Ramos's paper will help Mary frame her insights. This is where guidance is helpful – to create a learning milieu of high challenge and support (Johns, 2004).

One area of practice Chris could explore further with Mary is to challenge the way she views and knows a patient, given her tendency to view the person primarily in terms of presenting symptoms and that she values seeing the whole person.

Burford reflective and holistic model

One approach that may be useful to WiC practitioners is the Burford NDU Model: caring in practice. The model was constructed at Burford Community

The Learning Organization	A system for ensuring effective communication	
A system for operationalising the philosophy within each unfolding moment	Collaborative and valid vision for clinical practice	A system for ensuring staff are developed to use the model in effective ways
	A system to ensure the model realises effective practice.	Transformational leadership

Figure 11.1 Structural view of the Burford NDU Model: caring in practice (Johns, 2009)

hospital in 1990 as a way to structure clinical practice through holistic and reflective values. At its core is a valid and collaborative vision or practice (Figure 11.1). By valid, I suggest the vision pay attention to certain issues (Johns, 2009). By collaborative, I suggest Mary should work with her colleagues to construct a valid WiC vision.

The model then proposes four reflective systems to facilitate the vision being realised as a lived reality set against an organisational culture that values the learning organisation and transformational leadership (Johns, 2009).

A reflective system to operationalise the vision within each unfolding clinical moment

What sort of reflective cues might Mary ask to tune herself into her client and her desired holistic vision for practice? To achieve this, the Burford Model identifies one core question – what information do I require to nurse this person? It also includes nine reflective cues.

- Who is this person?
- What meaning does this illness/health event have for the person?
- How is this person feeling?
- How has this event affected their usual life patterns and roles?
- How do I feel about this person?
- How can I help this person?
- What is important for this person to make their health care experience comfortable?
- What support does this person have in life?
- How does this person view the future for themselves and others?

The practitioner internalises these cues as a natural way to view the person. The cues do not require concrete answers. They encourage reflection as something lived within practice itself.

Consider how these cues might influence Mary's approach to Ms. A. Would they benefit your own practice? Remember they are *only cues* to nudge you to pay attention to the whole person.

Note the cue – *how do I feel about this person?* As Mary's reflection informs us, how we feel about the person can dramatically influence the way we see and respond to them. The cue – *what is important for this person to make their health care experience comfortable?* – is significant when we consider how uncomfortable Ms. A seemed to be. Issues about support in life and viewing the future may at first glance seem outside the scope of WiC practice but may be vital.

A reflective system to ensure staff are developed to use the model in effective ways

At Burford, guided reflection was developed as the way to develop staff to reflect on and develop effective performance, as illuminated by the dialogue between Chris and Mary. Guided reflection has become formalised within organisations through clinical supervision defined as:

> a formal process of professional support and learning which enables individual practitioners to develop knowledge and competence, assume responsibility for their own practice and enhance consumer protection and safety of care in complex situations. It is central to the process of learning and to the expansion of the scope of practice and should be seen as a means of encouraging self-assessment and analytical and reflective skills. (Vision for the future – National Health Service Management Executive, 1993:3)

This definition is probably self-explanatory. However, the significance of the practitioner is emphasised assuming responsibility for her own practice and self-assessment. Anything less is not taking professional responsibility. Mary mentions courage to face herself and her practice – as uncomfortable as it might sometimes be to face up to the reality that we are not as effective as we might like to be. In this respect, her reflection is like a confession as if she trusts Chris. Of course, trust is vital to the guided reflection and clinical supervision relationship. If Mary did not trust Chris (and her trust is blind), then she might not reveal herself so easily, or be very guarded in what she does reveal in case of repercussion.

A reflective system to ensure the model realises effective practice

Whatever model we use, we need quality feedback loops to ensure effective practice is realised. This is reflected in the clinical governance agenda which has been described as a framework through which health service organisations are accountable for continuously improving the *quality* of their services and safeguarding high standards of care by creating an environment in which clinical excellence will flourish (NHSME, 1993).

Through guided reflection, Mary accepts this responsibility on an individual level. Systems such as clinical audit would enable her to work in a similar way with her colleagues on a formal basis.

Clinical audit is a clinically led initiative which seeks to improve the quality and outcome of patient care through structured peer review whereby clinicians examine their practices and results against agreed standards and modify their practice where indicated (National Health Service Executive, 1996).

Clinical audit is concerned with two questions.

- What is best practice?
- Do we realise best practice?

Typically, a clinical audit group would meet as a multi-professional group once a month to address these questions through the presentation of a reflective case study. As such, Mary might present Ms. A, raising significant issues and insights as gleaned through the reflective process.

These systems only really work when the organisation, as a whole, is committed to being a learning organisation – defined as 'one where people continually expand their capacities to create the results they truly desire, where new and expansive patterns of thinking are nurtured, where collective aspiration is set free, and where people are continually learning to learn together' (Senge, 1990:3).

Of course, all organisations should learn on both an individual and a collective level. So Chris might challenge Mary to what extent the organisation is a learning organisation and what she can do to create and sustain such a learning culture. This prompts her to focus not just on her relationships with clients, but also on her relationship with the organisation. As such, the effective practitioner is political and works to create the best environment whereby she can be most available to her clients.

Conclusion

In this chapter, dialogue has been used within e-mail-guided reflection to illustrate the potential of guided reflection to enable WiC practitioners to be concerned with monitoring and developing clinical effectiveness. This has been framed within the Burford Model – a reflective and holistic way to structure clinical practice that enables the development of the learning organisation of which guided reflection on both individual and organisational levels is integral to learning.

References

Bolton, S. (2000) Who cares? Offering emotion work as a 'gift' in the nursing labour process. *Journal of Advanced Nursing*, 32; 580–586.

James, N. (1989) Emotional labour: Skill and work in the social regulation of feelings. *Sociological Review*, 37(1); 15–42.

Johns, C. (2004) *Becoming a Reflective Practitioner*. 2nd edn. Oxford: Blackwell Publishing.

Johns, C. (2006) *Engaging Reflection in Practice: A Narrative Approach*. Oxford: Blackwell Publishing.

Johns, C. (2009) *Becoming a Reflective Practitioner*. 3rd edn. Oxford: Wiley/Blackwell.

Johnson, M. and Webb, C. (1995) Rediscovering unpopular patients: The concept of social judgment. *Journal of Advanced Nursing*, 21; 466–475.

National Health Service Executive (1996) *Clinical Audit in the NHS. Using Clinical Audit in the NHS: A Position Statement*. Leeds: NHS Executive.

National Health Service Management Executive (NHSME) (1993) *A Vision for the Future*. London: Department of Health.

NHS (2006) *Clinical Governance*. http://www.icservices.nhs.uk/clinicalgovernance/pages/default.asp (accessed 3 February 2009).

Ramos, M. (1992) The nurse – patient relationship: Themes and variations. *Journal of Advanced Nursing*, 17; 496–506.

Schön, D. (1983) *The Reflective Practitioner: How Professionals think in Action*. New York: Basic Books.

Schön, D. (1987) *Educating the Reflective Practitioner*. New York: Jossey Bass.

Senge, P. (1990) *The Fifth Discipline. The Art and Practice of the Learning Organisation*. London: Century Business.

Use of theory and 12
research to inform
practice

Jane Bickerton

Introduction

The aim of this chapter is to explore the effective use of evidence-based practice (EBP) and identify the kinds of activities and approaches that could encourage the active use of this process by nurse clinicians in clinical practice, such as practice nurses (PNs) and walk-in-centre (WiC) nurses. The new autonomous practitioner expanded roles sitting between nursing and medicine are being shaped by the dominant managerial, professional and medical discourses (Aranda and Jones, 2008). These approaches may undermine the ontological and epistemological nursing approaches to caring and are likely to be task driven and emphasise a standardised approach to health care (Malone, 2003). The application of theory and EBP to direct care can challenge this practice. Acquiring evidence allows the WiC nurse and PN to develop and implement the advanced nursing professional role as well as provide examples of evidence of the professional domains of practice that meet the Knowledge and Skills Framework (KSF) (DoH, 2004). The information and knowledge dimensions of evidence in particular require the practitioner to have the knowledge and skills to acquire, organise, provide and use knowledge and information. The practitioners provide examples of application in practice to meet the domains of practice and one such example might be qualitative and quantitative research (NMC, 2006; RCN, 2008).

Learning Outcomes

- To understand the professional role of first-contact nurse in a WiC and the PN as it relates to EBP
- To assess how qualitative and quantitative theory and research are used to support EBP

- ▪ To consider the role of research and audit on the care of patients accessing first-contact and long-term condition health care
- ▪ To identify evidence-based research and theory and its use in the WiC and general practice setting
- ▪ To consider the role of EBP in a patient-centred and patient-led health service.

Background

'Health care that is evidence-based and conducted in a caring context leads to better clinical decisions and patient outcomes'. (Fineout-Overholt et al., 2005:335)

EBP is concerned with changing clinical practice to improve patient care. It is a flexible, dynamic and non-linear approach to health care practice (Levin and Feldman, 2006). EBP evolved out of evidence-based medicine (EBM) introduced by Dr Archie Cochrane in 1972 and was further developed through the Cochrane Collaboration in 1993 (Cody and Kenney, 2006). In order to provide best EBP, it requires the following elements:

- ▪ conscientious use of current relevant, well-designed, patient – centred clinical research;
- ▪ clinical skills including past experience;
- ▪ patient preferences, concerns and expectations (Sackett, 2000; Craig and Smith, 2007).

Although Florence Nightingale based her nursing practice on evidence obtained in the Crimean War, nursing has tended to be involved with routine and tasks, and to be procedure driven based on opinions, tradition or habit rather than research and critical appraisal (Profetto-McGrath, 2005). More recently, the UK government has supported the Centre for Evidenced-based Nursing that has been identifying ways to improve nurses' utilisation of research information (Kronenfeld et al., 2007). Developing nurse research leaders is part of government strategy (DoH, 2000, 2002, 2007) and a robust evidence base is emphasised for practice (DoH, 1999). But even with continued efforts to encourage a research-based culture (Kitson et al., 1996 cited in McCormack et al., 2002; Rycroft-Malone et al., 2002), nurses have very little knowledge of how to base their practice on current evidence (Pravikoff et al., 2005). Therefore, it is essential for nurses to learn the steps on how to search for evidence effectively – as opposed to accepting the presented evidence without question (Burke et al., 2005) and learn how to integrate EBP into their caring practice (Fineout-Overholt et al., 2005). Refer to Figure 12.1.

Activity

Identify how you can use EBP to change your clinical practice and improve patient care.

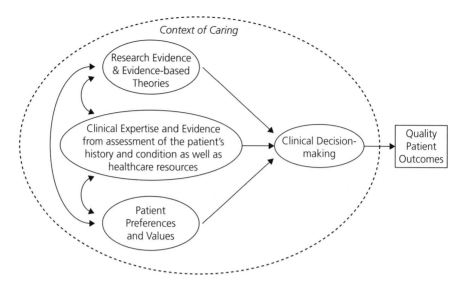

Figure 12.1 Evidence-based practice achieves the best outcomes when accomplished in a context of caring. Reprinted from Fineout-Overholt et al. (2005:10), with permission from Elsevier

Table 12.1 The RCN advanced nurse practitioner domain of competencies

Domain 4: professional role	NHS KSF dimension
Develops and implements the role	
1. Acquires and uses evidence and research to implement the role of the advanced nurse practitioner	IK3 L4
11. Uses information systems to support decision-making and to improve care	C5 and IK3 L4

(NMC, 2006).

Domain of practice

A competent practitioner practises autonomously, safely and effectively. These competencies are achieved through supervised practice-based learning and learning in an academic setting. Signoff mentors or practice teachers decide whether proficiency has been achieved in domains which require knowledge and skills of EBP. The Royal College of Nursing (RCN) advanced nurse practitioner (ANP) professional domain competencies that this chapter focuses on in particular (RCN, 2008) are shown in Table 12.1 but it is important to recognise that EBP is essential to all nursing practice.

The KSF provides dimensions and levels of evidence that workers are required to meet over time in order to meet their work bands and move up the banding scale. EBP provides the guide for continual learning and requires the use of an incremental model of a set of procedures where the corpus of nursing knowledge is continually revised (Trinder and Reynolds, 2000). In this chapter, the EBP process is used to satisfy the four levels of information and knowledge three at level four (refer to Table 12.1) and asks the reader to provide evidence for the five indicators (DoH, 2004).

Table 12.2 An Example of the Use of the PICO model

Patient population	Intervention of interest	Comparison of intervention or ground	Outcome
AND			
Acute stroke	Blood pressure reduction	No treatment	Secondary prevention
OR?			
Cerebrovascular accident	Anti-hypertensive agents	Placebo	Secondary prophylaxis
Cerebrovascular event	Hypertension – drug therapy diuretics, atenolol, etc.		Reduce mortality
Ischaemic stroke	Lowering blood pressure		Risk reduction

Adapted from NHS Thames Valley Health Libraries Network (2006).

The EBP process begins with a consideration of a clinical problem, as the model outlined identifies, and then evolves through five sequential steps (Trinder and Reynolds, 2000; Fineout-Overholt et al., 2005). These are:

1. Identify the problem presented by the patient and gap in knowledge.
2. Formulate structured, answerable question in PICO format:
   i. patient population;
   ii. intervention of interest;
   iii. comparison of intervention or ground;
   iv. outcome.
3. Search for information (evidence) to answer question and critical appraisal of the evidence.
4. Integrate evidence, clinical expertise and patient factors/preferences to implement a decision.
5. Evaluate outcome and process.

A study carried out with registered nurses in the USA (Pravikoff et al., 2005) found that nearly half were not familiar with EBP and that most nurses did not search information resources and only 27% had been taught about electronic databases. However, health consumers may have searched the Web for treatment information before attending a consultation (Mazurek-Melnyk and Fineout-Overholt, 2006). It is essential for nurses to be able to begin to discriminate between high- and poor-quality research but at present nurses' critical skills and expert nursing research are still limited (DoH, 1998; Pearson, 2003). Without critical skills, it is possible to complete a literature search using the PICO model (refer to Table 12.2) but not to make use of the knowledge.

Activity

Identify how the KSF is being met within your practice in order to meet your work band and move up the banding scale.

The five sequential steps for EBP are outlined in more detail below.

Health problem and gap in knowledge identified

A patient presents with a health concern in the urgent care setting. A few examples of health problems presented in the first-contact setting are presented in Table 12.2. EBP considers health issues presented by the health consumer population and flags up a lack of knowledge for the practitioner about particular health issues and health complaints. The practitioner has the difficult task of coming up with a research question that addresses the problem and that can be used to aid the search for information and evidence in health databases.

Formulate structured, answerable question in PICO format

There are different ways of formulating an answerable research question and, for the purposes of this chapter, a PICO format (NHS Thames Valley Health Libraries Network, 2006; Kronenfeld et al., 2007; O'Connor et al., 2008) is recommended and illustrated in Table 12.2.

This PICO format divides the research question into different areas of interest (search areas or concepts) and each concept can then be refined (e.g. listing all synonyms and alternative spellings); the terms are then structured in a search strategy to be used in literature databases (combined with Boolean operators). Librarians, usually in universities or hospitals, supporting a particular practice area can provide support to help learn how to develop a search strategy and the application of the PICO model throughout databases.

Search for information (evidence) to answer question and critical appraisal of the evidence

Search for information (evidence) to answer question

With the outcome from the PICO format, the practitioner is ready to search and organise the evidence into an organisational hierarchy of best evidence (Fineout-Overholt et al., 2005) that includes 'best evidence' for qualitative evidence (see Table 12.3).

Nursing research is often addressed using qualitative research, whereas medical research usually uses a quantitative methodology. The hierarchy of best evidence outlined above identifies systematic reviews of RCTs as the strongest level of evidence using quantitative rather than qualitative methodologies, but where the clinical question involves meaning and qualitative evidence a single descriptive or qualitative study represents the highest level of evidence (Fineout-Overholt et al., 2005).

Table 12.3 Ranking of Evidence

Ranking for quantitative research	Type of evidence	Ranking for qualitative research
1	Systematic review or meta-analysis of all relevant randomised controlled trials (RCTs)	5
2	Evidence-based clinical practice guideline based on systematic reviews of RCTs	6
3	Evidence obtained from at least one well-designed RCT	7
4	Evidence obtained from well-designed controlled trials without randomisation and from well-designed case–control and cohort studies	2
5	Evidence from systematic reviews of descriptive and qualitative studies	4
6	Evidence from a single descriptive or qualitative study	1
7	Evidence from opinion of authorities and/or reports of expert committees	3

Source: Adapted from Fineout-Overholt et al. (2005).

Qualitative research (Horsburgh, 2003; Burns and Grove, 2007) interprets a holistic world view with no single reality. The research data are interpreted through time and context and methodological approaches include phenomenology, grounded theory, ethnomethodology, ethnographic and historical. Qualitative research lends itself to the more individual and patient – centred aspects of health care.

Quantitative research (Burns and Grove, 2007) – on the other hand – is more measurable. It is a formal, objective, rigorous, controlled systematic process that can be descriptive, correlational, quasi-experimental or experimental.

For nurses working as a nurse practitioner, for example, extending their role requires a different focus of clinical skills with evidence-guiding practice (Cody and Kenney 2006). In everyday clinical practice, problems occur where there are gaps in nursing evidence that may be completed through the use of medical evidence. These types of problems and gaps in knowledge over time are resolved as nurses become researchers that are more expert.

Critical appraisal of the evidence

In order to clarify best practice, having searched databases, it is now essential to appraise the research to decide whether the studies or systematic reviews are valid, the findings significant and the results reliable and applicable for use in clinical practice with a particular patient population. The Critical Appraisal Skills Programme (CASP) approach provides tools and resources to critically appraise research (Public Health Resource Unit, 2006). Critical appraisal (Burns and Grove, 2007) includes analysing strengths, weaknesses, meanings and the significance of a study; Quantitative research includes understanding, comparison, analysis and evaluation whereas for qualitative research the parameters include descriptive vividness, methodological congruence, analytical and interpretative preciseness, philosophical or theoretical connectedness and heuristic relevance.

Qualitative data are holistic and dynamic, requiring an interpretative process to understand the context of the meaning, and the results are more difficult to justify than those of quantitative research. Schickler identifies a particular ability of nurses to listen and be with patients as they empathetically and caringly make sense of a patient's life, highlighting the importance of qualitative dimensions in nursing care; she summarises: 'The only way to find what a person thinks, believes and feels about health and illness is to ask them, to have conversation as one might in everyday life' (Schickler, 2004:184). Advanced nursing practice asks nurses to objectively assess the conversation in order to diagnose and treat. Nurse practitioners then use subjective and objective findings and critical thinking (CT) to synthesise nursing and medical evidence to provide best practice.

There are many contemporary examples of strategies and approaches that improve CT in order to better appraise the use of evidence. CT can be developed through participation in writing peer journal articles and reflective journals, role modelling and questioning, case presentations, journal clubs, clinical rounds and simulations, computer instructions and algorithms, as well as concept maps (Profetto-McGrath, 2005).

Integrate evidence, clinical expertise and patient factors/preferences to implement a decision

Evidence for the professional domains of practice requires that a primary care nurse working as an ANP meets specific indicators (DoH, 2004) such as gathers and evaluates information on the organisation's use of, and need for, knowledge and information resources and identifies any current or potential future issues and opportunities including the extent to which they support legislation, policies and procedures.

Table 12.4 develops examples following the *context of caring* in Figure 12.1 and includes research levels of evidence outlined in Table 12.2 with examples of databases searched such as CINAHL, Cochrane Register of Controlled Trials (CRCT), Cochrane Database of Systematic Reviews (CDSR), PsycINFO, National Library for Health (NLH), PubMed (Medline) and the Database of Abstracts of Reviews of Effects (DARE). The patient preferences and values as well as clinical decision-making are left blank for clinical reflection by the reader.

Integrating evidence to implement a decision

The WiC nurse and PN may not always have sufficient nursing research to make changes in practice (Closs, 2003). Research utilisation (RU) was developed prior to EBN to improve the use of research findings in practice (Rogers, 1995 cited in Burns and Grove, 2007). RU was often used for the development and implementation of protocols. More recently RU has been broadened in many cases to include the EBP process (Stetler and Caramanica, 2001; DiCenso et al., 2005; Fineout-Overholt et al., 2005).

Table 12.4 Examples of Context of Caring

Patient history and condition	Clinical expertise	Research evidence and evidence-based theories (accessed July 2008): quantitative research ranking (QnRR), qualitative research ranking (QLRR)	Patient preferences and values	Clinical decision-making
78-year-old woman with a simple urinary tract infection and no adverse reactions to medicines	3–6 or 7–14 days treatment as effective. Single-dose treatment not so effective but better accepted. Single studies on specific antibiotics needed	National Library for Health Cochrane Review: QnRR 1, QLRR 5 (Lutters and Vogt-Ferrier, 2002)		
6 years with acute otitis media × 2 days with symptoms improving	Antimicrobials provide small benefit and may cause diarrhoea, stomach pain and rash. Advise paracetamol or ibuprofen	CKS guidelines (2008): QnRR 2, QLRR 6		
25 years with Bell's palsy	Prednisolone within 24 h significantly improves recovery and acyclovir has no effect	NEJM Cochrane: QnRR 3, QLRR 7 database, DARE (Salinas et al., 2004)		
22-year-old unemployed man living in temporary accommodation diagnosed with tuberculosis	Risk assessment tool–prospective cohort tool. Social outreach model of care with emphasis on prevention and support reduces length of treatment	PubMed: QnRR 4, QLRR 2 (Craig et al., 2007)		
Using PDAs in clinical practice	Increases pharmacological and clinical contextual knowledge in nursing students	Cochrane: QnRR 5, QLRR 4 (Farrell and Rose, 2008)		
20-year-old patient with social problems	Social prescribing pathways could provide better care than from a general practitioner	PubMed (Medline) Cochrane: QnRR 6, QLRR 1 (Popay et al., 2007)		
Why do patient's attend Accident and Emergency and adjacent WiC services?	Majority saw health complaint as emergency and had no other ready access to health care	City University Report: QnRR 7, QLRR 3 (Procter et al., 2008)		

A protocol provides a detailed plan including health history, assessment of physical findings, performing diagnostic tests and plan of care to follow, and is used with patient group directions (PGDs). A protocol is more specific than a guideline, is not disease focused like a clinical guideline and is tailored to a particular population and practice situation. Clinical guidelines are systematically developed and are designed to help the practitioner and patient make appropriate decisions about health care and relate to global management of a disease as do the National Institute for Health and Clinical Evidence (NICE) diabetes mellitus and hypertension guidelines (Levin and Feldman, 2006; Rich and Newland, 2006). Protocols and guidelines are essential tools for the novice practitioner as well as important references for the expert practitioner to provide best practice and care in-line with other practitioners.

Nursing practice includes the evaluation of evidence that is provided by the government and the National Health Service (NHS). There is considerable guidance for clinical practice that includes essence of care benchmarking (DoH, 2001, 2003, 2007), NICE, Scottish Intercollegiate Guidelines Network (SIGN), Clinical Resource Efficiency Support Team (CREST) and Clinical Knowledge Summaries (CKS, formerly Prodigy), and, in addition, each trust may provide its own local guidelines. National Service Frameworks (NSFs) of evidence-based standards exist for major care areas and disease groups (DoH, 2000). Evidence generated from meta-analyses of several RCTs is used to develop evidence-based guidelines and EBM is often used in place of EBN. This is due in part to the fact that it is relatively new for nurses to work in the first-contact environment as autonomous practitioners. Many WiCs do use decision software developed specifically to aid nurses with the decision process that is supportive when nurses are novices in the first-contact environment (Hanlon et al., 2005).

Integrating clinical expertise to implement a decision

The first WiCs opened in 2000 and independent nurse prescribers gained access to all of the British National Formulary (BNF) in 2006 (BNF, 2008). These two events have changed the face of primary care nursing with their extension to include some of the GP's competencies. The practical issues related to evidence-based patient care fall between medicine and nursing and so current best practice may be medical and nursing evidence. With better access to Internet and the development of systematic databases which concentrate on unique problems for community nursing (Closs, 2003), problems of accessing information and research are being resolved. There is now the potential to improve patient outcomes, reduce errors and for nurses to increase satisfaction with their profession (Kronenfeld et al., 2007).

Prescribing rights for qualified independent nurse prescribers allows nurse prescribers to be more patient centred in their care. Other qualified nurses may prescribe using PGDs that offer a more prescriptive approach to health care and treatments but there is less flexibility of care using PGDs and patients' preferences are only possible within the bounds of the PGD. Independent non-medical pre-scribers require knowledge and skills competencies (NMC, 2006) to:

- assess a patient's clinical condition;
- undertake a thorough history including medical history, medication history and allergies, including over-the-counter medications and complementary therapies;
- decide on management and whether or not to prescribe medication;
- identify appropriate products if medication is required;
- advise patient on effects and risks;
- monitor response to medication and lifestyle choice.

Clinical expertise is learned through different forms of knowing that include empir-ical, ethical, aesthetic and personal knowing (Carper, 1978). Personal knowing for Carper is equivalent to the individual reflecting on how they influenced a situation (Johns, 1995). Other modes of knowing include a personal process of accumulating embodied practice expertise recognising expert intuitive practice as an important presence in decision-making (Benner, 1984). One writer has recently noted that evi-dence on the use of intuition in practice is not well researched but has generally been accepted as pivotal in decision-making (Livesley and Howarth, 2007). The process is a rapid unconscious process that is not explainable through cause-and-effect rela-tionships and builds on repeated practice situations (Greenhalgh, 2002). Other ways of gaining clinical expertise are through accumulating expertise, reflective practice, using expert opinion such as guidelines and reaching consensus, which could mean working with a role model and mentor (Livesley and Howarth, 2007). As clinical knowledge and expertise increase, clinicians rely less rigidly on applying rules to practice and are more able to make discretionary judgements (Greenhalgh, 2002). Clinical judgement is important in generating and using evidence and influences the evaluation of patient preferences as well as how patients enter into decision-making processes (Benner and Leonard, 2005).

Integrating patient factors/preferences to implement a decision

Involving patients in the EBP process requires the clinician to listen carefully to patient preferences and values, whilst being aware that patients may wish to be active and/or passive in the consultation and that this may affect the potential shared participation in decision-making (Mazurek-Melnyk and Fineout-Overholt, 2006; Stevenson, 2007). However, what receives less attention in publications and workshops than the other areas of EBP is the integration of the evidence along with the clinician's expertise and patient's preferences, and the values of patients in making the decision about the care that is delivered (Mazurek-Melnyk and Fineout-Overholt, 2006). The government and the NHS are slowly chang-ing this outcome. With a patient-led NHS, clinicians are expected to find ways to encourage patients to participate, if not lead, in making decisions on their health care (DoH, 2005). This means that it is essential to consider ways to improve the patient's health knowledge base, which is critical to shared decision-making.

The organisation of the meaning of involvement and participation into taxonomy highlights the complexity of the patient's choice in deciding their choice of interaction (Thompson, 2007). The patient's consensus and preference for treatment is an essential component of EBP. Stevenson et al. (2000) outline four conditions that lead to a successful consultation outcome. These conditions are that practitioners and patients:

- are involved in sharing information;
- build consensus on preferred treatment;
- agree on a treatment implement for the health complaint.

Within the professional domain of practice, one specific IK indicator (DoH, 2004) requires that a practitioner determines and implements appropriate ways of addressing issues and capitalising on opportunities. One example of evidence of this aspect of the dimension can be met through patient satisfaction surveys. The majority of patients attending urgent care services in the East End of London saw their health complaint as an emergency even though over 40% had discussed the health complaint with their GP and nearly as many were seeking reassurance and advice (Procter et al., 2008). The lay definition of emergency is different from the practitioner's definition. Lay experiences of health and illness offer other dimensions that are important to consider in EBP (Schickler, 2004). This highlights the importance of holistic health care in first-contact care that includes public health and health promotion.

Activity

Using the EBP diagram outline shown in Figure 12.2, identify the evidence-based process for a specific patient used to provide best practice care.

   Displaying examples of EBP in a central location in the workplace encourages other colleagues to consider examples of EBP. Can you identify areas within your workplace to display examples of EBP? Where are these located and who will see these?

Other ways to fulfil this specific indicator might be to scan the Web and identify useful information sites and integrate Web-based information into practice as a way for patients to understand choice and preferences. Sites that provide patient information sheets could also be considered.

Evaluate outcome and process

The audit process is used to evaluate outcomes and processes. NHS WiCs have been routinely audited by the government until recently to identify outcomes (Salisbury et al., 2002). The NHS pays GP practices through the Quality and Outcome Framework (QoF) points that are allocated by auditing practices.

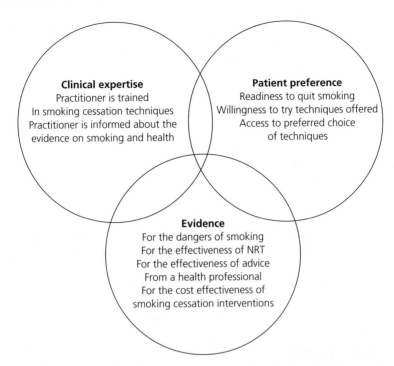

Figure 12.2   An example of the interrelationship of the elements of evidence-based nursing: smoking cessation (Bryan, R. and Griffiths, J.M. (2003) Practice development in community nursing: Principles and processes. *Hodder Education*). Reprinted with permission of Hodder & Stoughton Ltd.

Individual practitioners as well as services may provide their own audit to consider the success of evidence implementation. An audit cycle is presented as follows (Griffiths, 2003):

- evaluate clinical practice against standards;
- identify areas requiring change;
- set standards for good practice (EBP);
- evaluate practice and identify variations;
- develop an action plan;
- implement change.

An audit carried out in a systematic way aims to improve patient care by investigating the decision trail of performances and outcomes. Trusts usually have audit departments helpful in supporting auditing requests from services and practitioners. The audit process monitors standards and quality in practice and is repeated as often as is required to prove standards are met and improved. A recent audit of independent nurse prescribers found nurses are prescribing frequently using a range of advanced practice skills, although a comprehensive history was not always in evidence (Latter et al., 2007a). Nurses wrote accurate prescriptions, but did not necessarily include all the prescribing details in documentation showing that accurate documentation by managers and educationalists needs to be stressed (Latter et al., 2007a,b). Audits on prescribing practice also provide evidence that the non-medical prescriber scans the environment to identify new and emerging knowledge/information resources and technologies and evaluates their relevance and potential benefits to the organisation, in order to meet a specific dimension indicator (DoH, 2004).

Health care research in practice

Primary care nursing needs strategies to improve the current knowledge base and application of EBP. Fineout et al. (2005) identify key elements using the Advancing Research and Clinical Practice through Close Collaboration (ARCC) mentorship model that identifies elements for implementation of a successful learning culture. These include:

- EBP mentors;
- partnerships between academic and clinical settings;
- EBP champions;
- clearly written research;
- time, resources and administrative support.

EBP mentors support clinicians in involving patients in clinical decision-making that includes strategies valuing patient involvement, creating time in history taking to consider patient preferences and providing patients with health information leaflets, websites and videos about their health complaint. Involving universities in practice-based research provides academic support for practitioners and supports ring-fenced time so that clinicians develop EBP and clearly written research projects. EBP champions recognise how important clinicians' opinions are for patients and understand the importance of supporting EBP with time, resources and commitment. All these elements are identified as essential to cultivate shared consultation participation (Mazurek-Melnyk and Fineout-Overholt, 2006). Activities such as journal clubs, EBP clinical rounds, clinical mentorship, clinical supervision and reflective practice generate and sustain enthusiasm which in turn leads to EBP as a priority in patient care.

Evidence of professional development includes the specific indicator (DoH, 2004) that a nurse acquires additional knowledge/information resources and technologies and integrates them appropriately into the overall system/service.

An example of this is now given by the Acting Lead nurse of a WiC whose staff modified its practice by implementing a slot system.

At an East London Walk-in-Centre (WiC), there has been a growing awareness of the need for change over the past year. The WiC has been through a lot of upheaval not dissimilar to other departments within the NHS. These problems had been compounded by a vacancy in the lead nurse role over the past one-year.

It is a busy service and has been well used since its opening 5 years ago. Waiting times were consistently an issue. Our nurse consultant carried out a patient satisfaction survey earlier this year and waiting times was a big issue. People generally had to wait up to 2 hours to be seen by a clinician. The number of clinicians varied at any one time from 2 early in the morning to up to 5 at times during the day. There was a feeling generally that the queue was not being well managed and it was up to each individual clinician how fast or how slow they were. One of our regular GPs had long been suggesting change in the form of an appointment system; however, the Department of Health does not allow Walk-in Centres to have appointments.

The idea was discussed at various times with differing degrees of seriousness but never could be realised. In July 2006 he again suggested it and with the support of the acting lead nurse, admin manager for the Walk in Centre, Admin Manager for Urgent Care and the nurse consultant, it was decided to give it a go using a 'slot' time system. Patients walk in and are seen in time order. Rather than being given an appointment they are given an allocated slot, and an approximate idea of when they will be seen. So instead of having to wait in the WiC for up to 2 hours they could go shopping etc. Each nurse has 3 slots per hour and each GP has 4 slots per hour. There is a nurse in charge who together with the reception staff overseas the system and can help out any members who are falling behind. The workload is more evenly distributed and waiting times have reduced considerably. The success of this new 'slot' system reflects all the hard work of the staff at the WiC. A patient satisfaction survey April 2006 showed that patients would like a reduced waiting time. The 'slot' system started at the beginning of August this year has reduced the waiting times by approximately 30 minutes. (Mary Daly, Acting Lead nurse at the WiC in 2006)

There are different approaches to implementing EBP in practice. Bryar and Bannigan (2003) include a top-down model where leaders incorporate findings into policy such as guidelines and change is incorporated into every aspect of the organisation. Problems with this approach to change are that it fails to acknowledge the real world of clinical practice and can lead to unwillingness to engage in EBP. A bottom-up model implemented through interaction expects to minimise conflict and encourages practitioners to develop EBP strategies in practice settings. Finally, a strategic model implements change through an evolutionary approach and acknowledges aspects of both models outlined above and their limitations. Its focus is the creation of an organisational culture that facilitates learning.

Using the strategic model, one WiC successfully completed several research projects including publication of the results. A group expressing interest in research met with support from management and agreed to meet regularly. They were supported by academic researchers, including a research link worker, a professor of research, a statistician and a university librarian. Potential research projects were discussed and three research projects were submitted for grant funding, with two proposals approved. The group continued to meet irregularly, with various staff members attending if they expressed interest. With changing staff, the research projects took 5 years to complete. The processes included ethical approval, collecting and analysing the data and writing up the results for publication. There were many topics covered and included 'Patient identification and electronic healthcare systems' (Lichtner et al., 2008), 'Streaming A and E patients to walk-in centre services' (Bickerton et al., 2005), 'Evidence-based primary health care and local research: a necessary but problematic partnership' (Abbott et al., 2008) and a report on 'Streaming patients from A and E to primary care' (Procter et al., 2008). Other publications are expected to follow.

The final KSF specific dimension indicator asks that a worker promotes and facilitates the use of knowledge and information throughout the organisation.

One example could be the completion of a research project. In order to complete research in practice, support is required as well as the researcher's commitment. Where management is not supportive, research completion is unlikely to be successful, and research funding is unlikely to be approved. However, understanding the research process is an essential part of EBP. All research requires the practitioner to develop a research question and to complete a literature search. Experts are essential to support research, so, for example, it is appropriate to consult a dietician for research that is considering dietary habits, and a statistician for statistical analysis. The local Higher Education Institution and colleagues with a special interest in research can often assist in finding specialist support for research.

If funding is applied, then the funding sponsor will provide an application form that is filled out by the applicant and submitted. A successful applicant will normally receive part of the funding at the commencement of the study, part of the funding when the data have been collected and the final sum of money on completion of the study, having met the agreed goals throughout the research process. The research protocol will require ethical approval and the local ethics office will provide support and advice with completing the application. Make an appointment and visit the local office and ask for feedback prior to submitting the ethical approval application. The principal investigator will normally be invited to the ethics committee to answer specific questions. Note that it is rare that a protocol is approved without changes. After the data are collected and analysed, the results should be presented to all parties involved including colleagues so that they gain from experience. Write up and publish the results. Publishing in a peer-reviewed journal is an essential part of the process. However, practice research may be difficult to support in practice even though it begins to answer questions related to the local community (Abbott et al., 2008), namely that practice research is often small-scale, undertaken to answer local questions. From a formal research perspective, such studies, simply because of their scale, do not provide evidence that is robust by the standards of the Cochrane Library. In any case, the difficulties of carrying out research whilst also managing large clinical case-loads are considerable, whilst many NHS staff find it difficult to access expert research advice. Thus, many factors may limit the scientific value of local studies.

Specific factors include the use of a qualitative rather than a quantitative methodology, and another is the application of interdisciplinary methodologies (Smith et al., 2004). Nurses may use observing, listening and feeling as sources of evidence, and even though these factors are difficult to measure in terms of quantitative outcomes, they provide an opportunity to consider 'individual wisdom/experience, and the often hidden and unarticulated humanistic and relational elements of nursing practice' (Smith et al., 2004). EBP requires then a broader base bringing together both the 'external scientific and the internal, intuitive' (Rycroft-Malone et al., 2004:81).

Research may not be published for other reasons. For example, an interesting project carried out in the East End of London by a diabetic lead nurse, a GP and a nurse consultant (NC) focused on the young male population and set out to identify how young men's health needs could be better addressed in general practice (Bickerton et al., 2007). The study identified that young men were slightly anxious about health checks as well as illness, needing medicine, increasingly anxious about behaviour judged by a health care professional and very anxious about not being able to access their GP when they were ill. The practitioners were keen to write up and publish the results; however, clinical and management pressures took precedence for all practitioners, and the NC, whose remit had included leading on research projects in urgent care, was no longer needed in the trust. Where projects are supported by an academic institution or a research body as well as the NHS, they are more likely to receive the support essential to move a project from the beginning right through to writing up and publication.

Conclusion

EBP is identified in the professional domain of advanced nursing practice and levels and examples of practice are developed through the KSF with EBP underpinning all patient-led health care. Transforming EBP in primary care nurses (such as PNs and WiC nurses) through a leadership role requires sustained encouragement and empowerment (Mazurek-Melnyk and Fineout-Overholt, 2006).

Examples of how leaders of EBP can empower and support interdisciplinary staff are through supporting reflection on practice, time to explore EBP ideas, encouraging interdisciplinary staff to engage and participate in EBP projects, supporting clinical evidence in practice, welcoming ideas for practice improvement, encouraging the use of current literature to support change, citing evidence for practice or policy changes, involving interdisciplinary staff in reviews of policies, protocols and guidelines with reflection on the best available evidence, identifying priority clinical practice issues requiring EBP solutions, empowering interdisciplinary staff to gain confidence in their practice by being able to articulate best practice and, finally and most importantly, supporting an environment where patients are empowered to lead or at the very least have the knowledge and support to effectively share their own preferences in their own health care planning.

The main points of the chapter are as follows:

- The knowledge and skills to apply EBP are an essential part of primary care nursing and include both qualitative and quantitative approaches to evidence.

- EBN includes following evidence such as clinical guidelines and protocols based on someone else's research (e.g. NICE guidelines), critically appraising existing evidence for a particular clinical population, searching for evidence carried out on a practice population group as well as completing and publishing research projects that include questions relevant to the local population.
- Shared and patient – centred approaches to consultation practice are essential components of EBP.

Through the effective use of EBP, PNs and WiC nurses can engage in expanded roles that sit between nursing and medicine.

References

Abbott, S., Bickerton, J., Daly, M. and Procter, S. (2008) Evidence-based primary health care and local research: A necessary but problematic partnership. *Primary Care Research and Development*, 9(1); 191–198.

Aranda, K. and Jones, A. (2008) Exploring new advanced practice roles in community nursing: A critique. *Nursing Inquiry*, 15(1); 3–10.

Benner, P. (1984) *From Novice to Expert: Excellence and Power in Clinical Nursing Practice*. Menlo Park, CA: Addison-Wesley.

Benner, P. and Leonard, V. (2005) Patient concerns and choices and clinical judgment in EBP. In Melnyk, B. and Fineout-Overholt, E. (Eds.) *Evidence-based Practice in Nursing and Healthcare: A Guide to Best Practices*. Philadelphia: Lippincott.

Bickerton, J., Dewan, V., Allan, T. and Procter, S. (2005) Streaming A&E patients to walk-in centre services. *Emergency Nurse*, 13(3); 20–23.

Bickerton, J., Driver, R. and Reid, J. (2007) *Healthy Choices for Male College Students in Tower Hamlets Primary Care Trust*. London: City University London (unpublished research).

BNF (2008) *British National Formulary*. http://www.bnf.org/bnf/bnf/current/104945.htm (accessed 8 July 2008).

Bryar, R. and Bannigan, K. (2003) The process of change: Issues for practice development. In Bryar, R. and Griffiths, J. (Eds.) *Practice Development in Community Nursing: Principles and Processes*. London: Hodder and Stoughton.

Burke, L., Schlenk, E., Sereika, S., Cohen, S., Happ, M. and Dorman, J. (2005) Developing research competence to support evidence-based practice. *Journal of Professional Nursing*, 21(6); 358–363.

Burns, N. and Grove, S. (2007) *Understanding Nursing Research: Building an Evidence-based Practice*. Edinburgh: Saunders Elsevier.

Carper, B. (1978) Fundamental ways of knowing in nursing. *Advances in Nursing Science*, 1(1); 13–23.

CKS (2008) *Otitis Media – Acute – Management – Scenario: First-line Treatment*. http://cks.library.nhs.uk/otitis_media_acute/management/quick_answers/scenario_first_line_treatment (accessed 11 July 2008).

Closs, J. (2003) Evidence and community based nursing practice. In Bryar, R. and Griffiths, J. (Eds.) *Practice Development in Community Nursing: Principles and Processes*. London: Hodder and Stoughton.

Cody, W. and Kenney, J. (2006) *Philosophical and Theoretical Perspectives for Advanced Nursing Practice*. London: Jones and Bartlett Publishers.

Craig, G., Booth, H., Story, A., Hayward, A., Hall, J., Goodburn, A. and Zumla, A. (2007) The impact of social factors on tuberculosis management. *Journal of Advanced Nursing*, 58(5); 418–424 (doi: 10.1111/j.1365-2648.2007.04257.x).

Craig, J.V. and Smyth R.L. (Eds.) (2007) *The evidence-based practice manual for nurses*, Edinburgh, Churchill Livingstone.

Dicenso, A., Guyatt, G. and Ciliska, D. (2005) *Evidence-based Nursing: A Guide to Clinical Practice*. St. Louis, MO: Mosby.

DoH (1998) *Information for Health: An Information Strategy for the Modern NHS 1998005*. Department of Health. http://www.dh.gov.uk/en/Publicationsand statistics/Publications/PublicationsPolicyAndGuidance/DH_4007832 (accessed 12 July 2008).

DoH (1999) *Clinical Governance in the New NHS*. Department of Health. http://www.dh.gov.uk/en/Publicationsandstatistics/Lettersandcirculars/ Healthservicecirculars/DH_4004883 (accessed 12 July 2008).

DoH (2000) *Towards a Strategy for Nursing Research and Development Proposals for Action*. Department of Health. http://www.dh.gov.uk/en/Publicationsandst atistics/Lettersandcirculars/Professionalletters/Chiefnursingofficerletters/DH_ 4004641 (accessed 12 July 2008).

DoH (2001) *Essence of Care*. Department of Health. http://www.dh.gov.uk/en/ Publicationsandstatistics/Publications/PublicationsPolicyAndGuidance/DH_ 4005475 (accessed 12 July 2008).

DoH (2002) *Nurses' Use of Research Information in Clinical Decision Making: A Descriptive and Analytical Study*. Department of Health. http://www.dh.gov. uk/en/Researchanddevelopment/A-Z/Promotingimplementationresearchfindings /DH_4001837 (accessed 12 July 2008).

DoH (2003) *Essence of Care*. Department of Health. http://www.cgsupport.nhs.uk/ PDFs/articles/Essence_of_Care_2003.pdf, http://www.dh.gov.uk/en/Publications andstatistics/Bulletins/Alliedhealthprofessionalsbulletin/Browsable/DH_ 5816256 (accessed 12 July 2008).

DoH (2004) *The NHS Knowledge and Skills Framework (NHS KSF) and the Development Review Process*. Department of Health. http://www.dh.gov.uk/ en/Publicationsandstatistics/Publications/PublicationPolicyAndGuidance/DH_ 4090843 (accessed 12 July 2008).

DoH (2005) *Creating a Patient-led NHS: Delivering the NHS Improvement Plan*. Department of Health. http://www.dh.gov.uk/en/Publicationsandstatistics/ Publications/PublicationsPolicyAndGuidance/DH_4116716 (accessed 12 July 2008).

DoH (2007) *Towards a Framework for Post Registration Nursing Careers Consultation Document*. Department of Health. http://www.dh.gov.uk/en/ Consultations/Closedconsultations/DH_079911 (accessed 12 July 2008).

Farrell, M. and Rose, L. (2008) Use of mobile handheld computers in clinical nursing education. *The Journal of Nursing Education*, 47(1); 9–13.

Fineout-Overholt, E., Melnyk, B.M. and Schultz, A. (2005) Transforming health care from the inside out: Advancing evidence-based practice in the 21st century. *Journal of Professional Nursing*, 21(1); 335–344.

Fritsche, L., Greenhalgh, T., Falck-Ytter, Y., Neumayer, H.-H. and Kunz, R. (2002) Do short courses in evidence-based medicine improve knowledge and skills? Validation of Berlin questionnaire and before and after study of courses in evidence based medicine. *BMJ*, 325(7376); 1338–1341.

Greenhalgh, T. (2002) Intuition and evidence – Uneasy bedfellows? *British Journal of General Practice*, 52(478); 395–400.

Griffiths, J. (2003) Practice development: Defining the terms. In Bryar, R. and Griffiths, J.M. (Eds.) *Practice Development in Community Nursing: Principles and Processes*. London: Hodder and Stoughton.

Hanlon, G., Strangleman, T., Goode, J., Luff, D., O'Cathain, A. and Greatbatch, D. (2005) Knowledge, technology and nursing: The case of NHS Direct. *Human Relations*, 58(2); 147–171.

Horsburgh, D. (2003) Evaluation of qualitative research. *Journal of Clinical Nursing*, 12(2); 307–312.

Johns, C. (1995) Framing learning through reflection within Carper's fundamental ways of knowing in nursing. *Journal of Advanced Nursing*, 22(22); 226–234.

Kronenfeld, M., Stephenson, P.L., Nail-Chiwetalu, B., Tweed, E.M., Sauers, E.L., McLeod, T.C., Guo, R., Trahan, H., Alpi, K.M., Hill, B., Sherwill-Navarro, P., Allen, M.P., Stephenson, P.L., Hartman, L.M., Burnham, J., Fell, D., Kronenfeld, M., Pavlick, R., MacNaughton, E.W., Nail-Chiwetalu, B., Ratner, N.B. **(2007)** Review for librarians of evidence-based practice in nursing and the allied health professions in the United States. *J Med Libr Assoc*. 95(4); 394–407.

Latter, S., Maben, J., Myall, M., Young, A. and Baileff, A. (2007a) Evaluating prescribing competencies and standards used in nurse independent prescribers' prescribing consultations: An observation study of practice in England. *Journal of Research in Nursing*, 12(1); 7–26.

Latter, S., Maben, J., Myall, M., Young, A., Latter, S. and Maben, J. (2007b) Perceptions and practice of concordance in nurses' prescribing consultations: Findings from a national questionnaire survey and case studies of practice in England. *International Journal of Nursing Studies*, 44(1); 9–18.

Levin, R. and Feldman, H. (Eds.) (2006) *Teaching Evidence-based Practice in Nursing: A Guide for Academic and Clinical Settings*. New York: Springer.

Lichtner, V., Wilson, S. and Galliers, J. (2008) The challenging nature of patient identifiers: An ethnographic study of patient identification at a London walk-in centre. *Health Informatics Journal*, 14(2); 141–150.

Livesley, J. and Howarth, M. (2007) Integrating research evidence into clinical decisions. In Craig, J. and Smyth, R. (Eds.) *The Evidence-based Practice Manual for Nurses*. 2nd edn. Edinburgh: Churchill Livingstone.

Lutters, M. and Vogt-Ferrier, N. (2002) *Antibiotic Duration for treating Uncomplicated, Symptomatic Lower Urinary Tract Infections in Elderly Women.*

The Cochrane Collaboration. http://pharmacoclin.hug-ge.ch/_library/pdf/cochrane 2008.pdf (accessed 21 April 2009).

Malone, R. (2003) Distal nursing. *Social Science and Medicine*, 56(11); 2317–2326.

Mazurek-Melnyk, B. and Fineout-Overholt, E. (2006) Consumer preferences and values as an integral key to evidence-based practice. *Nursing Administration Quarterly*, 30(2); 123–127.

Mccormack, B., Kitson, A., Harvey, G., Rycroft-Malone, J., Titchen, A. and Seers, K. (2002) Getting evidence into practice: The meaning of 'context'. *Journal of Advanced Nursing*, 38(1); 94–104.

NHS Thames Valley Health Libraries Network (2006) *The Literature Review Process: Recommendations for Researchers*. http://www.oxfordradcliffe.nhs.uk/ research/researchers/news/documents/LiteratureSearchingGuidelinesChecklist. pdf (accessed 11 July 2008).

NMC (2006) *Framework for the Standard for Post Registration Nursing*. http:// www.nmc-uk.org/aArticle.aspx?ArticleID=2038 (accessed 2 June 2008).

O'Connor, D., Green, S. and Higgins, J. (2008) *Cochrane Handbook for Systematic Reviews of Interventions Version 5.0.0 [updated February 2008]*. The Cochrane Collaboration. www.cochrane-handbook.org (accessed 1 July 2008).

Pearson, A. (2003) Guest editorial: Liberating our conceptualization of 'evidence'. *Journal of Advanced Nursing*, 44(55); 441–442.

Popay, J., Kowarzik, U., Mallinson, S., Mackian, S. and Barker, J. (2007) Social problems, primary care and pathways to help and support: Addressing health inequalities at the individual level. Part II: Lay perspectives. *Journal of Epidemiology and Community Health*, 61; 972–977.

Pravikoff, D., Tanner, A. and Pierce, S. (2005) Readiness of U.S. nurses for evidence-based practice: Many don't understand or value research and have had little or no training to help them find evidence on which to base their practice. *American Journal of Nursing*, 105(9); 40–51.

Procter, S., Bickerton, J., Allan, T., Davies, H. and Abbott, S. (2008) *Streaming to Streaming Emergency Department Patients to Primary Care Services: Developing a Consensus in North East London*. London: City University London Press.

Profetto-Mcgrath, J. (2005) Critical thinking and evidence-based practice. *Journal of Professional Nursing*, 21(6); 364–371.

Public Health Resource Unit (2006) *Critical Appraisal Skills Programme (CASP)*. http://www.phru.nhs.uk/Doc_Links/Qualitative%20Appraisal%20Tool.pdf, http://www.phru.nhs.uk/Pages/PHD/resources.htm (accessed 8 July 2008).

RCN (2008) *RCN Competencies: Advanced Nurse Practitioners: An RCN Guide to the Advanced Nurse Practitioner, Competencies and Programme Accreditation*. London: Royal College of Nursing.

Rich, E. and Newland, J. (2006) Creating clinical protocols with an Apgar of 10. In Levin, R.F. and Feldman, H.R. (Eds.) *Teaching Evidence-based Practice in Nursing: A Guide for Academic and Clinical Settings*. New York: Springer.

Rycroft-Malone, J., Seers, K., Titchen, A., Harvey, G., Kitson, A., McCormack, B. (2004) What counts as evidence is evidence-based practice? *Journal of Advanced Nursing*, 47(1); 81–90.

Rycroft-Malone, J., Kitson, A., Harvey, G., Mccormack, B., Seers, K., Titchen, A. and Estabrooks, C. (2002) *Ingredients for Change: Revisiting a Conceptual Framework*. http://qhc.bmj.com/cgi/content/full/11/2/174 (accessed 1 July 2008).

Sackett, D. (2000) *Evidence-based Medicine: How to Practice and Teach EBM*. Edinburgh: Churchill Livingstone.

Salinas, R., Alvarez, G. and Ferreira, J. (2004). *Corticosteroids for Bell's Palsy (Idiopathic Facial Paralysis)*. http://www.mrw.interscience.wiley.com/cochrane/clsysrev/articles/CD001942/frame.html (accessed 11 July 2008).

Salisbury, C., Chalder, M., Manku-Scott, T., Ruth, N., Deave, T., Noble, S., Pope, C., Moore, L., Coast, J., Anderson, E., Weiss, M., Grant, C. and Sharp, D. (2002) *National Evaluation of NHS Walk in Centres*. London: Department of Health.

Schickler, P. (2004) Lay perspectives and stories – Whose health is it anyway? In Smith, P., James, T., Lorentzon, M. and Pope, R. (Eds.) *Shaping the Facts: Evidence-based Nursing and Health Care*. Edinburgh: Churchill Livingstone.

Smith, P., James, T., Lorentzon, M. and Pope, R. (Eds.) (2004) *Shaping the Facts: Evidence-based Nursing and Health Care*. Edinburgh: Elsevier Science.

Stetler, C. and Caramanica, L. (2001) Evaluation of an evidence-based practice initiative: Outcomes, strengths and limitations of a retrospective, conceptually-based approach. *Worldviews on Evidence-Based Nursing*, 4(1); 187–199.

Stevenson, F. (2007) What is a good consultation and what is a bad one? The patient perspective. In Collins, S., Britten, N., Ruusuvuori, J. and Thompson, A. (Eds.) *Patient Participation in Health Care Consultations: Qualitative Perspectives*. Maidenhead: Open University Press.

Stevenson, F.A., Barry, C.A., Britten, N., Barder, N., Bradley, C.P. (2000) Doctor-patient communication about drugs: the evidence for shared decision making. *Social Science & Medicine*, 50(6); 829–840.

Thompson, A. (2007) The meaning of patient involvement and participation in health care consultations: A taxonomy. In Collins, S., Britten, N., Ruusuvuori, J. and Thompson, A. (Eds.) *Patient Participation in Health Care Consultations: Qualitative Perspectives*. Maidenhead: Open University Press.

Trinder, L. and Reynolds, S. (2000) *Evidence-based Practice: A Critical Appraisal*. Oxford: Blackwell Science.

Domain 5

Managing and Negotiating the Health Care Delivery System

Collaboration and working with the multidisciplinary team and agencies

13

Kathryn Waddington

Introduction

The aim of this chapter is to provide some guiding principles and exposure to theoretical perspectives that will promote flexibility of thought, and will both refresh and challenge professional issues in primary care nursing. In doing so, the chapter addresses three broad areas:

- key concepts that inform collaborative working in health and social care;
- theoretical perspectives with which to understand interprofessional partnerships, conflict and teamwork;
- critical reflective practice at individual, relational and organisational levels of analysis.

The intention is to provide an interdisciplinary range of theoretical and research-based perspectives from sociology, organisational theory, work and organisational psychology and psychodynamic and systems theories. Whilst the focus here is predominantly confined to the UK health and social care practice and primary care nursing, many issues also have relevance and application in other sectors. In order to get the most from this chapter, you should read it, talk about it and reflect on the implications for your own practice, either alone or with colleagues. You can then decide what actions and changes you might make in your own thinking, behaviour and work/organisational setting to promote effective collaborative practice.

Learning Outcomes

- To define collaborative working and understand the differences that exist between other forms of working (i.e. interprofessional, interagency, multi-agency and partnership)
- To appreciate how the use of metaphors can lead to greater understanding of how individuals collaborate
- To identify the importance that clear and concise verbal communication has in creating an environment that promotes collaborative working
- To appraise factors that inhibit collaborative working
- To critically analyse and synthesise the factors necessary to promote an effective collaborative working environment.

Background

Partnerships, multi-agency working and collaborative care have been part of government rhetoric since the 1990s, and have become part of the vocabulary and discourse of professional and interprofessional practice (DoH, 1998, 2000; Butt et al., 2008). Current European Union (EU) and World Health Organisation (WHO) European Region policy mandate the need for collaborative interagency, interprofessional and intersectoral practice (WHO, 2006; Yan et al., 2007). There is also an abundance of support for the inherent value of collaborative, interagency working, as the inclusion of this chapter in *Professional Issues in Primary Care Nursing* testifies. However, public inquiries, for example, into the tragic deaths of Victoria Climbié and 'Baby P', continue to find failures in collaboration between practitioners, and failures in organisations and agencies that do not coordinate their work with each other (Laming, 2003; Department for Children, Schools and Families, 2008).

Collaboration is a multidimensional and complex activity, involving nurses, doctors and other health and social care practitioners working together in the provision of services and care for individual patients, families and communities. One of the consequences of the reconfiguration of health care provision away from acute/hospital settings is that collaboration is also an expanding concept. There is now a need for wider partnerships, for example, with environmental, transport and agriculture directorates whose policies impact on a much broader conceptualisation of health and well-being (Tope and Thomas, 2007; Harvey and McMahon, 2008). The traditional boundaries of health and social care practice are shifting, and the multidisciplinary team may now include architects, engineers, teachers, community leaders and commissioners, as well as artists and poets-in-residence (Barr et al., 2005; Behan, 2006; Foureur et al., 2007). Ultimately, collaborative partnerships look set to change the way that health services are delivered, yet relatively little is known about their impact on patients and health economies. The evidence base for interagency collaboration is both limited and emergent. In other words, it is not necessarily the case that collaboration and partnership working is unsuccessful. Rather we do not know because of the paucity of empirical work in the field, and further research is necessary.

This then is the paradoxical landscape of collaboration facing primary care practitioners, patients and communities. There is no 'one-size-fits-all' solution to the challenges that this landscape of collaboration presents, although flexibility of thought, an open mind and self-awareness are important practitioner attributes.

Key concepts and definitions

In the first instance, it is important to find, and use, shared language and frameworks to describe and understand collaborative practice and patient – centred services (Reder and Duncan, 2003; Gilbert, 2005; Reeves and Sully, 2007). This is necessary to ensure that approaches to the assessment, planning, implementation and evaluation of collaborative care are appropriately aligned. However, this is not always an easy task and the field of collaboration and multidisciplinary teamwork is laden with terminological confusion. On the one hand, some authors note that the terms collaboration, partnership teamwork, interdisciplinary and interprofessional are used interchangeably (Curran, 2004; Butt et al., 2008). This can be confusing. On the other hand, broad conceptual distinctions between interprofessional, interagency, multi-agency and partnership approaches have also been discerned (Rushmer and Pallis, 2002; Anning et al., 2006; Stepney and Callwood, 2006; Curran, 2007), for example:

- *Interprofessional*: It involves professionals from different disciplinary backgrounds (e.g. nursing, social work, medicine and physiotherapy) working together more effectively, often in teams, to improve the quality of care provided to individuals, families and communities.
- *Interagency*: It involves more than one agency (e.g. social services, primary health care services and housing) working together in a planned and formal way, which can be at different levels either strategic or operational, and may be concurrent or sequential.
- *Multi-agency*: It involves more than one agency working with an individual, family or project, but not necessarily jointly.
- *Partnership*: It indicates the collaborative nature of the above processes.

A related concept is that of *collaborative care*, defined as:

'A patient/client-centred process in which two or more professions/disciplines *interact* to share knowledge, expertise and decision-making in the interest of *improved* patient/client care'. (Curran, 2007:vii; emphasis added)

The crucial elements of Curran's definition for patients, practitioners and researchers are: (i) the quality and frequency of interaction, (ii) the impact and outcomes of collaboration and (iii) the way criteria for judging improved care are described and agreed. Sustainability is also an important aspect of collaborative care, and

Table 13.1   Factors influencing Collaboration

	Domain Five: Managing and Negotiating Health Care Delivery Systems
Attitudes	
• Readiness to exchange viewpoints and share information about structures and processes	• 6.5, 6.7, 6.17
• Willingness to share or relinquish responsibility	• 6.6, 6.7, 6.12
• Trust and respect for each professional	• 6.10, 6.12, 6.16
Knowledge	
• Understanding of own and others' roles and responsibilities	• 6.1, 6.2, 6.9
• Understand national and local contexts facilitating or inhibiting collaboration	• 6.4, 6.8, 6.13, 6.14
• Understand a variety of strategies to improve collaboration and underpinning change models	• 6.10, 6.14
Skills	
• Negotiate effectively with other professionals and agencies	• 6.10, 6.12
• Assess own work/practice context to identify and act on areas for collaborative development	• 6.1, 6.2, 6.3, 6.15
• Select and adapt appropriate and responsive strategies for improving collaboration	• 6.8, 6.13, 6.14, 6.17
Organisational factors	
• Co-location of services	• 6.2, 6.3, 6.10, 6.17
• Ability to share patients/clients	• 6.2, 6.11, 6.17
• Regular face-to-face contact	• 6.10, 6.12
• Joint work on local projects or specific topics	• 6.6, 6.7, 6.10, 6.15
• Support from senior management	• 6.6, 6.9

Freeth et al. (2005) usefully outline a number of factors which support such an approach. Table 13.1 summarises the factors influencing collaboration, mapped against the NMC competencies within Domain Five: '*Managing and Negotiating Heath Care Systems*'.

Effective communication is an essential aspect of all of the above factors, although it is often assumed that this is 'given', for example, that co-location of services and regular face-to-face contact will result in the sharing of information. However, inquiries into organisational failures and human tragedy all too often reveal that this is sadly not the case (Laming, 2003).

Communication and partnership working

Reder and Duncan's (2003) review of communication problems between professionals in fatal child abuse cases draws upon the words spoken by the fictional character of 'Alice' in Lewis Carroll's *Alice in Wonderland* at 'A Mad Tea Party':

'Then you should say what you mean', the March Hare went on.

'I do', Alice hastily replied, 'at least – at least I mean what I say – that's the same thing, you know'. 'Not the same thing a bit!' said the Hatter. (Gardner, 1970:95)

The above quote illustrates important issues in interprofessional communication regarding the discrepancy between what we *think* we mean how we communicate this meaning verbally and non-verbally and how our meanings might be perceived and understood *differently* by others. An example from my own experience, described in Box 13.1, illustrates this point.

Box 13.1   Talking about Transitions

I was participating in a meeting to discuss the launch of an interprofessional organisational change project within a Primary Care Trust and Social Services Directorate. I was representing the university who were an academic partner in this project. Around the table were practitioners from health and social care who worked with children and families, and those who worked with adults; there were also senior managers and other university colleagues. The discussion moved to themes for the launch of the change project, and the concept of 'transitions' was agreed. Enthusiastic nods and brief-aside conversations took place around the table. However, it quickly became apparent that we were all thinking about the concept of transitions from very different perspectives. I was considering the impact of change on service delivery and associated organisational transitions. Others were thinking about the impact of role change on practitioners, and individual and team transition processes. Another meaning, reflected in the experience and thinking of practitioners attending the meeting, was that of service users' transitions from children's to adult services. There was a moment of tangible confusion, followed by clarification of our different perspectives, and then the talk moved on.

Activity (Points for Reflection)

- What are the risks associated with misunderstanding what other people mean?
- How can these risks be minimised and managed?
- How do you feel when you are misunderstood?

Context, perceptions and experience all impact on how meanings are construed. For example, my use and understanding of the term 'academic', as used in Box 13.1, reflects particular values associated with rigour, scholarship, critical thought, theoretical perspectives and their pragmatic application to practice. There are, however, other contexts where the term 'academic' may be used differently, for example, to illustrate a foregone conclusion, or as an ironic term of abuse or mockery. It is vital then that shared language and understandings are given the opportunity to develop in practice; however, misunderstandings are all too commonplace.

(Continued)

In a primary care context, interprofessional working between health and social care practitioners is often fraught by misunderstandings of professional roles and functions (Devla et al., 2008; McDonald et al., 2008). There are also fundamentally different perceptions, for example, relating to concepts of time and urgency as Kharicha et al.'s (2005:401) research demonstrated: 'When the doctor says immediate he means now, when a social worker says immediate or urgent he means in three weeks, and I'm not being funny'. Misunderstanding of meaning can result in conflict in professional relationships, leading to gaps between policy, practice and professional discourses. Unless these gaps are exposed and understood, there is a risk that integrated teamwork and provision of collaborative care will remain an 'unachievable rhetoric' (Stark et al., 2002:11).

Interprofessional discourses

The term *discourse* can be used in at least two ways: as a verb meaning to talk about and as a noun that describes particular ways of talking about something expressed through words. Discourse forms reflect different ways of being in the world, combining words, actions, beliefs, values, social and professional identities based in language.

Barr et al. (2005) argue that *all* health and social care professionals should be aware of the key discourses and their role in professional and interprofessional communications. Tension and conflict can arise *between* professions employing different discourses and value bases, for example, relating to managerialism, professionalism and inspection. Competing discourses may simultaneously define patients as: (i) individuals whose concerns set the agenda for consultation, (ii) objects of pursuit in terms of their contribution to targets or (iii) customers whose complaints and waiting times have become a yardstick of satisfaction and quality (Weir and Waddington, 2008). Conflict can also arise *within and across* professions as new discourses, for example, of business efficiency and social enterprise emerge (Parkinson and Howorth, 2007; McDonald et al., 2008). Discursive conflict, if unresolved, can result in professional resentments, blame cultures and toxic 'them and us' scenarios. The toxicity arising from unresolved conflict can inhibit effective collaborative working and interprofessional practice. So what factors promote effective collaboration?

Factors promoting effective collaboration

Research conducted by the National Audit Office (NAO, 2006) suggests that successful collaborative relationships need flexibility of thought, which implies versatility and the capacity to change in response to new conditions. Flexibility of thought also involves the ability *and confidence* to move beyond linear, reductionist models of thinking which have dominated theories and practice discourses of health science and organisational change (Ashworth et al., 2001; Thomas, 2006; Canam, 2008). However, this may not be an easy or straightforward journey for some practice nurses, general practitioners and managers whose education and knowledge base may be firmly rooted in the comfort zones of linear thinking. Ultimately, linear thinking can lead to a blinkered approach which stifles the development of creative collaboration and innovative practices.

For example, linear thinking might mean viewing collaboration as something that occurs at a micro-level between patients, practitioners, professions and agencies, ignoring macro-level organisational issues, for example, relating to power, politics and organisational culture. Yet shifting the focus of attention to inter-organisational working may overlook the importance of interprofessional relationships. Therefore, according to D'Amour et al. (2005), the most *complete* models of collaboration attend to both micro- and macro-levels of analysis, and are grounded in a strong theoretical background of organisational theory and research, and these are considered next.

Organisational theories and collaboration

This section draws from the literature relating to organisation theory in general and psychodynamic and systems theories in particular, and is necessarily selective. The rationale for selecting these particular perspectives is that they build a strong conceptual model to guide critical reflection into individual, relational and organisational aspects of collaboration.

Broadly speaking, organisational theory draws upon the sciences, arts and humanities and brings with it the challenges of thinking in interdisciplinary ways. Rather like nursing theory, it takes inspiration from diverse fields of study that include human understanding, scientific explanation and artful appreciation (Hatch and Cunliffe, 2006). Organisation theory is a practical and social activity which seeks to answer questions such as:

- What exactly do people do when they work together in organisations?
- How are policy objectives set, by whom and with what consequences?
- What is the impact of history on organisational structures, processes and relationships?

These are big questions which address big ideas and issues, and organisation theory is relevant to the macro-health care organisational context of primary care and practice nursing and also to the experience of the micro-practitioner–patient relationship and care environment. It is now widely accepted that metaphor plays an important role in organisational theory and research, as a way of thinking differently in order to see and understand situations in new ways (Morgan, 1997; Cornelissen et al., 2005). Therefore, using metaphor is also a potentially useful method and approach to better understand and enhance collaborative working and interprofessional teamwork.

Using metaphor to understand collaborative working

Metaphor consists of giving a name to an aspect of experience that belongs to, or can be described as, something else. Using metaphor is one way of enabling practitioners to reflect on aspects of individual, team and organisational aspects of their practice (Morgan, 1997; Bolton, 2005; Ghaye, 2005, 2008). This can yield insights into practice, and is a way of encouraging professionals to observe how they might be perceived and experienced by others – including patients and service users – in order to reveal that which may be hidden (Bolton, 2005).

Morgan (1997) provides a number of metaphorical 'images' of organisations, two of which are particularly pertinent to health care organisations and working collaboratively: (i) organisations as political systems that reflect diverse interests, power distribution and conflict and (ii) organisations as psychic prisons that contain conscious and unconscious traps and barriers to change. These two metaphorical images are now explained and explored further from the theoretical standpoint of psychodynamic and systems theories.

Organisations as political systems

This metaphor is based on the assumption that individuals in organisations will fight for their particular interests and positions. Politics in organisations has been defined as 'those activities carried out by people to acquire, enhance, and use power and other resources to obtain preferred outcomes in situations where there are disagreements' (McKenna, 2006:699). The metaphor of organisations as political systems also assumes that conflict is *always* present, the outcome of which will depend on the power relations between individuals and groups. For instance, the outcome of conflict is not always negative, and if managed constructively, can be a source of excellence, quality and creativity (West, 2004). At the same time, however, interpersonal conflict can be harmful and unhealthy for the individuals and teams concerned. This can lead to rivalry and competition, rather than collaboration, between professions, organisations and agencies, which leads to 'turf wars', territorialism, protection of vested interests and gossip (Waddington, 2005; Waddington and Fletcher, 2005).

Thinking about organisations as political systems in an interprofessional context enables practitioners to consider explicitly the relationship and impact of power and conflict. It enables us to examine and evaluate interests, power-bases and relationships, and to critically reflect on how we individually and professionally develop skills of political awareness and leadership (which are addressed more fully in Chapter 12 – Use of theory and research to inform practice). A systems approach also provides a sound theoretical base for the understanding and development of collaborative working:

> Von Bertalanffy (1971) and his successors developed the concept of 'system' as an antidote to the limitations of specialist disciplines in addressing complex problems. It could be applied across all disciplines, from physics and biology, to the social and behavioural sciences, seeing wholes as more than the sum of their parts, interactions between parties as purposeful, boundaries between them as permeable, and cause and effect as interdependent not linear . . . Intervention by one profession at one point in the system affects the whole in ways that can only be anticipated from multiple professional perspectives. (Barr et al., 2005:131)

Therefore a systems approach integrates multiple perspectives, avoiding linear cause–effect relations that can lead to the creation and reinforcement of blame cultures. For example, when examining and reflecting on a particular incident or episode of communication, it may be tempting to resort to explanations such as 'they are a fragmented team', or that 'this general practitioner is always difficult'. However, such explanations are limited, providing solutions that identify and fix the dysfunctional part, but fail to address the wider organisational whole (Obholzer and Roberts, 1994; Huffington et al., 2004).

Organisations as psychic prisons

This metaphor comes from Plato's *Republic* (Morgan, 1997; Bolton, 2005), which pictures prisoners chained in a cave, unable to turn around. All they can see is a wall in front of them, whilst a fire burns behind them, casting light on the wall. There is also a ledge behind the prisoners, along which puppeteers can walk and hold up puppets that cast shadows on the wall in front of the prisoners. The prisoners can only see and hear shadows and echoes cast by objects which they cannot see. The imprisoned cave dwellers equate the images cast as shadows with the reality of the external world.

The relevance of this particular metaphor may not be immediately apparent; however, Morgan (1997:215) extends the imagery of Plato's cave to that of a 'psychic prison'. In this sense, organisational structures and shared meanings can become conscious and unconscious traps and barriers to change, acting as defences that keep external reality denied or at an objectified distance (Menzies, 1970). Individuals, professions and organisations can become 'imprisoned' in favoured ways of thinking and perceiving through education and socialisation processes. They may become trapped by and collude with these perceptions, which results in an understanding of reality which is both limited and potentially flawed. An awareness and appreciation of these often unconscious processes can enable individuals to see beyond the surface, to what lies beneath (Obholzer and Roberts, 1994; Huffington et al., 2004), and freeing them from their metaphorical shackles.

Theoretically, as Morgan (1997) illustrates, the metaphor of organisations as psychic can be understood from a psychodynamic perspective, which places a strong emphasis on unconscious psychological conflicts and processes that operate at individual, group and organisational levels of analysis. For example:

> In organizations that project a team image, various kinds of splitting mechanisms are often in operation, idealizing the qualities of team members whilst projecting fears, anger, envy, and other bad impulses onto persons and objects that are not part of the team. (Morgan, 1997:235)

In an interprofessional context, splitting and projection involves practitioners displacing their anxieties, envy and resentments onto other practitioners and professions. This may be manifest in gossip and anecdotes about the behaviour and practice of others, used as social defence as a means of expressing and managing strong emotions associated with distressing and stressful aspects of practice (Waddington and Fletcher, 2005). The role of emotion is not always fully appreciated in interprofessional practice, and this can compromise team effectiveness. Interprofessional teams require time and space in a safe environment where anxieties and issues can be expressed and explored without retrenchment to defensive positions and group dysfunction. Therefore, we now turn to the factors that impact on the creation of effective interprofessional teams.

Creating effective interprofessional teams

A significant challenge facing health and social care practitioners is how to create, within the existing and future workforce, teams that are capable of effective and sustainable collaboration. Research findings from primary care teams, as well as other organisational contexts and industries (West, 2004; D'Amour et al., 2005; NAO, 2006; West et al., 2006; Delva et al., 2008), indicate the following overarching themes/issues:

- Promoting effective interprofessional collaboration in the delivery of health and social care may contribute to improved teamwork, increased job satisfaction and a reduction in patient morbidity.
- The effect of multidisciplinarity is contingent on the quality of team processes such as reflexivity, commitment to high performance and task orientation.
- Leadership is an important factor in the development of effective collaborative relationships (see also Chapter 14, this volume).
- Investment in the development of strong collaborative relationships leads to enhanced quality of service provision.
- Measuring and reflecting on relationships can help underpin effective collaborative working, for example, with regard to trust and support, goals, learning, roles, communication and managing conflict.
- Constructive team conflict when managed effectively can be a source of creativity, excellence and quality.

▪ Best practice follows clear principles – listening and talking to a wide range of stakeholders and service users, reviewing the messages and meanings communicated, and joint commitment to action.

Future research is likely to be guided by extended community and patient participation models and national frameworks for interprofessional education and practice, which in turn require mechanisms for multiple funding and accountabilities. However, researchers and practitioners alike may face similar difficulties with working collaboratively. As we have seen, these are often the result of deep-rooted professional, interpersonal and organisational defences, rivalries, resentments and resistance to modernising policies and interprofessional practice. We will now return to two issues introduced earlier in the chapter, namely metaphor and *Alice in Wonderland* (Gardner, 1970) in order to explore some of these issues further.

Using metaphor to promote team reflexivity

As we have seen, metaphors can create different ways of shaping our experience in organisations and teams, but paradoxically they may also act as barriers to seeing the whole system. Metaphors can create powerful insights that can also become distortions, and no single metaphor will ever give a perfect all-purpose viewpoint.

Therefore, it is important to use a range of metaphors within a framework of critical reflection and reflexivity. Critical reflection has been defined as:

> A process (and theory) for unearthing individually held social assumptions in order to make changes in the social world . . . reflection is more than simply thinking about experience. (Fook and Gardner, 2007:14)

Reflexivity differs from reflection in the way that it 'embraces subjective understanding of reality in order to think more critically about one's values and the *effect of one's actions on others*' (Gray, 2007:505, emphasis added). Insight and understanding of the effect of one's actions on others are crucial elements of collaborative working, which is reflexivity at the individual/practitioner level of analysis. At a team level, West (2004) argues that in order to function effectively, teams need to regularly and systematically focus on their objectives and ways of working, which he refers to as *task reflexivity*. In addition, in order to promote individual and team well-being, West argues that teams also need to reflect on support structures, conflict resolution and the overall social climate of the team, which is referred to as *social reflexivity*.

One way of promoting task and social reflexivity in teams is to use metaphor, asking if this team were something else, then what would it be? For example, would it be a diverse and vibrant multicultural community? A pack of wolves? A smooth running environmentally friendly vehicle? Box 13.2 contains an extract from *Alice in Wonderland* (Gardner, 1970:93) with some associated questions for reflection. This extract, from 'A Mad Tea Party', has been chosen primarily to provoke thought and reflection about interprofessional defences, teamwork, meetings and team reflexivity. It is also used to raise issues of professional invisibility, silence and the challenges of dealing with absences/non-attendance at multidisciplinary team meetings (Canam, 2008; Delva et al., 2008).

Box 13.2   A Mad Tea Party

'There was a table set out under a tree in front of the house, and the March Hare and the Hatter were having tea at it: A Dormouse was sitting between them, fast asleep, and the other two were using it as a cushion, resting their elbows on it, and talking over its head. 'Very uncomfortable for the Dormouse', thought Alice, 'only as it's asleep, I suppose it doesn't mind'. The table was a large one, but the three were all crowded into a corner of it. 'No room! No room!' they cried out when they saw Alice coming. 'There's *plenty* of room!' said Alice indignantly, and she sat down in a large arm-chair at one end of the table'. (Gardner, 1970:93)

Activity (Points for Reflection)

- What does the extract given in Box 13.2 make you feel and think about regarding your experience of working collaboratively?
- What might the statement 'No room! No room!' suggest about professional boundaries and defences?
- How frequently do you ask questions such as: 'what is the task/purpose of this meeting?' or 'how might we work better together?'

The extract given in Box 13.2 and the above points for reflection may, or may not, have enabled you to think differently about your own experience of teamwork and collaboration. It is included here to provide an example of how metaphor can be invoked to understand complex and paradoxical aspects of organisational life and interprofessional practice.

Putting it all together

Following the *Bristol Inquiry* (Kennedy, 2001) and other subsequent tragic failures of communication between professionals, the discourse of interprofessional practice has gained currency as a response to the realities of fragmented health care practices. One of the challenges for interprofessional practice is that of how different professional territories are being carved out in the changing landscape of contemporary policy and practice (D'Amour et al., 2005). D'Amour and Oandasan (2005) have advanced the concept of *interprofessionality* as a frame of reference within which to understand the emergence of a more cohesive picture of interprofessional practice. They define interprofessionality as 'the development of a cohesive practice between professionals from different disciplines' (D'Amour and Oandasan, 2005:9), and which:

- is a process by which professionals reflect on and develop ways of practicing that provide an integrated answer to the needs of the client/family/population;
- is guided by the need for professionals to reconcile their differences and sometimes opposing views;
- involves continuous interaction and knowledge sharing amongst multiple stakeholders.

Interprofessionality is an important concept in understanding effective collaboration because it concerns the political, organisational and professional processes and determinants that influence interprofessional practice and education initiatives. The concept of interprofessionality also addresses the need for collaboration between practitioners, researchers, educators, policy-makers and the public.

Conclusion

In summary, collaboration is commonly defined through the underlying concepts of: (i) sharing, (ii) partnership, (iii) power, (iv) interdependency, (v) process and (vi) outcomes. Organisational, professional and systemic factors such as structure, communication, boundaries, socialisation, values, cultural ideals and beliefs have the potential to either enhance or inhibit collaborative relationships and interprofessional practice. There is no 'one-size-fits-all' solution to the challenges of collaborative practice, which has wide-ranging parameters and meaning. On one hand, it may be a brief and short-term interaction between two practitioners exchanging patient-related information. On the other hand, it may involve sustained episodes of formal and informal interprofessional and interagency engagement and teamwork. Despite advances in 'joined-up working', failure and tragedy are likely to persist unless we continue to address both micro- and macro-aspects of collaborative practice. At a macro-level, collaboration involves professions and agencies working together across organisational boundaries and cultures, for example, in health, education and social services. At a micro-level, collaboration involves practitioners working in a nimble-footed way in public and private sectors with statutory and voluntary organisations. Gilbert (2005) offers some salient reminders for good practice:

- Focus always on the patient/client and the place of the patient/client in their community.
- Understand the way the provision of health and social care is conducted within the policy domains of governments.
- Recognise diversity in any consideration of interprofessional patient – centred collaborative care.

▪ Understand and make explicit that all participants in the education of health and human service professionals will have their own aims, objectives, priorities and philosophical positions which result in different approaches and perspectives on what is judged as quality care.

Finally, Stepney and Callwood (2006) suggest that three scenarios for the future can be constructed. The first is an optimistic vision of creative collaborative interprofessional practice, supported by a substantive evidence base and properly funded system of accessible care. The second, a more pessimistic view, is that funding will be inadequate and unable to sustain research, collaboration and interagency working, and old 'Berlin wall' divisions and mistrust between professionals will continue. This will result in 'pseudo-collaboration' masquerading as genuine partnership working and interprofessional practice in order to meet government targets and 'flavour-of-the-month' policy initiatives. The third scenario lies somewhere between these two extremes, where collaborative practice evolves flexibly to meet the diverse and changing needs of patients and practitioners in different cultural and organisational contexts.

References

Anning, A., Cotterell, D., Frost, N., Green, J. and Robinson, M. (2006) *Developing Multiprofessional Teamwork for Integrated Children's Services: Research, Policy and Practice.* Maidenhead: Open University Press.

Ashworth, P.D., Gerrish, K. and McManus, M. (2001) Discourses underlying the attribution of master's level performance in nursing. *Journal of Advanced Nursing*, 34(5); 621–628.

Barr, H., Koppel, I., Reeves, S., Hammick, M. and Freeth, D. (2005) *Effective Interprofessional Education: Argument, Assumption and Evidence.* Oxford: Blackwell Publishing.

Behan, D. (2006) *Facing the Evidence: Successes and Failures in Integrated Care.* Key Note Speech to Care and Health Conference, 19 April 2006, Civil Partnerships: Joint Commissioning for the Individual – Implementing the Health and Care White Paper, http://www.csci.org.uk/docs/Care_and_Health_Final_20060419%20.doc (accessed 1 August 2008).

Bolton, G. (2005) *Reflective Practice: Writing and Professional Development.* 2nd edn. London: Sage.

Butt, G., Markle-Reid, M. and Browne, G. (2008) Interprofessional partnerships in chronic illness care: A conceptual model for measuring partnership effectiveness. *International Journal of Integrated Care*, 8; 1–14, http://www.ijic.org/ (accessed 1 June 2008).

Canam, C.J. (2008) The link between nursing discourses and nurses' silence: Implications for a knowledge-based discourse for nursing practice. *Advances in Nursing Science*, 31(4); 296–307.

Cornelissen, J.P., Kafouros, M. and Lock, A.R. (2005) Metaphorical images of organization: How organizational researchers develop and select organizational metaphors. *Human Relations*, 58(12); 1545–1578.

Curran, V. (2004) *Interprofessional Education for Collaborative Patient – centred Practice: Research Synthesis Paper*, http://www.hc-sc.gc.ca/hcs-sss/hhr-rhs/strateg/interprof/synth-eng.php (accessed 18 July 2008).

Curran, V. (2007) *Collaborative Care*. Ottawa: Health Canada Publications.

D'Amour, D., Ferrada-Videla1, M., San Martin Rodriguez, L. and Beaulieu, M.-D. (2005) The conceptual basis for interprofessional collaboration: Core concepts and theoretical frameworks. *Journal of Interprofessional Care*, Supplement 1; 116–131.

D'Amour, D., and Oandasan, I. (2005) Interprofessionality as the field of interprofessional practice and interprofessional education: An emerging concept. *Journal of Interprofessional Care*, Supplement 1; 8–20.

Delva, D., Jamieson, M. and Lemieux, M. (2008) Team effectiveness in academic primary health care teams. *Journal of Interprofessional Care*, 22(6); 598–611.

Department for Children, Schools and Families (DCSF) (2008) *Ofsted Joint Area Review of Haringey*, http://www.dcsf.gov.uk/haringeyreview/ (accessed 20 December 2008).

DoH (1998) *Partnership in Action: New Opportunities for Joint Working between Health and Social Services – A Discussion Document*. London: Department of Health.

DoH (2000) *The NHS Plan*. London: Department of Health.

Fook, J. and Gardner, F. (2007) *Practising Critical Reflection: A Resource Handbook*. Maidenhead: Open University Press.

Foureur, M., Bush, R., Duke, J. and Walton, C. (2007) Poetry: A reflective practice tool for nurses and midwives. *Practice Development in Health Care*, 6(4); 203–212.

Freeth, D., Hammick, M., Reeves, S. and Barr, H. (2005) *Effective Interprofessional Education: Development, Delivery and Evaluation*. Oxford: Blackwell Publication.

Gardner, M. (1970) *The Annotated Alice: Alice's Adventures in Wonderland and through the Looking Glass by Lewis Carroll*. London: Penguin.

Ghaye, T. (2005) *Developing the Reflective Healthcare Team*. Oxford: Blackwell Publishing.

Ghaye, T. (2008) *Developing the Reflective Organisation*. Oxford: Blackwell Publishing.

Gilbert, J. (2005) Interprofessional learning and higher education structural barriers. *Journal of Interprofessional Care*, 19(S1); 87–106.

Gray, D. (2007) Facilitating management learning: Developing critical reflection through reflective tools. *Management Learning*, 38(5); 495–517.

Harvey, S. and McMahon, L. (2008) *Shifting the Balance of Health Care to Local Settings: The SeeSaw Report*. London: The Kings Fund.

Hatch, M. and Cunliffe, A. (2006) *Organization Theory: Modern, Symbolic and Postmodern Perspectives*. 2nd edn. Oxford: Oxford University Press.

Huffington, C., Armstrong, D., Halton, W., Hoyle, L. and Pooley, J. (2004) *Working below the Surface: The Emotional Life of Contemporary Organizations*. London: Karnac.

Kennedy, I. (2001) *Learning from Bristol: The Report of the Public Inquiry into Children's Heart Surgery at Bristol Royal Inquiry 1984–1995*. London: The Stationary Office.

Kharicha, K., Iliffe, S., Levin, E., Davey, B. and Fleming, C. (2005) Tearing down the Berlin wall: Social workers' perspectives on joint working with general practice. *Family Practice*, 22(4); 399–405.

Laming, H. (2003) *The Victoria Climbié Inquiry: Report of an Inquiry by Lord Laming*. Norwich: HMSO.

McDonald, R., Harrison, S. and Checkland, K. (2008) Identity, contract and enterprise in a primary care setting: An English general practice case study. *Organization*, 15(3); 355–370.

Meads, G., Ashcroft, J., Barr, H., Scott, R. and Wild, A. (2005) *The Case for Interprofessional Collaboration: In Health and Social Care*. Oxford: Blackwell Publishing.

Menzies, I. (1970) *The Functioning of Social Systems as a Defence against Anxiety: A Report on a Study of a Nursing Service of a General Hospital*. London: Tavistock.

McKenna, E. (2006) *Business Psychology and Organisational Behaviour: A Student's Handbook*. 4th edn. Hove: Psychology Press.

Morgan, G. (1997) *Images of Organization*. Thousand Oaks, CA: Sage.

NAO (2006) *Good Governance: Measuring Success through Collaborative Working Relationships*. London: National Audit Office.

Obholzer, A. and Roberts, V. (1994) *The Unconscious at Work: Individual and Organizational Stress in Human Services*. London: Routledge.

Parkinson, C. and Howorth, C. (2007) *The Language of Social Entrepreneurs*. Lancaster University Management School Working Paper 2007/032, http://www.lums.lancs.ac.uk/publications/viewpdf/005135/ (accessed 1 August 2008).

Reder, P. and Duncan, S. (2003) Understanding communication in child protection networks. *Child Abuse Review*, 12(2); 82–100.

Reeves, S. and Sully, P. (2007) Interprofessional education for practitioners working with the survivors of violence: Exploring early and longer-term outcomes on practice. *Journal of Interprofessional Care*, 21(4); 401–412.

Rushmer, R. and Pallis, G. (2002) Inter-professional working: The wisdom of integrated working and the disaster of blurred boundaries. *Public Money and Management*, 23(1); 59–66.

Stark, S., Warne, T. and Street, C. (2002) Practice nurses and integrated care examined. *Primary Health Care Research and Development*, 3; 11–21.

Stepney, P. and Callwood, I. (2006) *Collaborative Working in Health and Social Care: A Review of the Literature*. Wolverhampton: University of Wolverhampton. http://wlv.openrepository.com/wlv (accessed 18 July 2008).

Thomas, P. (2006) *Integrating Primary Health Care: Leading, Managing, Facilitating*. Oxford: Radcliffe Publishing Ltd.

Tope, R. and Thomas, E. (2007) *Health and Social Care Policy and the Interprofessional Agenda. The First Supplement to creating an Interprofessional Workforce: An Education and Training Framework for Health and Social Care in England*, http://www.caipe.org.uk/silo/files/cipw-policy.pdf (accessed 18 July 2008).

Waddington, K. (2005) Behind closed doors: The role of gossip in the emotional labour of nursing work. *International Journal of Work, Organisation and Emotion*, 1(1); 35–47.

Waddington, K. and Fletcher, C. (2005) Gossip and emotion in nursing and health-care organizations. *Journal of Health Organization and Management*, 19(4/5); 378–394.

Weir, H. and Waddington, K. (2008) Continuities in caring? Emotion work in a NHS Direct call centre. *Nursing Inquiry*, 15(1); 67–77.

West, M. (2004) *Effective Teamwork: Practical Lessons from Organizational Research*. 2nd edn. Oxford: The British Psychological Society/Blackwell.

West, M., Guthrie, J., Dawson, J., Borrill, C. and Carter, M. (2006) Reducing patient mortality in hospitals: The role of human resource management. *Journal of Organizational Behavior*, 27(1); 983–1002.

WHO (2006) *World Health Report 2006: Working Together for Health*. Geneva: World Health Organization.

Yan, J., Gilbert, J. and Hoffman, S. (2007) World Health Organization study group on interprofessional education and collaborative practice. *Journal of Interprofessional Care*, 21(6); 588–589.

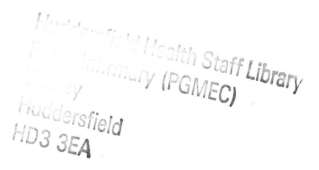

Leadership and organisational decision-making: the nurse's role in implementing policy and practice

14

Kathryn Waddington

Introduction

The overall aim is to promote a critical approach to leadership, policy, organisational decision-making and practice. This is a wide-ranging remit, as these are all huge topics, informed by theoretical perspectives that include psychology, sociology, political science and economics. Word limit has precluded inclusion of detailed practical examples and readers are encouraged to use the material in this chapter to critically reflect on aspects of their own current/future role and practice, for example, with regard to:

- leading practice, teams and services in transition;
- developing, supporting and sustaining effective leadership in self and others;
- balancing between leadership and management, professional values and the business of care, and power, politics and organisational culture;
- influencing organisational decision-making and policy development.

Learning Outcomes

- To critically explore the characteristics of critical thinking and why these are fundamental in dealing leadership skills
- To advocate the necessity for nurses to advance and promote nurse-led practices from practitioner level to policy-making level

- ■ To identify ways in which nurses can effectively engage in the policy-making process
- ■ To encourage nurses to become more active in the political process.

Background

'Nursing careers must respond to the profound changes taking place in the structure of health care delivery and the need for nurses to exercise leadership to bring about change'. (DoH, 2006:3)

Leadership has risen to a prominent position in health care policy and professional practice, as illustrated by the above extract from *Modernising Nursing Careers* (DoH, 2006). The leadership and managerial environment in which nurses and health care professionals work is changing, all the time and quickly. Practice nurses (PNs) and walk-in-centre (WiC) nurses, therefore, face many new challenges that will call for new ways of thinking about leading and advancing practice. The focus of this chapter is primarily geared towards practitioners who lead teams and services, although the theoretical perspectives and approaches introduced clearly also have a wider application.

The big picture

In an era of increasing globalisation and international health system reform, governments are revising health policies and making radical, transformational changes to organisational structures and methods of service delivery. In this broad context, nurses have a pivotal, but still relatively under-developed, role to play in the health policy arena (International Council of Nurses (ICN), 2005). Nurses work collaboratively with other health care professionals, teams and agencies (see Chapter 11) and are often closely involved with communities, patients/clients, their families and carers. This is a 'horizontal' approach to the complex interactions involved in integrating and delivering services which can be set alongside a complementary 'vertical' approach which prioritises integration of services around care pathways for named conditions. In the latter, policy tends to be dominated by the medical model, whereas nurses are particularly well placed to lead and influence policy that addresses the horizontal integration of care (Thomas and While, 2007).

In the UK, new patterns of health care provision and practice-based commissioning (PBC) require PNs to have a shrewd understanding of the organisational and political context of 'the business of care' (Burdett Trust for Nursing, 2006:1; DoH, 2008a). Lord Darzi's *NHS Next Stage Review* (DoH, 2008b,c) marks a critical moment in health care policy in England. Ambitious plans include empowerment of frontline staff to lead change and improve the quality of care for patients, conceptualised around the principles of patient safety, patient experience and effectiveness of care. Nursing is at the forefront of these health care reforms, and the vision of the nurse of the future is one of practitioner, partner and *leader* (Maben and Griffiths, 2008). This presents unique opportunities for nurses working in primary care (e.g. PNs or WiC nurses) to advance their practice in WiCs, nurse-led community services and general practitioner (GP)-led health centres.

Arguably however, primary care nursing faces particular challenges in responding to and implementing this next tranche of policy initiatives and health care reforms. First, there are significant gaps in knowledge in relation to primary care workforce data and subsequent difficulties in constructing a national picture of career pathways and opportunities in primary care and community settings (Storey et al., 2007; Drennan and Davis, 2008). Second, there is a risk that well-intentioned 'nurse-led' initiatives may not achieve their full potential unless wider issues of organisational power and professional cultures are addressed. According to Redfern (2008), the NHS has been criticised as being over-managed but under-led, and this was borne out in Weir and Waddington's (2008) examination of emotion work in a NHS call centre.

Finally, a recent survey of 1,400 primary care nurses conducted in the UK (Linnane, 2008) suggested that nurses are significantly under-represented in the PBC arena, which poses a significant threat to the survival of nursing values. Strong clinical, professional and educational leadership is needed at all levels, from the point of patient contact to board level and beyond. This is vital to ensure that primary care nursing responds promptly and politically to the challenges ahead, and this chapter is written with these challenges in mind.

A critical approach

This section outlines the broad foundations of a critical approach, which is then applied and developed further in subsequent sections of the chapter. When thinking about leadership, being critical involves taking a 'more radical, reflective and marginal stance, in contrast to taking a more mainstream, positivistic or rationalistic perspective' (Western, 2008:8). Adopting a critical approach to the material in this chapter will involve the reader engaging actively with the text, reflecting, arguing with the concepts and ideas presented, and searching for better arguments and evidence with which to advance practice.

Broadly speaking, a critical approach entails critical thinking, which requires individuals to move beyond the linear thinking that has traditionally informed, but also constrained, professional and managerial practices (Thomas, 2006; Thomas and While, 2007). The ability to think critically is expected and often assumed, particularly as nursing shifts to becoming an all graduate profession. However, philosophers, educationalists, students and practitioners alike often struggle – in their own various ways – to articulate precisely what critical thinking entails.

Therefore, as a reminder, Box 14.1 outlines some of the key characteristics of critical thinking that underpin this chapter.

Box 14.1 The Characteristics of Critical Thinking

- *Having an open mind*: appreciating alternative perspectives, understanding different cultural/professional values to gain insight into self and others.
- *Being inquisitive*: curious and enthusiastic, seeking to know how systems work even if the application or relevance is not immediately apparent.
- *'Truth' seeking*: being courageous about asking difficult questions, and hearing answers, obtaining new/different knowledge and perspectives.
- *Using critical analysis*: appraising verifiable information from multiple sources, application of reason and evidence.
- *Being systematic*: appreciating a focused and rigorous approach to problems at multiple levels of complexity.
- *Challenging*: questioning and unsettling values, assumptions, power bases and ways of thinking.
- *Self-confidence*: trusting one's own reasoning, skills, insights and judgements.

Adapted from Banning (2004).

Critical thinking is an essential aspect of the nurse's role in implementing policy and practice, which changes at a bewildering rate. The speed of altered priorities, targets and detailed directives creates a relentless pace of work that leaves practitioners feeling overwhelmed by bureaucracy and paperwork, with little time for reflection (Davies, 2003; Fook and Gardner, 2007). The pace and volume of change is such that Light (2008:210) has coined the term 'redisorganisation' to describe the continual and costly pattern of change. The effects of such change could, arguably, be located along (at least) two dimensions of:

- anticipated outcomes of responsive, adaptive, advanced practice;
- experienced outcomes of change-fatigued practitioners and services.

The organisational symptoms of change fatigue include low morale and motivation, stress, sickness absence, poor staff retention, resistance to planned change and sabotage (Obholzer and Roberts, 1994; Fook and Gardner, 2007; Light, 2008; Linnane, 2008). However, adoption of a critical approach allows practitioners to work creatively in the space between change fatigue and advanced practice because, as Fisher and Owen (2008:2065) note:

> Practitioners move continuously between the discourses of public policy and experiential knowledge; much of their work involves mediating between these areas.

Adopting a critical approach to policy and practice requires us to inform change agents and policy makers of the likely, and experienced, consequences of their policies. It also requires practitioners to question the motives behind policy decisions and to work with uncertainty and complexity. Competencies within Nursing and Midwifery Council (NMC, 2005) Domain 3 of Practice and the Royal College of Nursing (RCN, 2008) Domain 1: *Managing and Negotiating Health Care Delivery Systems* include advocating for increasing access to health care and participating in legislative and policy-making activities and advocating for culturally sensitive policies and those that reduce environmental health risk (6.15, 6.16 and 6.17). This requires an understanding of the principles of policy formulation, implementation and analysis, which are considered next.

Activity

Consider how you employ a critical approach to your practice.

- How much of your practice involves linear thinking?
- Have you identified constraint in your professional and managerial practice? If so, what should you be doing about this constraint?

Policy formation, implementation and analysis

Critical thinking and questioning are essential aspects of policy formation and analysis, addressing broad topics such as the role of the state in the policy process, the role of citizens and experts in the public sphere, the social construction of policy targets and cultural pluralism (Fischer, 2003). However, the exact nature of social policy is difficult to define, its scope is very broad and health policy is just one aspect. Peckham and Meerabeau (2007:15, citing Baldock et al.) suggest that there are three broad domains of social policy: '(i) the intentions and objectives that lie behind policies; (ii) the administrative and financial arrangements used to deliver policies; and (iii) the outcomes of policies, particularly in terms of who gains and loses'. These domains influence the allocation of resources for health, which, according to Daniels and Sabin (2008), relies on fair processes of decision-making. In order to gain visibility and influence in the policy-making arena, nurses need to understand the processes of organisational decision-making.

Policy and organisational decision-making

The focus here is on decision-making in an organisational context, rather than clinical decision-making (see Chapter 5), although clearly there are similarities in terms of the cognitive processes and critical thinking skills used. The main difference is one of *context*; when individuals are involved in organisational decision-making, it is often as part of a team, committee or board, and a theoretical understanding of processes of groupthink and power dynamics are helpful here.

According to McKenna (2006), groupthink is the outcome of group pressure, impeding the efficient execution of members' mental faculties and interfering with members' ability to test reality and preserve their judgement. Groupthink amounts to an unintentional erosion of one's critical faculties as a result of adopting group norms. It can lead to uncritical acceptance of the status quo, and reluctance to 'rock the boat'. This can lead to a number of difficulties ranging from 'over-optimism and lack of vigilance to ineffectiveness and lack of realism in the formulation and implementation of policy' (McKenna, 2006:337). The implications for primary care nursing are that practitioners need the confidence and skills to challenge, and also support and follow through, policy-related organisational decisions. This involves detailed analysis and challenge of all the evidence, robust debate and careful consideration of criteria and metrics (measures) relating to:

- acceptability and accessibility;
- clinical sustainability and delivery;
- health outcomes;
- financial and workforce implications.

Arguably the nurses' leadership role in policy and practice in the future will be to influence the language and discourse of the 'business of caring' (Burdett Trust for Nursing, 2006). Nurses will also need to develop a deeper understanding of the sources and dynamics of power, and these issues are considered next.

The sources and dynamics of power

Power is relational, dynamic and multifaceted, and manifests in at least three dimensions that can be considered in any organisational and policy analysis. First, the macro-level is a systemic dimension encompassing *who* has power over others, and the visible structures and processes such as positional authority, formal and informal organisational hierarchies, policies and procedures. Second, the discourse of power analyses *how* power is used to shape perceptions and belief systems, and is ideological and interpretative. Finally, the informal exercise of power at the micro-political, local level emphasises *where* and *how* power circulates in everyday organisational practices, networks, hidden agendas and invisible structures (Foucault, 1982; McKenna, 2006).

Foucault's analysis of power is important, extensive and complex, centred on the premise that power is not a 'thing' or a 'capacity' which can be owned either by governments, social class or particular individuals' (O'Farrell, 2005). This analysis falls within poststructuralist inquiry, which draws attention to the relationship between power and knowledge, where the production of knowledge is seen as an exercise of power and where only some voices are heard. Government policies have a significant impact on health care provision and professional practice, and it is critically important that nursing voices are heard at every level from practitioner to policy makers in order to advance nurse-led practice.

However, as Hart (2004) points out, nurses are trapped within insidious power structures that not only damage their interests, but also rob them of the authority and confidence to resolve the problems they face in their daily work. In a primary care nursing context, historical 'baggage' and organisational cultures may impede practitioners' confidence and ability to raise potentially difficult issues. For example, McKenna et al.'s (2004) study into perceptions of nursing leadership in primary care in Northern Ireland revealed a perceived inability to nurture strong leaders. This was attributed to the 'traditional subservient culture of community nursing' (McKenna et al., 2004:69). Clearly these findings are not necessarily generalisable or applicable to all practitioners or primary care nursing environments. Nevertheless, they raise important issues relating to power dynamics, professional cultures and the nurse's role in policy, all of which are relevant to the current policy environment. Box 14.2 therefore contains suggestions for ways that practitioners can effectively engage in the policy process.

Box 14.2   Strategies for Effective Engagement in the Policy Process

1. *Keep up-to-date with policy developments*: know what is happening locally and in the wider political/professional arenas. Access policy reviews and analyses from a range of sources, for example, professional and academic journals, and develop a critical and factual base for your opinions to ensure an informed debate.

2. *Write and publish*: well-placed articles can help influence opinion; seek advice from and write with others, for example, advanced practitioners, university lecturers, GPs.

3. *Awareness of professional/academic associations and networks*: your contribution might be more effective if channelled through a larger group, for example, the Association of Advanced Nursing Practitioner Educators (http://www.aanpe. org/)and the Royal College of Nursing Practice Nurses Association (http://www. rcn.org.uk/).

4. *Know who holds key nursing positions*: these may be both strategic and local, for example, nurses in executive positions with influence at board level, as well as PN forums; nurses also work in influential positions outside of nursing, for example, in voluntary organisations, social enterprises and non-governmental organisations (NGOs). These practitioners have access to other sources of support and influence.

5. *Communicate your position*: this can be achieved by ongoing representation on policy-making committees or boards, lobbying, meeting with people in positions of influence and actively using your professional networks.

Source: Adapted from ICN (2005) Guidelines for developing Effective Health Policy.

The strategies outlined in Box 14.2 call for nurses to develop a political voice and presence in the policy-making arena, but so far this has been lacking. This has resulted in the announcement of hugely important health policies without meaningful professional involvement, consultation or piloting. The lack of nurses' engagement in policy has been compounded by the historical lack of a real career framework for nursing and a general lack of political awareness or 'savvy'. In the past, nurses had little knowledge, motivation, direction or support in getting into a position of clinical or political leadership. However, the nursing profession cannot afford to ignore, or neglect, the need to become more political and lead health care reforms. Arguably the current policy environment offers significant opportunities for PNs to develop their practice.

Activity

What are the sources of power within your practice setting?

■ How will you shed the 'historical baggage' within your practice setting if present?

The current policy environment

Current broad policy themes that are relevant to primary care nursing include:

■ growing empowerment of patients and service users, and people with long-term conditions will be encouraged to have greater control over their care;
■ initiatives designed to integrate the policies of the Department of Work and Pensions (DWP), Social Care, the NHS and education in the pursuit of population health and welfare;
■ development of a greater range and volume of care and services that can be delivered 'closer to home' and 'out-of-hospital';
■ a shift from provision to commissioning of services, from an increasingly diverse range of providers, including private and not-for-profit organisations.

Modernising Nursing Careers (DoH, 2006) and the *Next Stage Review* (DoH, 2008b) look set to dominate policy and practice in the short to medium term, and one of the many implications for nursing in general and primary care nursing in particular is leadership – again?

Looking back at leadership in the NHS

The current leadership development agenda can be traced back to the NHS Plan (DoH, 2000) which pointed to the need for first-class leadership to deliver radical change and modernised health care services. We are now entering what has been described as arguably the most difficult yet potentially most exciting period of transformation (Maben and Griffiths, 2008). The new strategic plan for the NHS in England states: 'Leadership has been the neglected element of the reforms of recent years. That must now change' (DoH, 2008c:66). However, this statement appears to overlook the significant investment that has been made into leadership development over the past 10 years.

Following the introduction of the NHS Plan, £4 million was invested in nursing leadership development and subsequent research into leadership development initiatives demonstrated positive change in clinical leadership capability and competence (Hancock et al., 2005; Large et al., 2005). However, change at the individual level of capability and competence without associated change in organisational and professional cultures to support and embed leadership development is a recipe for failure. Looking back, it is apparent that sustainable leadership development was elusive, often despite significant financial investment, indicating the need for future research into cost analysis and return on investment (Large et al., 2005).

The early part of the 21st century also witnessed many other local and national leadership initiatives. These included the short-lived NHS University (NHSU), the NHS Modernisation Agency and the Leadership Development Centre with associated frameworks, toolkits, change agents, transition teams and taskforces. All of these bodies have since been merged or subsumed into the *current* NHS Institute for Innovation and Improvement (previously known as the NHS Institute for Learning, Skills and Innovation). Changes in policy appear to beget new organisations and agencies which are set up quickly, and then disappear equally quickly. This leads to a sense of fads, fashions and flavour of the month – here today but gone tomorrow – and practitioners seeking continuing personal development (CPD) opportunities need to negotiate their way through a plethora of leadership development initiatives.

The future is likely to continue to see a growth in the business of leadership education, coaching, training and development, particularly within primary and integrated care (DoH, 2009). PNs and WiC nurses seeking to advance their leadership skills and the managers and leaders who support and guide them will be faced with a vast array of local and national initiatives. Therefore, there are two key questions facing primary care nursing. The first is quite simply: What will we do this time round – more of the same, or something different? The second is: What theories, frameworks and skills are needed to enable PNs and WiC nurses to advance in their role as practitioners, partners and leaders?

New leadership agendas for PNs – linking theory and practice

A critical approach to leadership is important because 'critical thinking skills are *the* pre-requisite leadership skills required to promote sustainable emancipatory change within organizations' (Western, 2008:9, emphasis added). When thinking about leadership development to support advanced practice then, the discerning practitioner should ask the question: What is the evidence base for this programme/framework/intervention?

A number of leadership frameworks have emerged over the past 10 years, with the *NHS Leadership Qualities Framework* as one example (http://www.nhsleadershipqualities.nhs.uk/). Such frameworks mark an important transition in the understanding of leadership in health care. There are, however, two critical points to note. First, it has been argued that such competency frameworks are either too conceptually/methodologically flawed or too simplistic to be of any significant benefit on their own (Alimo-Metcalfe and Alban-Metcalfe, 2006; Bolden et al., 2006). Second, leadership competencies and development programmes are either theoretical or grounded uncritically in theoretical perspectives that may not necessarily be wholly relevant to health care (Gilmartin and D'Aunno, 2007).

For example, a quick glance at 'general' leadership theories shows that these are still dominated by Western male heroic stereotypes of 'great' military, political and sports leaders (McKenna, 2006). This is not necessarily helpful or relevant for either PN or WiC nursing which is a predominantly female, culturally diverse workforce. Leadership is a hugely researched yet poorly understood topic, and the *essence* of leadership is that it is a process of social influence between individuals and/or groups within a particular context.

Turning to leadership research and theoretical developments that specifically address health care and nursing contexts (Alimo-Metcalfe and Alban-Metcalfe, 2006; Alimo-Metcalfe et al., 2007; Gilmartin and D'Aunno, 2007; Shaw, 2007), a number of critical themes can be discerned:

- leadership is a social process of engaging others as partners in the development and achievement of shared goals and visions;
- leadership is associated with individual and group satisfaction, retention and performance;
- there is a need to develop conceptually strong leadership models that also go *beyond* individuals and groups;
- nurse leaders require a critical understanding of the broader health and social systems within which nursing operates;
- transformational and transactional leadership theories comprise the largest subset of research on leadership in health care.

Transformational and transactional leadership

Transformational and transactional leadership has dominated the literature for over 30 years, envisioned in the work of Burns (1978) and Bass (1985) (cited in Western, 2008). Briefly, transactional leadership is based on the idea that the relationship between leaders and followers is based on the exchange of some reward, such as recognition, praise, pay or performance ratings. It is a managerially focused approach that involves leaders clarifying goals, communicating these goals and the planning and organising of tasks and activities necessary to ensure that goals are met. This is a control model of leadership. On the other hand, transformational leadership works on the principles of collaboration rather than direct control, and is concerned with establishing a long-term vision, motivating, enabling and developing individuals in pursuit of achieving change.

The development of services based solely on transformational leadership vision risks failure if transactional controls, such as paying attention to competitor analysis, are not addressed. It is also important that the current focus on clinical leadership does not lose sight of the management task, which may be perceived as less attractive than leadership but which is also necessary to improve the quality of care. The current policy emphasis is on bringing leadership to frontline services where *everyone* has a role to play in the 'process of leadership' and delivery of quality care. This approach draws attention to the critical importance of followers in the leadership process, because without followers there cannot be leaders (Kellerman, 2008).

Leading advanced practice in primary care

Box 14.3 summarises some of the leadership elements of the vision of the future registered nurse, which chimes with Thomas and While's (2007) argument that nurses are particularly well placed to lead and influence policy that addresses the horizontal integration of care.

Box 14.3   Nurses as Practitioners, Partners and Leaders

The practitioner, partner and leader model is at the heart of care. It involves coordinating multiprofessional teams and resources, across care settings and agencies. *The leadership component of this model envisages individuals who are:*

- continually challenging and improving care quality and championing the experience of people who receive services;
- coordinating resources and skills to deliver high-quality care;
- responsible for an effective care delivery;
- ambitious for nursing as a profession;
- confident innovators, keen for the nursing contribution to be demonstrated;
- exerting influence and credibility from point of care to board room;
- supervising, monitoring, teaching and mentoring health care assistants' practice to support excellent patient care delivery.

Source: Adapted from Maben and Griffiths (2008).

Whilst all the elements in Box 14.3 are important, arguably a crucial aspect is that of 'coordinating resources and skills to deliver high-quality care', and much can be learned and transferred from the field of interprofessional practice and interagency working (see Chapter 11). However, what appears to be missing from the leadership elements of the model in Box 14.3 is authority, and without this the coordination of care can be ultimately frustrating and time-consuming (Obholzer and Roberts, 1994). It is also vitally important that the role elements align in order to avoid role and interpersonal conflict. In other words, the leadership element, which may also include managerial and financial responsibility, should not conflict with the partnership element of working collaboratively with colleagues and other professionals.

The 'dark side' of practice

PNs and indeed WiC nurses seeking to advance their practice and develop their leadership skills need to be mindful of two critically important points to avoid potential failure and frustration. The first is that it is vital that if leadership is to be sustained, it *must be embedded* in the organisational culture (Alimo-Metcalfe and Alban-Metcalfe, 2006). This is easier said than done, and the second critically important point is that there are distinct and typical cultural patterns and dynamics that exist across all the helping professions which may act as barriers to advanced practice (Hawkins and Shohet, 2006). This is the 'dark side' of practice, where gossip, strong emotions, hidden agendas, rivalries, resentments and power struggles lurk in the 'unmanaged spaces' of organisations, such as car journeys, coffee rooms and corridors (Waddington, 2005). Unless these dysfunctional cultural patterns are exposed, understood and shifted, the dark side of practice remains a hidden – and sometimes not so hidden – threat to sustained leadership and practice development.

Shifting dysfunctional cultural patterns

Hawkins and Shohet (2006) report a number of dysfunctional patterns that are found in the organisations in which care and services are delivered. These 'cultural dynamics' (Hawkins and Shohet, 2006:196) include:

- *Hunt the personal pathology*: this culture is based on seeing all problems as located in the personal pathology of individuals, and has also been referred to as 'the troublesome individual in the troubled institution' (Obholzer and Roberts, 1994).
- *Strive for bureaucratic efficiency*: this culture is high on task orientation and low on personal relatedness (Menzies, 1970); there are policies and protocols to cover all eventualities, but little understanding in the rush to find tidy answers.
- *Watch your back*: this culture emerges in highly politicised, highly competitive environments, and 'good behaviour' is rewarded; this involves putting a good gloss on individual and corporate image, whilst covering up or failing to admit difficulties, inadequacies or problems (Kahn, 2005).

Steps to shift dysfunctional cultural patterns begin with awareness. The activities below outline questions that can tap into underlying patterns, enabling practitioners and teams to move towards a more embedded learning culture of sustained leadership development.

Activity (Reflecting on Cultural Patterns)

The following questions are intended to help you access and understand the cultural patterns and context of your current role:

- What behaviours are rewarded by the organisation and what typical patterns of behaviour do you notice at meetings?
- What stories and gossip are circulating in the 'unmanaged spaces', for example, tales of the unexpected heroes, villains and fools?
- What metaphors are used to describe the culture, for example, this place is like . . . (see Chapter 11)?
- What/who would be included in the 'unofficial induction programme'?
- What are the 'organisational secrets' – the things that most people know, but which cannot be talked about openly? Why are these issues not confronted?

The next set of questions can be used as a team reflexivity exercise (see Chapter 13):

- What needs to be safeguarded, nurtured and preserved?
- What 'excess baggage' is slowing down change?
- What no longer fits and can be discarded?
- What needs to be incorporated, acquired or done differently?

Source: Adapted from Hawkins and Shohet (2006).

Reflecting on cultural patterns is the first step in culture change, but shifting long-held, ritualised and sometimes cherished patterns of behaviour and relating is not easy. In real terms, this will involve team, organisational *and* individual transition, evoking the image of a changing practitioner practising in a changing environment. An understanding of the concept of professional development across the lifespan, and the importance of managing transitions, is highly relevant here.

Managing transitions

The questions in Box 14.4 address the organisational and team context of cultural change and development. At the individual level, transition theories can help practitioners understand the experience of role change (Glen and Waddington, 1998; http://www.eoslifework.co.uk/transprac.htm). Adapting to transitions involves a change in behaviour and thinking, which can be both exciting and also disruptive to the individual's peace of mind, competence, performance and relationships. Transition psychology has its origins in studies of grief, loss and bereavement, and the various models of transition try to explain how individuals respond to change in terms of their thoughts, feelings and actions. Transitions involve both serious hazards and enormous opportunity for growth, and according to Nicholson (McKenna, 2006) the *transition cycle* consist of four discrete stages:

- preparation;
- encounter;
- adjustment;
- stabilisation.

These stages are interdependent, and what happens in one stage will influence what happens in the next, which may also be influenced by where you see yourself in terms of overall career development. The age profile of the primary care workforce (Drennan and Davis, 2008) is such that some practitioners are likely to be in the *maintenance* phase of their career, or looking towards decreasing involvement, *disengagement* and retirement. On the other hand, more recently qualified practitioners will be at the *establishment* phase of their career. The important point to note is that policy-driven professional and organisational change and role development can be experienced by practitioners as intense personal loss and/or threat to their established or emerging professional identities. The equally important question is: 'what helps?', and the enabling factors in transitions include:

- *supportive work environment*: high respect/low control culture, good team morale, clear role and contract terms, work-life boundaries respected;
- *transition support*: briefing, monitoring issues, practical support, life-career planning, tolerance, dignity, valuing the past, coaching and mentorship, and freedom/recognition for new ideas (Glen and Waddington, 1998; McKenna, 2006).

Conclusion

New terms to describe the emerging landscape of NHS reform and leadership development include: *co-production*, which means that all parts of the system need to work together on shaping and implementing change, and *subsidiarity* which means ensuring that decisions are taken at the right level of the system, which is as close to the patient as possible (DoH, 2009). These are wise words with huge implications for patients and professionals, but as Western (2008) warns, there is still a tendency for organisations to 'drift blindly and unknowingly towards seductive but dangerous totalizing cultures' (Western, 2008:200). 'Totalising cultures' are characterised by *uncritical* adoption and conformist commitment, often reflected in 'management-speak' and jargon, which can lead to 'counter-cultures' of destructive gossip and sabotage (Obholzer and Roberts, 1994; Weir and Waddington, 2008). It is probably too early to tell what extent this will happen, or not, in the health care environments of the future, whether that is a WiC, GP-led health centre, social enterprise, supermarket, investor-owned or privately held company. However, PNs and WiC nurses have a critical role to play in ensuring nursing values and voices inform and lead future policy and practice.

References

Alimo-Metcalfe, B. and Alban-Metcalfe, J. (2006) More (good) leaders for the public sector. *International Journal of Public Sector Management*, 19(4); 293–315.

Alimo-Metcalfe, B., Alban-Metcalfe, J., Samele, C., Bradley, M. and Mariathasan, J. (2007) *The Impact of Leadership Factors in implementing Change in Complex Health and Social Care Environments*. Department of Health NHS SDO, Project 22/2002. London: Department of Health.

Banning, M. (2004) Nursing research: Perspectives on critical thinking. *British Journal of Nursing*, 15(8); 458–461.

Bolden, R., Wood, M. and Gosling J. (2006) Is the NHS Leadership Qualities Framework missing the wood for the trees? In Casebeer, A.L., Harrison, A. and Mark, A.L. (Eds.) *Innovations in Health Care: A Reality Check*, pp. 17–29. Houndsmills: Palgrave Macmillan.

Burdett Trust for Nursing (2006) *Who Cares, Wins: Leadership and the Business of Caring*, http://www.burdettnursingtrust.org.uk/docs/5719_burdett_trust_who_cares_wins_031006.pdf (accessed 6 January 2009).

Daniels, N. and Sabin, J.E. (2008) *Setting Limits Fairly: Learning to share Resources for Health*. 2nd edn. New York: Oxford University Press.

Davies, C. (2003) Introduction: A new workforce in the making? In Davies, C. (Ed.) *The Future Health Workforce*, pp. 1–13. Basingstoke: Palgrave Macmillan.

DoH (2000) *The NHS Plan: A Plan for Investment, A Plan for Reform*. London: Department of Health.

DoH (2006) *Modernising Nursing Careers setting the Direction*. London: Department of Health.

DoH (2008a) *Practice-based Commissioning (PBC) Implementation Progress Report*. Department of Health. http://www.dh.gov.uk/en/Publicationsandstatistics/Publications/DH_077742 (accessed 6 January 2009).

DoH (2008b) *High Quality Care for All: NHS Next Stage Review Final Report*. Cm 7432, http://www.dh.gov.uk/en/Publicationsandstatistics/Publications/PublicationsPolicyAndGuidance/DH_085825 (accessed 6 January 2009). London: Department of Health.

DoH (2008c) *NHS Next Stage Review: Our Vision for Primary and Community Care*, http://www.dh.gov.uk/en/Publicationsandstatistics/Publications/Publications PolicyAndGuidance/DH_085937 (accessed 6 January 2009). London: Department of Health.

DoH (2009) *Inspiring Leaders: Leadership for Quality*, http://www.dh.gov.uk/en/Publicationsandstatistics/Publications/PublicationsPolicyAndGuidance/DH_093395 (accessed 24 January 2009). London: Department of Health.

Drennan, V. and Davis, K. (2008) *Trends over Ten Years in the Primary Care and Community Nurse Workforce in England*. London: St. Georges, University of London and Kingston University.

Fischer, F. (2003) *Reframing Public Policy: Discursive Politics and Deliberative Practices*. Oxford: Oxford University Press.

Fisher, P. and Owen, J. (2008) Empowering interventions in health and social care: Recognition through 'ecologies of practice'. *Social Science and Medicine*, 67(12); 2063–2071.

Fook, J. and Gardner, F. (2007) *Practising Critical Reflection: A Resource Handbook*. Maidenhead: Open University Press.

Foucault, M. (1982) The subject and power. In Dreyfus, H.L. and Rabinow, P. (Eds.) *Michel Foucault: Beyond Structuralism and Hermeneutics*. 2nd edn., pp. 208–226. Chicago: University of Chicago Press.

Gilmartin, M. and D'Aunno, T. (2007) Leadership research in healthcare: A review and roadmap. *The Academy of Management Annals*, 1; 387–438.

Glen, S. and Waddington, K. (1998) Role transition from staff nurse to clinical nurse specialist: A case study. *Journal of Clinical Nursing*, 7(3); 283–290.

Hancock, H., Campbell, S., Bignell, P. and Kilgour, J. (2005) The impact of leading empowered organisations (LEO) on leadership development in nursing. *International Journal of Health Care Quality Assurance*, 18(3); 179–192.

Hart, C. (2004) *Nurses and Politics: The Impact of Power and Practice*. Basingstoke: Palgrave Macmillan.

Hawkins, P. and Shohet, R. (2006) *Supervision in the Helping Professions*. 3rd edn. Maidenhead: Open University Press.

International Council of Nurses (ICN) (2005) *Guidelines on shaping Effective Health Policy*. Geneva: ICN.

Kellerman, B. (2008) *Followership*. Boston, MA: Harvard Business School.

Kahn, W. (2005) *Holding Fast: The Struggle to create Resilient Caregiving Organizations*. Hove: Brunner-Routledge.

Large, S., Macleod, A., Cunningham, G. and Kitson, A. (2005) *A Multiple-case Study Evaluation of the RCN Clinical Leaders Programme in England*. London: Royal College of Nursing.

Light, D. (2008) Will the NHS strategic plan benefit patients? *British Medical Journal*, 337; 210–212.

Linnane, E. (2008) A message to the Minister: The NiP survey results. *Nursing in Practice*, (January/February), 40(1); 16–24.

Maben, J. and Griffiths, P. (2008) *Nurses in Society: Starting the Debate*. London: Kings College.

McKenna, E. (2006) *Business Psychology and Organisational Behaviour: A Student's Handbook*. 4th edn. Hove: Psychology Press.

McKenna, H., Keeney, S. and Bradley, M. (2004) Nurse leadership within primary care: The perceptions of community nurses, GPs, policy makers and members of the public. *Journal of Nursing Management*, 12(1); 69–76.

Menzies, I. (1970) *The Functioning of Social Systems as a Defence against Anxiety: A Report on a Study of a Nursing Service of a General Hospital*. London: Tavistock.

NMC (2005) *Annex 1 – Domains of Practice and Competencies, NMC Consultation on a Proposed Framework for Post-registration Nursing*. London: Nursing and Midwifery Council.

Obholzer, A. and Roberts, V. (Eds.) (1994) *The Unconscious at Work: Individual and Organizational Stress in Human Services*. Milton Park: Routledge.

O'Farrell, C. (2005) *Michel Foucault*. London: Sage.

Peckham, S. and Meerabeau, L. (2007) *Social Policy for Nurses and the Helping Professions*. 2nd edn. Maidenhead: Open University Press.

RCN (2008) *Competencies. Advanced Nurse Practitioners – An RCN Guide to the Advanced Nurse Practitioner Role, Competencies and Programme Accreditation*, https://www.rcn.org.uk/__data/assets/pdf_file/0003/146478/003207.pdf (www.rcn.org.uk) (accessed 1 October, 2008). London: Royal College of Nursing.

Redfern, L. (2008) The challenge of leadership. *Nursing Management*, 15(4); 10–11.

Shaw, S. (2007) *Nursing Leadership*. Oxford: Blackwell Publishing Ltd.

Storey, C., Ford, J., Cheater, F., Hurst, K. and Leese, B. (2007) Nurses working in primary and community care settings in England: Problems and challenges in identifying numbers. *Journal of Nursing Management*, 15(8); 847–852.

Thomas, P. (2006) *Integrating Primary Health Care: Leading, Managing, Facilitating*. Oxford: Radcliffe Publishing Ltd.

Thomas, P. and While, A. (2007) Should nurses be leaders of integrated care? *Journal of Nursing Management*, 15(6); 643–664.

Waddington, K. (2005) Behind closed doors – The role of gossip in the emotional labour of nursing work. *International Journal of Work, Organisation and Emotion*, 1(1); 35–47.

Waddington, K. and Michelson, G. (2009) *Gossip and Organizations* (Routledge Studies in Management, Organizations and Society). Milton Park: Routledge.

Weir, H. and Waddington, K. (2008) Continuities in caring? Emotion work in a NHS Direct call centre. *Nursing Inquiry*, 15(1); 67–77.

Western, S. (2008) *Leadership: A Critical Text*. London: Sage.

Domain 6

Monitoring and Ensuring Quality of Health Care Practice

Implications of the new GMS contract

15

Marie C. Hill

Introduction

The aim of this chapter is to explore the implications of the new General Medical Services (new GMS) contract and how this has changed the day-to-day working life of the practice nurse (PN). The different types of services that the new GMS contract provides, the reasons why some practices decide to opt out of these services and whether the Quality and Outcome Framework (QoF) is meeting the needs of patients since the implementation of the new GMS contract in 2004 will be explored. Throughout the chapter, narratives will be provided by PNs on their experiences of the new GMS contract.

Learning Outcomes

- To assess how the new GMS contract has changed the working lives of PNS
- To explore whether the new GMS contract has enabled PNS to develop and provide new services in primary care
- To assess the effectiveness of the new GMS contract and the QoF since 2004
- To explore working opportunities for PNS due to the new GMS contract.

Background

The new GMS contract: essential, additional and enhanced services

The new GMS contract was implemented in April 2004. Some of the main characteristics of this new contract have already been explored in Chapter 2 to explain how this new contract has influenced the changing role of the PN. The new GMS contract is a contract between an individual practice and a primary care organisation (PCO) (Drennan and Goodman, 2007).

All partners in the practice have to sign the practice contract, but only one partner has to be a general practitioner (GP). The list of services that a practice can provide falls into three distinct areas: essential, additional and enhanced services.

All practices who enter into a contractual agreement with their PCO must deliver essential services. These essential services consist of:

- day-to-day medical care of their practice population including management of minor and self-limiting illness and referral to secondary services;
- care of the terminally ill;
- chronic disease management (Drennan and Goodman, 2007).

Practices can opt out of providing 'additional services' and consequently receive reduced funding. This can be on either a temporary or a permanent basis. These services include: cervical screening, providing contraceptive services, immunisations, childhood health surveillance (excluding the neo-natal check), maternity services (excluding intra-partum care) and minor surgery procedures of curettage, cautery, cryocautery of warts and verrucae and other skin lesions (Drennan and Goodman, 2007). For example, if Practice A decided not to provide childhood and adult immunisations, the PCO would have to ensure that these services are provided locally by another practice for the population of Practice A. In this case, the PCO must ensure that access to services would be available so that patient service would not be compromised, which would have a detrimental effect on the quality of service provided.

Enhanced services are commissioned by the PCO. These services have been defined as:

> Services not provided through essential or additional services, or essential and additional services delivered to a higher specified standard. They were negotiated into the GMS contract as a key tool to help Primary Care Trusts (PCT) reduce demand on secondary care. Their main purposes are to expand the range of local services to meet local need, improve convenience and choice, and ensure value for money. They were designed to provide a major opportunity to expand and develop primary care, and give practices greater flexibility and the ability to control their workload. (www.dh.gov.uk, 2008a:1)

In addition, enhanced services would be the services not provided in certain practices (i.e. those practices that opt out of these services). These could include services that address specific local health needs or requirements. Examples of these services include anticoagulant monitoring and care for the homeless.

What are the implications for general practice? The contract has far-reaching implications for practice and will.

- Allow practices a greater flexibility to determine the range and breadth of services that they wish to provide for their practice population, which would include opting out of additional services and out-of-hours care.
- Reward practices for delivering clinical and organisational quality though the evidence-based QoF and for improving patient experience.
- Allow practices to be responsive to the different needs of GPs depending on their location, for example, in deprived parts of the country or in rural and remote areas.

- Facilitate the modernisation and development of the practice to include the premises and information technology (IT) of the practice.
- Allow practices to provide guaranteed levels of investment through a Gross Investment Guarantee.
- Allow practices to support the delivery of a wider range of higher quality services for patients and empower patients to make best use of primary care services.
- Simplify how contractual mechanisms work (BMA, 2003).

The new GMS contract recognises the need for GPs to have a balance between their work and personal commitments, as well as opting out of additional services. Practices could opt out of providing out-of-hours services. In this case, by the end of December 2004, all PCOs should have taken full responsibility for out-of-hours services using other health care providers and professionals such as NHS Direct, NHS walk-in-centres, pharmacists and paramedics to name some examples. The guidance from the British Medical Association (BMA) on out-of-hours service provision has acknowledged that different models of care will need to be developed in different areas to suit the local population's needs.

Opting out of services

The initial guidance on the new GMS contract (BMA, 2003) acknowledged that some practices would not wish to provide or indeed be in a position to deliver some services and would choose to opt out (on either a temporary or a permanent basis), only providing certain additional services. Among reasons that could influence a practice's decision to opt out of some services are the following:

- workforce shortages would prevent some practices providing certain services;
- the practice has never provided such a service (i.e. even under the previous GMS scheme) and would not wish to start providing this service;
- lack of skill in the practice to provide certain services;
- the practice does not wish to provide a service on conscientious grounds;
- the practice is not fulfilling its obligations for that additional service under the new GMS contract and there is a lack of practice commitment to solving the problem (BMA, 2003).

Domain of practice area content with specific competencies

The sixth Domain of Practice: '*Monitoring and Ensuring Quality of Health Care Practice*' is relevant to all PNs to ensure that they meet the required competencies of the Knowledge and Skills Framework (KSF) (DoH, 2004). Job descriptions of many PNs will be adhering to the recommendations of the KSF.

Initially, the review of the seven Domains of Practice for advanced nursing practice was driven by the requirements to implement the KSF, the debate about

Table 15.1   Domain 6: Core Competencies

Ensuring quality

1. Incorporates professional/legal standards into advanced clinical practice
2. Acts ethically to meet the needs of the patient in all situations, however complex
3. Assumes accountability for practice and strives to attain the highest standards of practice
4. Engages in clinical supervision and self-evaluation and uses this to improve care and practice
5. Collaborates and/or consults with members of the health care team about variations in health outcomes
6. Promotes and uses an evidence-based approach to patient management that critically evaluates and applies research findings pertinent to patient care management and outcomes
7. Evaluates the patients' response to the health care provided and the effectiveness of the care
8. Interprets and uses the outcomes of care to revise care delivery strategies and improve the quality of care
9. Accepts personal responsibility for professional development and the maintenance of professional competence and credential

Monitoring quality

10. Monitors quality of own practice and participates in continuous quality improvement
11. Actively seeks and participates in peer review of own practice
12. Evaluates patient follow-up and outcomes, including consultation and referral
13. Monitors current evidence-based literature in order to improve quality of care

RCN (2008:18).

what constituted advanced nursing practice and the need for the Nursing and Midwifery Council (NMC) to develop a competency framework for advanced nurse practitioners and importantly to enhance public protection (RCN, 2008). Although it could be argued that this is nurse practitioner driven, it relates to the ability of a practitioner (e.g. a PN) to be able to work to high standards of quality care. The next section of this chapter will emphasise the key role that the PN will play in assessing quality care in general practice as assessed by the QoF. Therefore, it is essential that a PN is working to these quality standards to be able to meet the requirements of the QoF to both ensure and monitor quality (Table 15.1).

Table 15.1 lists the 13 competencies that are related to Domain 6, many of which are core competencies.

Activity

After you have read Table 15.1, write your answers to the following:

What competencies are you currently meeting in relation to Domain 6 as a PN?
What evidence do you have that you are meeting these competencies? List this evidence.
How do you ensure your competency in this domain?
What competencies have you not met from Domain 6?
How do you plan to meet these? Include a time frame to meet these competencies.

PNs and the new GMS contract

The role of the PN in the new GMS contract has been cited as key to the delivery of services (BMA, 2003). With the PN taking on more advanced and specialists' roles, the following should apply:

- All employed PNs should be supported to participate in clinical supervision and appraisal and to have access to professional advice, continuing professional development and information, management and technology (IM&T).
- New advanced and specialist roles in first-contact, chronic disease management and preventive services will need to be supported by the necessary skills and knowledge provided by training and education and an understanding of the nurse and their employer of the NMC's *Code of Professional Conduct* (NMC, 2008). This relates to the professional accountability of the nurse regardless of who delegates roles.
- The skills and expertise of nurses working in general practice working at a more specialised level will be developed (BMA, 2003).

The concept of the PN taking on more advanced and specialists' roles has been supported by other policy documents such as *The NHS Plan* (DoH, 2000) and *Liberating the Talents: Helping Primary Care Trusts and Nurses to deliver the NHS Plan* (DoH, 2002).

Liberating the Talents has emphasised the growing importance of primary care services where '90% of patient journeys begin and end . . . and it is where most contacts with the NHS take place' (DoH, 2002:3). Furthermore, this paper acknowledges the importance that nursing will play in meeting some of the key requirements of the NHS plan such as: becoming non-medical prescribers, reducing waiting times so that patients will be able to have an appointment with a primary care professional (e.g. a PN) within 24 hours of making an appointment, increasing and improving primary care in deprived areas, introducing screening programmes for women and children and providing smoking cessation services (DoH, 2000). In order for nurses to be able to meet the NHS plan, 10 key roles have been identified to enable them to undertake a wide range of specialist and advanced nursing clinical tasks. These are:

- ordering diagnostic investigations such as pathology tests and X-rays;
- making and receiving referrals directly (e.g. to a therapist or pain consultant);
- admitting and discharging patients with specified conditions and within agreed-to protocols;
- managing patient caseloads (e.g. diabetes mellitus (DM) or rheumatology);
- running clinics (e.g. ophthalmology or dermatology);
- prescribing medicines and treatments;
- carrying out a wide range of resuscitation procedures including defibrillation;
- performing minor surgery and outpatient procedures;
- triaging patients using the latest IT to the most appropriate;
- leading in the organisation and running of local health services (DoH, 2002).

It would seem that the new GMS contract along with these health policy documents is opening up new opportunities for nurses and particularly PNs to develop skills and expertise to meet the NHS plan. However, central to this role expansion is education, which has been addressed in Chapter 2. The new Code of Professional Conduct provides guidance that it is a nurse's responsibility to take part in appropriate learning and practice that both maintains and develops professional competence and performance (NMC, 2008).

The QoF

QoF is a key feature of the new GMS contract, as practices will be rewarded on the basis of the quality of care that is provided, rather than the numbers of patients that are treated (White et al., 2004). The QoF will provide a quantitative way of assessing aspects in quality in general practice (DoH, 2005). It will link up to 25% of the practice's income to performance and this will be measured against 146 clinical and organisational quality indicators (Guthrie et al., 2006). The QoF has four areas of care referred to as domains. The domains comprise areas relating to: clinical, organisation, additional services and patient experience (Hall, 2004). Practices will be assessed though an annual audit of specific indicators and financially rewarded if points are achieved. Undertaking audits has been cited as one of the roles of a PN (Drennan and Goodman, 2007).

The clinical standard maximum points are 550 covering 10 specific areas: coronary heart disease (CHD), strokes, hypertension, diabetes (mellitus), chronic obstructive pulmonary disease, epilepsy, hypothyroidism, cancer, mental health and asthma (Hall, 2004). The maximum points for administration are 500, with a total maximum QoF score of 1,050 (Morgan and Beerstecher, 2006). The role of PNs will be crucial in achieving these points, considering that many have previously been involved in managing long-term conditions.

The following extract from a PN gives a personal account of how her role has adapted to the new GMS contract and in meeting the QoF:

> Since the new GMS contract came into existence, my role has changed a great deal. Previously my role consisted more of treatment room procedures, travel and childhood immunisation and little involvement with managing long term conditions. However, after 2004, I have had to undertake training to acquire new skills, which put me in a better position to assume skills which ordinarily would have been performed by doctors. My IT skills improved a great deal from barely using templates to consultation with EMIS, using population manager to track patients and manage quality outcome frame figures. Also, I have more autonomy with managing long term conditions.
>
> The Quality and Outcome Framework (QoF) set out clinical indicators according to disease categories that must be monitored. With higher standards being progressively required by government and expected by patients, it is certain that the domains of QoF will continue to change as nurses become more involved with managing long term conditions.

The domains have continued to expand each year. For example, hypothyroidism, sexual health and learning difficulties were added recently. This has resulted in the expansion of my responsibilities. I must now make a conscious effort to keep a disease register, a call and recall system and ensure that patients do not slip through the system. This was not the case before the new GMS contract. Annual reviews are now conducted with follow up of these patients. The different domains in the clinical indicators must be achieved for the practice to make financial gain. It could be argued that the aim is to provide holistic evidence-based care to the patients, while at the same time rewarding the practice for providing such services.

The bulk of the work relating to the new GMS contract is undertaken by nurses. This leaves me stressed towards the end of the financial year, struggling to meet QoF points. This must apply to many other Practice Nurses.

The government is stressing the importance of meeting patients' needs more than before and surgeries are now required to provide services at convenient times. The surgery where I work like many others, now opens on Saturdays and early weekday mornings from 7–8.30 am providing opportunities for early consultations and 6.30–8 pm for late consultations principally for those who are employed. This means I now work on Saturday mornings. One of the reasons why I left secondary care was not to work unsocial hours! Once again I am required to work unsocial hours, which we were not required to do so before the new GMS contract.

More recently, governmental policy on improving patient access that patients should be able to consult a health professional within 24 hours and GP within 48 hours means I have to provide more access to patients' and more sessions created by me. Telephone nurse triage was introduced to reduce face to face consultations, provide fast access and reduce waiting time for patients' to be seen. I had to undertake training to acquire new skills to triage. I also enrolled to study for a MSc in Primary Care (Nurse Practitioner programme) to equip myself with the necessary skills, knowledge and competencies required for the challenges that the new GMS contract has brought'. (Winnifred Egemonye, PN)

The above extract has highlighted the importance of the clinical and managerial input and indeed the expertise from a PN to achieve the financial rewards with respect to the clinical domain of the QoF (Derrett and Burke, 2006). Indeed, it can be argued that the importance of having robust administrative support mechanisms in practice is to ensure that practices are equipped to meet the demands of QoF. Some writers have acknowledged that the new contract is an opportunity for nursing to take a strategic role within primary care (Robinson, 2003; White et al., 2004). What do practices need to provide to meet the QoF relating to the original 10 clinical specific areas? There are slight variations with respect to what is required to meet the 10 clinical areas. Two examples now follow, which relate to the original clinical domain points in 2004.

Box 15.1   Example 1: Clients with a Diagnosis of Hypertension

This example demonstrates the importance of how this condition is documented and who provides the service. Points are awarded for having a register of all hypertensive clients, a register of their diagnosis and treatment and a register of their ongoing disease management. Key to achieving the maximum number of points and with this greater financial remuneration is five quality indicators:

1. Records:
   i. BP 1: The practice can produce a register of patients with established hypertension.
2. Diagnosis and initial management:
   i. BP 2: The percentage of patients with hypertension whose notes record smoking status at least once.
   ii. BP 3: The percentage of patients with hypertension who smoke, and whose notes contain a record that smoking cessation advice has been offered at least once.
3. Ongoing management:
   i. BP 4: The percentage of patients with hypertension in which there is a record of the blood pressure in the last 9 months.
   ii. BP 5: The percentage of patients with hypertension in whom the last blood pressure (measured in the last 9 months) is 150/90 or less.

Box 15.2   Example 2: Clients with a Diagnosis of DM

As the reader will note, much more is expected of the practice to provide an expected level of care with 18 quality indicators:

1. Records:
   i. DM 1: The practice can produce a register of all patients with DM.
2. Ongoing management:
   i. DM 2: The percentage of patients with diabetes whose notes record BMI in the previous 15 months.
   ii. DM 3: The percentage of patients with diabetes in whom there is a record of smoking status in the previous 15 months except those who have never smoked where smoking status should be recorded once.
   iii. DM 4: The percentage of patients with diabetes who smoke and whose notes contain a record that smoking cessation advice has been offered in the last 15 months.
   iv. DM 5: The percentage of diabetic patients who have a record of HbA1c or equivalent in the previous 15 months.
   v. DM 6: The percentage of patients with diabetes in whom the last HbA1C is 7.4 or less (or equivalent test/reference range depending on local laboratory) in the last 15 months.
   vi. DM 7: The percentage of patients with diabetes in whom the last HbA1C is 10 or less (or equivalent test/reference range depending on local laboratory) in the last 15 months.

vii.   DM 8: The percentage of patients with diabetes who have a record of retinal screening in the previous 15 months.

viii. DM 9: The percentage of patients with diabetes with a record of presence or absence of peripheral pulses in the previous 15 months.

ix.   DM 10: The percentage of patients with diabetes with a record of neuropathy testing in the previous 15 months.

x.   DM 11: The percentage of patients with diabetes who have a record of the blood pressure in the last 15 months.

xi.   DM 12: The percentage of patients with diabetes in whom the last blood pressure is 145/85 or less.

xii.   DM 13: The percentage of patients with diabetes who have a record of micro-albuminuria testing in the previous 15 months (exception reporting for patients with proteinuria).

xiii. DM 14: The percentage of patients with diabetes who have a record of serum creatinine testing in the previous 15 months.

xiv.   DM 15: The percentage of patients with diabetes with proteinuria or micro-albuminuria who are treated with ACE inhibitors (or A2 antagonists).

xv.   DM 16: The percentage of patients with diabetes who have a record of total cholesterol in the previous 15 months.

xvi.   DM 17: The percentage of patients with diabetes whose last measured total cholesterol within previous 15 months is 5 or less.

xvii. DM 18: The percentage of patients with diabetes who have had influenza immunisation in the preceding 1 September to 31 March.

The workload for providing the quality of service for all DM clients has implications for the practice in how this is provided (i.e. in specific clinics and/or opportunistically), who provides this service (i.e. relating to the skill mix of the practice) and how frequently a diabetic service needs to be provided. In some cases, depending on local population demographics, the frequency of the service will be dictated by the ethnicity of the population due to some groups' predisposition to DM, the number of diabetic clients and their diabetic control. An example of how demographics can influence the prioritisation of diabetes services follows. The prevalence of DM in the borough of Tower Hamlets is 5% (www.thpct.nhs.uk, 2008) while the prevalence for England in 2006 cited was 3.55% (www.gpcontract.co.uk, 2008). Therefore, in Tower Hamlets there will be a greater demand for diabetic service provision and for practices to utilise skill mix (i.e. GP, PN and Health Care Support Workers) to deliver these services.

Another factor that emerges from the quality indicators that needs to be met for clients with DM is the implications for the clinical laboratory and the increase in laboratory requests (e.g. measurement of lipids and HBA1c). Beastall (2005) has commented on the increase in laboratory requests noticeable from the outset of the new GMS contract, with a mean increase in requests of 18% in the first 3 months of 2004 compared with the corresponding period in 2003.

How have the additional requirements of the QoF influenced a PN's day-to-day professional life? The following extract reveals how this PN has adapted to the new QoF focusing specifically on meeting the required targets for hypertension and DM services:

> In the clinical role, I think definitely QoF made us more audit focused and what surprised me was that you actually realised how many patients were slipping through the net. When you look at your appointment page you are always extremely busy, you are always seeing lots of patients. But it really makes you sit up and think about those patients you do not see. I think because there is money attached to it, it makes you act upon it . . .
>
> Before (i.e., prior to the new GMS contract) we were very patient focused on the patients that you managed to see. I think what you are doing in hypertension and diabetes has not changed, but it makes you look at the patients that you are not seeing and also that you are being stricter. Because it says that your cholesterol has to be below 5, so you are making sure that you are going to hit those targets. I think it makes you drive yourself a bit harder. (Sabine Lenny, Nurse Practitioner, reflecting on the impact that the new GMS contract made on her workload as a PN from 2004 to 2006)

The new GMS contract: is it working?

A question that many PNs and indeed other health professionals will ask is whether the QoF is providing a quality service for patients and if this is cost-effective. What is the evidence to date? Three studies (Guthrie et al., 2006; Morgan and Beerstecher, 2006; Wang et al., 2006) will now be critically discussed. These focus on:

- effectiveness of funding and the impact on quality;
- workload and payment in the QoF;
- exploring the relationship between practice size points attained in the QoF.

Morgan and Beerstecher (2006) conducted an observational study to determine whether there was a relationship between funding, contract status and the QoF score. This study wished to explore whether differences in funding and contract status affected quality in primary care. The sample involved 164 practices in England, covering six Primary Care Trusts (PCTs). All the PCTs had differing socio-economic demographics using the Index of Multiple Deprivation 2004. Practice data of all 164 practices were collated for contract status and income. The outcome measure was the QoF score for 2004–2005. Data were analysed statistically.

It is important to differentiate the different funding sources in primary care that this study examined, which are GMS, Personal Medical Services (PMS) and finally Employed Medical Services (EMS). The GMS contract is a contract between the practice and PCO (Drennan and Goodman, 2007).

Table 15.2 Practice Funding and QoF points for 2004/2005v Morgan and Beerstecher (2006).

Contract status	Funding (per patient per year, £)	QoF points
GMS	62.51	942.4
PMS	87.38	942.4
EMS	105.37	757.9

PMS contracts, begun in April 1998, offer practices a locally negotiated contract to meet population-specific heath care needs. The key aims of PMS when it was introduced were to:

■ provide greater freedom to address the primary care needs of patients;
■ enable flexible and innovative ways of working, encouraging greater skills mix and a team-based approach to managing patient care;
■ address recruitment problems by providing a GP salaried option and supporting an enhanced role for nurses (e.g. PNs) within general practice;
■ tackle issues of under-resourcing by attracting GP and nurses to previously under-resourced areas (www.dh.gov.uk, 2008b).

The third type of contract – EMS – refers to the employment status of the GP and this could be with a PMS or a PCT.

The results revealed that contract status had an impact on contract funding with levels of funding for PMS and EMS practices greater than for GMS practices. In addition, there were differences between the QoF scores of GMS and PMS compared to EMS practices (Table 15.2).

The results demonstrated that GMS practices were the most efficient in terms of value for money and the resultant QoF outcomes. However, the authors recommended that further research needed to be undertaken to examine what other variables could influence practice performance in terms of efficiency and increased quality, as measured by the QoF.

Guthrie et al. (2006) examined the decision to use the adjusted disease prevalence factor (ADPF), rather than true prevalence, as a method of payment for prevalence of disease in practices. The argument for using the ADPF was that the small percentage of practices with low disease prevalence would not be financially penalised compared to practices with high disease prevalence. The use of the ADPF was primarily to reduce variation in payment. The authors compared the use of the ADPF with a rejected payment system – the true disease prevalence factor (TDPF). Their paper wished to examine whether the ADPF succeeded in its stated aims of:

■ reducing variation in overall payment compared to TDPF;
■ maintaining a fair link between payment and workload;
■ helping to tackle health inequalities.

The sample was 903 general practices in Scotland and covered the financial payments for 2004–2005. The data were publicly available; therefore, ethnical approval was not required. The ADPF succeeded in its first aim by reducing variation in total practice income. However, this was achieved at a cost of up to a 44-fold variation in payment per patient for the same level of achievement. The authors concluded that the second aim of this paper of ensuring fairness between workload and payment was not achieved. An example was cited of two practices with similar QoF points relating to the clinical domain of CHD. One practice has a higher than average prevalence rate of CHD, whilst the larger practice in terms of population has a lower prevalence rate. Using ADPF, the larger practice earned considerably more (£25,063) compared to the smaller practice (£850). However, both practices would have earned the same using the TDPF. Finally, the authors concluded that the use of the ADPF did not tackle health inequalities, as this financial system favoured the more affluent areas. The authors recommended that payment systems should be rigorously tested before implementation.

Wang et al. (2006) explored the relationship with practice size and the number of QoF points attained. The sample was 638 urban practices in Scotland comprising of single-handed practices to small-, medium- and large-sized practices. The categorisation of practices was according to the number of their whole time equivalents (WTE) GP principles.

The results showed that smaller practices received fewer QoF points compared to larger practices, but this was because of lower points received by the smaller practices for the organisational domain. There were no statistical differences in QoF points for the other domains that related to clinical or holistic care. The mean values of the other domains (i.e. additional services and patient experience) were the same, if not similar, across all four practice groups. The authors suggest that smaller practices may require increased resources to meet the organisational domain requirements of the QoF.

Practice nursing and the new GMS contract: implications of role development and expansion

A number of studies have been explored that examine the effectiveness of the new GMS contract in terms of cost-effectiveness and its impact on quality, equity of payment related to workload and the effect on a practice's size compared to the number of QoF points attained. A key question is how do these changes affect the PN and what opportunities are available for role expansion?

The RCN (2004) recommends that nurses can extend their interest within the general practice setting in a number of ways, such as:

- becoming more involved in the business aspects of the practice;
- taking a strategic role within primary care;
- becoming partners within the practice.

Within clinical practice, PNs could become sub- or specialist providers of services, such as sexual health, minor surgery and immunisations (Robinson, 2003).

Therefore, PNs along with other community nurses could set up their own limited company and become a provider of additional services to local practices that had decided to opt out of providing these services. Indeed for the more entrepreneurial PN, a keen understanding of the different contractual arrangements (as previously discussed) within primary care is essential with the opportunities that are possible if a PN is part of a PMS practice or indeed becomes a practice partner within a GMS practice. Over 40% of GPs in England now work within a PMS contract arrangement (www.dh.gov.uk, 2008b).

The new GMS contract emphasises the general practice team and rewards more effective skill mix within the practice. Nursing teams (e.g. a group of primary care nurses, including PNs) are able to access resources that will help to provide more integrated and effective patient care. Certainly, the emphasis on collaborative working will not be a new concept to a PN as guidelines within the Code of Professional Conduct are explicit in supporting such partnership working with other members of the multidisciplinary team: '. . . work with others to protect and promote the health and wellbeing of those in your care, their families and carers, and the wider community . . . you must work cooperatively within teams and respect the skills, expertise and contributions of your colleagues' (NMC, 2008:1, 5). What will be very different will be the opportunities that are available for PNs to lead on service provision. It has been suggested that the growing emphasis on team working will encourage practices to make better use of skill mix (Robinson, 2003). This would suggest that practices would examine their pre-existing workforce structures and examine ways in which certain roles and responsibilities could be delegated to other members of the practice team, for example, a Health Care Support Worker undertaking new patient registrations rather than a PN, thus freeing the PN time to address the clinical standards that need to be met in the new GMS contract.

The new GMS contract generates new opportunities for nurses to work in different ways, taking on extended roles such as proactive chronic disease management and minor surgery. This has implications for the practice to increase income generation. This raises the importance of not only education, but also mentorship of PNs in order to achieve the diversity of service provision. Therefore, PNs must be supported and trained and have access to the requisite training and professional support to enable them to take on these new roles. All nurses, midwives and specialist community public health nurses are professionally accountable for their practice (NMC, 2008). This is regardless of who the employer is (i.e. whether a GP or GP/nurse partnership or a PCO). Young's (2008) commentary emphasises that in order for nursing to achieve its potential in improving health and social care, nurses must be educated, rewarded, supported, valued and respected. However, for nursing to become increasingly professionalised, relevant education must be the key to this development and indeed nurses must articulate the need for this to their employing organisations. Change is inevitable in today's health care economy, particularly in primary care. Indeed, this is all too apparent with the QoF requirements, as these have been revised in 2006. In comparison to the QoF requirements in 2004, there are now five domains with the latest addition being the holistic care domain, which can achieve a maximum of 20 points (www.qof.ic.nhs.uk, 2008). Other changes to the QoF in 2006 were the nine extra clinical indicators as follows:

- atrial fibrillation;
- chronic kidney disease;
- dementia;
- depression;
- heart failure;
- learning disabilities;
- obesity;
- palliative care;
- conditions assessed for smoking (www.isdscotland.org, 2008).

How has this increasing workload affected quality, morale and team working in general practice? A qualitative study by Edwards and Langley (2007) in 14 practices in South Wales revealed that the increased workload of the new GMS contract affected team working and morale. Although the majority of teams accepted change, team incentives were found to be motivational in some practices. In some other practices, some staff perceived these incentive schemes as unfair and this contributed to some staff leaving their practice. However, Edwards and Langley (2007) found that for some teams, the increasing team size, involvement of the team in change and good leadership were found to motivate the team and this was perceived to have improved quality of care. Although these findings cannot be viewed as representative for all practices in Wales, the main findings demonstrate the importance of change implementation within a practice team and strong leadership to initiative this change.

Conclusion

This chapter has examined the impact that the new GMS contract has had and indeed is still continuing to have on the PN. Narratives from PNs have illustrated how their roles and responsibilities have changed as a result of the implementation of the new GMS contract since 2004. Contemporary studies have demonstrated that GMS practices are more cost-effective and efficient compared to differently funded practices, although PMS practices are as efficient compared to the QoF points achieved.

PNs are in a state of role transition and it may be argued that this will continue to be so, as the QoF continues to expand. This brings both opportunities and challenges for PNs. For example, one opportunity is the increasing management of clients with long-term conditions. The associated challenge is to ensure that they have the necessary competencies and skills to manage such clients. With this diverse role come challenges in how the PN meets the requisite skills required to practice competency at this level. The ageing nursing workforce in primary care and the increasing number of Health Care Support Workers may potentially erode some of the work previously undertaken by the PN. However, this need not be a threat to PNs, as long as PNs can articulate, promote and justify their unique role and contribution they make to primary care and ultimately to the public they serve.

References

Beastall, G.H. (2005) The new General Medical Services contract: Opportunity or threat? *Annals of Clinical Biochemistry*, 42(1); 3.

BMA (February 2003) *Investing in General Practice: The New General Medical Services Contract*. London: British Medical Association.

Derrett, C. and Burke, L. (2006) The future of primary care nurses and health visitors. *British Medical Journal*, 331(December); 1185–1186.

DoH (2000) *The NHS Plan: A Plan for Investment, A Plan for Reform*. London: Department of Health.

DoH (2002) *Liberating the Talents: Helping Primary Care Trusts and Nurses to deliver The NHS Plan*. London: Department of Health.

DoH (2004) *The NHS Knowledge and Skills Framework and the Development Review Process*. London: Department of Health.

DoH (2005) *Standard General Medical Services Contract*. London: Department of Health.

Drennan, V. and Goodman, C. (2007) *Oxford Handbook of Primary Care and Community Nursing*. Oxford: Oxford University Press.

Edwards, A. and Langley, A. (2007) Understanding how general practices addressed the Quality and Outcomes Framework of the 2003 General Medical Services contract in the UK: A qualitative study of the effects o quality and team working of different approaches used. *Quality in Primary Care*, 15(5); 265–275.

Guthrie, B., McLean, G. and Sutton, M. (2006) Workload and reward in the Quality and Outcomes Framework of the 2004 general practice contract. *British Journal of General Practice*, 56(532); 836–841.

Hall, G. (2004). The new GMS contract: Gathering points and improving care in diabetes. *Practice Nurse*, 28(1); 11–16.

Morgan, C. and Beerstecher, H. (2006) Primary care funding, contract status, and outcomes: An observational study. *British Journal of General Practice*, 56(532); 825–829.

NMC (2008) The Code: *Standards of Conduct, Performance and Ethics for Nurses and Midwives*. London: Nursing and Midwifery Council.

RCN (2004) *Nurses employed by GPs. RCN Guidance on Good Employment Practice*. London: Royal College of Nursing.

RCN (2008) *Advanced Nurse Practitioners: An RCN Guide to the Advanced Nurse Practitioner Role, Competencies and Programme Accreditation*. London: Royal College of Nursing.

Robinson, F. (2003). The GMS contract and you. *Practice Nurse*, 26(2); 11–13.

Wang, Y., O'Donnell, C., Mackay, D. and Watt, G. (2006) Practice size and quality attainment under the new GMS contract: A cross sectional analysis. British *Journal of General Practice*, 56(532); 830–835.

White, E., Singer, R. and McQuarrie, R. (2004) An opportunity for community nurses? *Community Practitioner*, 77(4); 129–130.

www.dh.gov.uk/en/HealthcPrimarycare/are/Primarycarecontracting/PMS/index. htm (2008a) *Personal Medical Services* (PMS) (accessed 23 April 2008).

www.dh.gov.uk/en/Publicationsandstatistics/Publications/PublicationsPolicyAnd Guidance/DH_4066930 (2008b) *Sustaining Innovation through New Personal Medical Services* (PMS) *Arrangements* (accessed 23 April 2008).

www.gpcontract.co.uk/browse.php?year=5 (2008) (accessed 21 April 2008).

www.isdscotland.org/isd/3363.html (2008) *General Practice Quality and Outcomes Framework. Clinical Domain Points Available 2004/05–2006/07* (accessed 24 April 2008).

www.qof.ic.nhs.uk/search.asp (2008) *Quality and Outcomes Framework 2006/07 Online GP Practice Results Database* (accessed 24 April 2008).

www.thpct.nhs.uk/uploads/LongTermConditions/(MISC)_LTC%20strategy. pdf.TowerHamlets:LongTermConditions:AnnuaReportSeptember2005- September2006 (2008) (accessed 19 March 2008).

Young, L. (2008) Incompetence and empty pockets: All in a day's work. *British Journal of Nursing*, 17(1); 6.

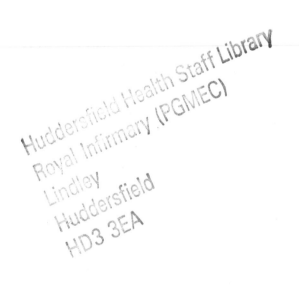

Art and science of providing quality nursing care in general practice and WiC settings

16

Carol L. Cox

Introduction

The aim of this chapter is to reflect on the provision of general practice (GP) and walk-in-centre (WiC) nursing that reflects the highest standards. Without question, this must be the aspiration of all nurses working within these health care settings. Being able to demonstrate that you have the knowledge and skills to deliver care of a uniformly high standard is an essential requirement of the Nursing and Midwifery Council (NMC) and is fully described within its Council Code of Conduct (NMC, 2008). The NMC (2008:1) indicates that 'people in your care must be able to trust you with their health and wellbeing'. You are personally accountable for your actions and omissions and must always act lawfully and be able to justify your practice decisions.

Learning Outcomes

- ▦ To focus on some of the core attributes and knowledge that are required to provide high-quality care
- ▦ To reflect on the art and science of practice
- ▦ To consider a framework for describing and providing high-quality care.

Background

In the 21st century, we face radically different requirements in the provision of nursing care and yet, the foundations of our practice, regardless of whether it is in the GP setting or WiC, remain the same. The Department of Health is pushing forward initiatives to modernise nursing careers (DoH, 2006a). The four UK Chief Nursing Officers established the modernising nursing careers initiative in 2005/2006. *Modernising Nursing Careers: Setting the Direction* (DoH, 2006a) forms part of an overarching programme designed to restructure all of the professions providing aspects of care throughout the UK.

In this report, it is indicated that:

> No one can doubt that health care services across the United Kingdom are going through a period of profound change. More change will be needed if we are to continue to provide a health service that is free according to need and that keeps the trust and support of the public. Wherever they work, nurses will be aware of how health care is changing and wondering what it all means for their careers. (DoH, 2006a:3)

The priorities delineated in the report focus on the careers of registered nurses. It is recognised that nurses do not work in isolation and nursing teams include more than registered nurses. However, it could be argued that the caring (caring-healing according to Watson, 1999) practices of nursing have been on the margins in recent history. According to Watson (1999), nursing caring theory (which underpins our practice) is calling for a new caring knowledge and practice that is informed by human values and an ethos of caring. Certainly this reverberates with the NMC (2008) perspective that the care of people is your first concern and that you must treat them all as individuals respecting their dignity. This is a moral obligation that can only be accomplished through the integration of the art and science of nursing within your practice setting.

The art of nursing and caring is integral to the applied science of nursing practice. This is evident in the way in which care is delivered and the way in which nurses relate with their patients, their carers and other health care professionals. Hand in hand with the idea of nursing being an art is the importance of nursing being a science. A caring theory, such as the theory articulated by Watson (1999) or other nurse theorists, provides the theoretical underpinnings that are important for effective, professional nursing care delivery. In the narrative that follows, you will be introduced to the sources of knowledge that may be used to inform your practice, caring relationships and caring behaviours.

In 1978, Carper's seminal research was published in a research article titled 'Fundamental Patterns of Knowing in Nursing'. Carper's four fundamental patterns of knowing are empirical (scientific) knowledge, aesthetic (art) knowledge, personal knowledge and ethical knowledge. The combination of these ways of knowing provides nurses with a sound basis for nursing practice.

Empirical knowing is synonymous with science, which in nursing is scientific knowledge associated with evidenced-based practice. Empirical knowledge may be equated with formal research-based knowledge that describes, explains or predicts natural and social phenomena. Empirical knowledge is related to factual evidence which can be used to inform clinical decision making. It is objective, obtained through the senses and can be verified and quantified. Inductive and deductive reasoning are logical thought processes involved in the discernment of empirical knowledge.

Activity

Identify how empirical (scientific) knowledge is used in your practice. Explain how this promotes high-quality care.

Aesthetic knowing is associated with the art of nursing. Aesthetic knowledge contributes to our understanding of how nursing is undertaken. It involves an expression of skill and the personal qualities of caring that lead to a difference in the patient's health. According to Carper (1978), the art of nursing is based on actual experience. Carper (1978:16) indicates that aesthetic knowledge begins with the 'singular, particular, subjective expression of imagined possibilities'. Therefore, the art of nursing is expressed through creativity and style in planning and providing care that is both effective and satisfying to the patient and nurse alike. The nurse's skilful delivery of care is provided in partnership with the patient and reflects a holistic and problem-solving nursing process.

Activity

Articulate how you act as an advocate for those in your care and help them to access relevant health and social care, information and support as specified by the NMC (2008).

Personal knowledge involves a 'knowing, encountering and actualising of the concrete individual self' (Carper, 1978:18). Through the discovery of self, reflection and synthesis of perceptions of what the nurse knows from life experience, a nurse can establish a satisfactory nurse–patient relationship. Personal knowing is associated with the inner experience of becoming an aware being. In the process of establishing the nurse–patient relationship, efforts of authenticity, rather than detachment, in interpersonal relations occur on the part of the nurse, resulting in an experience of interconnectedness between the nurse and patient. Personal knowing allows the nurse to be able to see the patient holistically; subsequently, the relationship with the patient becomes therapeutic.

Activity

Reflect on how your personal knowing allows you to create a relationship with patients that acknowledges their strengths and knowledge and enables them to address their needs (Domain 2: The Nurse–Patient Relationship; RCN, 2008).

Ethical knowledge involves the moral component of knowing. Ethics maintain a focus on 'matters of obligation or what ought to be done' (Carper, 1978: 20). It involves 'all voluntary actions that are deliberate and subject to the judgment of right and wrong' (Carper, 1978:20). In relation to nursing, ethical knowing involves making moral choices even when value judgements may conflict. Cultural and spiritual/religious beliefs that confront the nurse in day-to-day practice within a multi-cultural society may challenge the nurse's assumptions about moral and ethical behaviour. Therefore, it is important to recognise that ethical knowing is subject to personal knowing as well as empirical evidence. Ethical knowledge influences the way we live in the world and nurses are responsible for the choices they have made.

Activity

Consider your responsibility to be open and honest, act with integrity and uphold the reputation of your profession (NMC, 2008).

Acknowledge that you must always act lawfully, whether those laws relate to your professional practice or personal life (NMC, 2008).

Carper's (1978) four fundamental patterns of knowing are woven into the narrative of the chapters that follow. As you consider the empirical, aesthetic, personal and ethical knowledge conveyed in this section, you will gain a sound foundation on which to base your nursing practice.

A framework for practice

Frameworks have been developed by different professional and government organisations within the UK. One of these is a toolkit for benchmarking the fundamentals of care (DoH, 2001, 2003, 2006b). This document has been, since its inception, the foundation for clinical audit within nursing's clinical governance structure. The intention of developing the toolkit was to enable health and social care personnel to use the benchmarking document to address issues of concern within their areas of work in order to improve services already provided as well as to monitor existing practices. The Department of Health (DoH, 2003:2) noted that 'the benchmarks are relevant to all health and social care settings . . . and can be used in primary, secondary and tertiary' *care settings*. They are applicable to all patient/client/carer groups. What is of primary concern is that all health care practitioners engaged in benchmarking, including patients and carers, where involved, should agree with the indicators that demonstrate best practice within their area of care. The importance of getting these fundamental aspects of care right is essential if patient/client/carer care is to improve. Getting the fundamentals right was reinforced in the NHS Plan (2000) to improve the patient experience. It is so important that since the introduction of the NHS Plan (2000) and the Essence of Care

(DoH, 2001, 2003, 2006b), many health care organisations have begun special programmes designed to ensure staff have the necessary skills and knowledge to guarantee high standards of care. According to the Department of Health:

> The Essence of Care has been designed to support the measures to improve quality, set out in 'A First Class Service', and will contribute to the introduction of clinical governance at local level. The benchmarking process outlined in 'The Essence of Care' helps practitioners to take a structured approach to sharing and comparing practice, enabling them to identify the best and to develop action plans to remedy poor practice. (http://www.dh.gov.uk/en/ Publicationsandstatistics/Publications/PublicationsPolicyAndGuidance/ DH_4005475)

The Essence of Care toolkit (DoH, 2001, 2003, 2006b) is one strategy introduced throughout England to provide health care practitioners with a framework to take a patient-focused structured approach to sharing and comparing practice. It enables health care practitioners to identify best practice and to develop action plans that can improve care. The benchmarks that have been developed by the Department of Health (DoH, 2001, 2003, 2006b) cover 10 essential areas of patient care. These are:

1. continence and bladder and bowel care;
2. personal and oral hygiene;
3. food and nutrition;
4. pressure ulcers;
5. privacy and dignity;
6. record keeping;
7. safety of clients with mental health needs in acute mental health and general hospital settings;
8. principles of self-care;
9. communication between patients, carers and health care professionals;
10. promotion of health (DoH, 2006b).

You can find the Essence of Care benchmarks (DoH, 2003) which are nursing's primary caring framework on the Department of Health website: www.publications. doh.gov.uk/essenceofcare. This framework is focused on three levels: individual patients, communal/community and government activity/action.

The Essence of Care benchmarking toolkit includes an overall patient-focused outcome statement and factors related to the outcome for each benchmark. Overall patient-focused outcomes express what patients and/or carers want from care in a particular health care setting. Factors that need to be considered in order to achieve the overall patient-focused outcome consist of a patient-focused benchmark statement of best practice, a scoring process on a continuum between poor and best practice and indicators for best practice that have been identified by patients, carers and professionals that support the attainment of best practice. Within the toolkit, there is information on how to use the benchmarks and forms to facilitate documentation. The benchmarking process is closely associated with the Modernisation Agency's clinical governance agenda. In the discussion that follows, a synopsis of each benchmark is presented.

Continence and bladder and bowel care

Continence care is the 'total care package tailored to meet the individual needs of patients with bladder and bowel problems' (DoH, Continence and bladder and bowel care, 2003:1). This could include strategies to prevent incontinence, assessment investigation, conservative and surgical intervention and methods to manage intractable incontinence. The patient-focused outcome is achieved when accountable practitioners and professionals ensure practice demonstrates the benchmarks of best practice and all carers demonstrate commitment to the provision of quality patient/client care. Therefore, patients/clients and/or carers should have free access to evidence-based information about bladder and bowel care that is individualised to patient/client needs and/or those of their carer. In addition, patients/clients must have direct access to professionals who can meet their continence needs and ensure that services are actively promoted for the benefit of patients/clients. The effectiveness of patient/client bladder and bowel care should be continuously evaluated so that it leads to either effectively meeting their needs or modifying the plan of care such as in referral to other specialists. According to this benchmark, patients/ clients are assessed and have their care planned by health care professionals who have received specific training in bladder and bowel care. In addition, these professionals are continuously updating their knowledge in the area of continence care. Patients also have care provided by carers who have undertaken continence care training that includes ongoing updating. Those who give care have their training needs assessed. How carers provide care and service user views and expectations are determined (by you and other health care practitioners) and included in the training programmes including links with self-help or user support groups.

Professional advice on continence care must be available locally, including specific strategies to access local communities. In addition, all opportunities should be taken that can promote continence and healthy bladders and bowels amongst patients/clients in the wider community. Users should always be involved in the planning and evaluating of services and the input they provide should be acted upon. As such, they should 'have access to appropriate 'needs specific' supplies and services that assist in the management of incontinence' (DoH, Continence and bladder and bowel care, 2003:3). Clinical audit is therefore undertaken and results are disseminated and inform practice development.

Activity

Consider how you provide evidence-based information about bladder and bowel care that is individualised to patient/client needs and/or those of their carer.

Personal and oral hygiene

Personal hygiene is the 'physical act of cleansing the body to ensure that the skin, hair and nails are maintained in an optimum condition' (DoH, Personal and oral hygiene, 2003:1). Oral hygiene is the 'effective removal of plaque and debris to ensure the structures and tissues of the mouth are kept in a healthy condition' (DoH, Personal and oral hygiene, 2003:1). In addition, a healthy mouth is a mouth that is 'clean, functional, comfortable and free from infection' (DoH, Personal and oral hygiene, 2003:1). Therefore, all patients must be assessed to identify the advice and care required to maintain and promote personal hygiene. The care that the patient receives should be negotiated with the patient and/or carers and is based on the individual needs of the patient. Patients should have access to the level of care they require in order to meet their hygiene needs. Furthermore, the care that the patient receives in relation to hygiene should be continuously evaluated, reassessed and, where required, the plan of care renegotiated with the patient/ client/carer(s).

Activity

Explain how patients within the context of your practice setting have access to the level of care they require in order to meet their hygiene needs. Indicate how and by whom the care that patients receive in relation to hygiene is continuously evaluated and reassessed and, where required, their plan of care is renegotiated with the patients/clients/carers.

Food and nutrition

Food means substances eaten or drunk or absorbed for the growth and repair of organisms and the maintenance of life. Nourishment is taken in solid as opposed to liquid form and is related to substances that sustain organisms and keep them active (DoH, Food and nutrition, 2003). Nutrition is the aggregate of all the processes by which food is assimilated, growth is promoted and waste is repaired in living organisms. Patients should be 'enabled to consume food (orally) which meets their individual need' (DoH, Food and nutrition, 2003:1). Therefore, nutritional screening must be undertaken on all patients identified at risk and their plan of care based on an ongoing nutritional assessment. The plan of care you devise is implemented and evaluated regularly.

The environment in which food is taken should be 'conducive to enabling the individual patient to eat' (DoH, Food and nutrition, 2003:1). Additionally, patients should have set meal times and offered a replacement meal if a meal is missed as well as have access to snacks at any time. All food that is provided by the service organisation should meet the individual needs of the patient and should be presented in a way that takes into account what appeals to the patient as an individual.

The 'amount of food patients actually eat should be monitored, recorded and lead to action when cause for concern' arises (DoH, Food and nutrition, 2003:2). Finally, all opportunities should be used 'to encourage patients to eat to promote their own health' (DoH, Food and nutrition, 2003:2). Best practice involves assessment occurring at the time of initial contact with the patient, and the need for reassessment of the patient should be continuously considered.

Activity

Consider how you teach carers to assess the amount of food the patient actually eats and how to monitor and record this information so that action can be taken when there is a cause for concern.

Pressure ulcers

A pressure ulcer, which is also referred to as a pressure sore/bed sore or decubitus ulcer, is a damage to an individual's skin due to the effects of pressure together with, or independently from, a number of other factors, for example, shearing, friction and moisture (DoH, Pressure ulcers, 2003). Patients/clients should be assessed by practitioners who have the required specific knowledge and expertise to assess and plan care. These practitioners should have ongoing updating. Patients/clients identified as being 'at risk' (DoH, Pressure ulcers, 2003:1) must receive screening that is adequate. This screening progresses to further assessment and is recorded. An individualised evidence-based documented plan of care that reflects current evidence should be agreed with the multi-disciplinary team in partnership with patients/clients/carers. There is evidence of ongoing assessment of patients within your GP practice or WiC setting.

According to the Department of Health (DoH, 2003), the patient's/client's need for repositioning is assessed, documented, met and evaluated. The patient's/client's comfort is assessed and assured. Patients/clients that are at risk of developing pressure ulcers are cared for on pressure-redistributing support surfaces that meet their individual needs. In addition, patients/clients should have all the equipment that they require in order to meet their individual needs and information about the equipment and specific care is provided in a format that meets patients'/clients' cultural needs such as language, tapes, videos and leaflets. There is an evidence-base for the information that is provided within your practice setting. There is documented evidence by health care professionals that the patient/client/carer has understood the information that has been provided as well as choices that have been made. Finally, infection control policies are in place and their relevance to surface cleaning is evident. A process for ordering, delivering and monitoring support surfaces for patients/clients is in place and followed. Clinical audit that assesses and informs practice is undertaken and ongoing.

Activity

Identify the updating you have received in relation to pressure ulcer management. Consider when you last undertook a continual professional development (CPD) course on tissue viability.

Privacy and dignity

Privacy involves 'freedom from intrusion and dignity is associated with being worthy of respect' (DoH, Privacy and dignity, 2003:1). Therefore, care is focused on respect for the individual patient/client. As such, patients/clients should 'feel that they matter at all times and they experience care in an environment that actively encompasses individual values, beliefs and personal relationships' (DoH, Privacy and dignity, 2003:1). Personal space is actively promoted by all health care personnel and communication between health care personnel and patients/clients takes place in a manner which respects their individuality. In relation to privacy, the patients'/clients' personal boundaries must be identified and communicated to others (e.g. using the patient's/client's own language). Strategies are put in place to prevent disturbing or interrupting patients/clients (e.g. knocking before entering a room) and privacy is effectively maintained by using curtains, screens, walls, rooms, blankets, appropriate clothing and appropriate positioning of the patient/client. Patient information is shared to enable care with the patient's/client's consent. Care actively promotes privacy and dignity and protects modesty. Furthermore, patients/clients and/or carers can access an area that safely provides privacy and modesty is achieved for patients/clients moving between differing care environments.

Health care personnel display good attitudes and behaviour towards patients/clients; good attitudes and behaviour are promoted and assured, including consideration of non-verbal behaviour and body language. Issues about attitudes and behaviour towards minority patient/client groups are addressed with individual staff using, for example, induction programmes. Stereotypical views are challenged and valuing of diversities is demonstrated. Individual patient/client needs and choices are ascertained and continuously reviewed.

The name that the patient wants to be called is identified, agreed and used. Where necessary, access to translation and interpretation services is made available and a determination is made about the quality of the service to the patient/client. Information is, therefore, adapted to meet the individual needs of patients/clients and appropriate records of communication exchanges and information provided are maintained.

The patient's/client's informed consent is sought when special measures are required to overcome communication barriers (e.g. when using trained interpreters) and precautions are taken to prevent information being shared inappropriately (e.g. telephone conversations being overheard, computer screens being viewed or white boards being read). Therefore, procedures are in place for sending and receiving information about patients/clients (e.g. handover, consultant and/or teaching rounds, admission procedures, telephone calls and breaking bad news).

Activity

Explain how your care actively promotes privacy and dignity and protects modesty.

Record keeping

The benchmarks delineated in the Essence of Care toolkit in relation to record keeping are applicable to any health care setting and within any health care delivery system (DoH, Record keeping, 2003:1). A health record is defined in Section 68(2) of the Data Protection Act (1998) and consists of:

a. any information relating to the physical or mental health of condition of an individual;
b. any information that has been made by, or on behalf of, a health professional in connection with the care of that individual and has been checked and found to be correct (DPA, 1998; DoH, Record keeping, 2003).

It is accepted practice that health records are legible, accurate, signed with the designation of the practitioner/patient/client/carer, dated, timed, contemporaneous, provide a chronology of events and contain only agreed international abbreviations. It is further accepted practice that patients are able to access all their current records if and when they choose to, in a format that meets their individual needs, and that patients/clients and/or carers are actively involved in continuously negotiating and influencing their care (DoH, Record keeping, 2003:2). In addition, patient records should be integrated, single and lifelong, which means that patients/clients have a single, structured, multi-professional and agency record that supports integrated care. An evidence-base should be used to guide and detail best practice; this should be demonstrated in the record and additionally that documented evidence of an active and timely review process of the care that the patient/client receives occurs. Where there is a variation to what is required according to best practice, this should be documented with an explanation in the health record.

Patient/client records should be safeguarded through explicit measures and again should have an active and timely review process. Confidentiality should always be maintained to protect the patient/client. Effective systems must be in place for the storage and retrieval of records. Evidence of discussions or negotiations should be recorded and evidence should be provided in the record that reflects discussions have influenced actions. Rationale for care and its consequences and alternatives should also be documented as being explained to patients/clients and carers.

In relation to best practice, a clear indicator in the record-keeping section of the toolkit (DoH, Record keeping, 2003:5) is that 'records should be user friendly' and it should be documented whether any special needs of the patient/client are or have been met. This means that documents are jargon free, abbreviation free and unambiguous. Furthermore, relevant stakeholders should be identified in the record as well as their involvement in care and how it is achieved.

A systematic review process must be used to ensure guidance remains based on the latest evidence and that robust and rigorous audit reviews are undertaken. This may involve peer review of quality and content of documentation. You should note that 'record keeping is an integral part of practice' (DoH, Record keeping, 2003:10) and that it should not be viewed as something separate from the caring process, and not an optional extra that is to be fitted in if circumstances allow.

The legal obligations of how health care professionals deal with confidential information provided by patients are now codified by statute. The introduction of the Data Protection Act (1998) that implements the 1995 European Community Data Protection Directive means that the use of personal information held on either paper/manual or computer records is governed by statute. Therefore, patients/clients must be made aware that NHS staff and sometimes staff from other types of agencies will have strictly controlled access to information about them and that this will be anonymised wherever possible in order to plan, deliver and manage services effectively. In some circumstances, it may be necessary for health care personnel to disclose or exchange information about a patient/client. This must be in accordance with the Data Protection Act (1998). Therefore, patients/clients should be made aware of the purposes to which information about them may be used so that they can exercise choice about how and whether this information is disclosed or exchanged.

Activity

Identify whether patients within your practice setting are able to access all their current records if and when they choose to, in a format that meets their individual needs, and whether patients/clients and/or carers are actively involved in continuously negotiating and influencing their care.

Safety of clients with mental health needs in acute mental health and general hospital settings

The client-focused outcome for the safety of clients with mental health needs in acute mental health and general hospital settings is that 'everyone feels safe, secure and supported with experiences that promote clear pathways to well being' (DoH, Safety of clients with mental health needs in acute mental health and general hospital settings, 2003:2). For the purpose of the benchmark:

a. safe means 'freedom from physical, mental, verbal abuse and or injury to self and others';
b. secure means 'emotional safety';

c. relational security means that 'clients needs are met through the development of trusting and genuinely therapeutic relationships with the client by members of the care team within safe and fully explained boundaries';

d. engagement means clients 'have staff who connect with them continuously, in an atmosphere of genuine regards, instilling feelings of well being, safety, security and sanctuary';

e. harm means to 'injure, hurt or abuse' (DoH, Safety of clients with mental health needs in acute mental health and general hospital settings, 2003:2).

In order to achieve the safety of clients with mental health needs, they must be fully orientated to the health care environment. They should have a comprehensive ongoing assessment of risk to themselves with full involvement of themselves in order to reduce potential harm to themselves and others. The environment in which care is provided should balance safe observations and privacy. Additionally, clients must be regularly and actively involved in identifying care that meets their safety needs. Therefore, there must be a 'no blame' culture that allows for a vigorous investigation of complaints and adverse incidents and near misses and also ensures that lessons are learnt and acted upon.

A full orientation including making the client familiar with and helping them understand the philosophy, staff, services, environment, policies/processes/procedures and physical layout of the health care setting and how to access their key worker including relevant information should occur. The orientation should focus around the client groups' cognitive skills. A specific person should be responsible for orientating the client to the health care setting (e.g. ward). This can include staff and also on occasion, other clients. A specific person should explain what will happen to the client and who will initially be looking after them. Specific action must be taken to ensure women and other vulnerable service users feel safe and secure within the health care setting. Therefore, specific booklets, tapes and videos may be used to promote orientation. Appropriate topics can then be addressed during the orientation.

Clients must have a comprehensive ongoing assessment of risk to themselves with full involvement of themselves in order to reduce the potential for harm. The key indicators of risk must be included in the risk assessment tool that is used. Knowledge of the client's history, social context and significant events should be ascertained, recorded and shared with the health care team. Assessment must further be undertaken by inpatient and community teams prior to discharge and it should be documented as to whether this includes assessment of risk and joint case review that also involves discharge planning. Users should be involved in the training of staff in order to ensure that assessment and management of clients is appropriate and sensitive to specific needs (e.g. religion, culture, age-related needs, human rights, child protection and previous history of life events).

In regard to self-harm, staff attitudes to self-harm should be ascertained, measured and supported. Outside user agencies that are being or have been used to act as support or information for clients who self-harm, such as the National Self-harm Network or Black and minority ethnic voluntary organisations, should be noted. Procedures should be in place to ascertain the presence of, and/or to identify misuse of, alcohol and drugs. Support services such as Rape Crisis, Incest Survives and the Samaritans should be made available to clients. An up-to-date observation policy should be in place. Documentation of observations should include who is involved (e.g. the multi-disciplinary team) and who observes the client and their qualifications (qualified or unqualified). Safety needs and how it is ensured that observations are supportive and therapeutic and maintenance of the privacy and dignity should also be documented in the plan of care.

Finally, as in other benchmarks, audit is essential. Systems should be in place for staff, practitioners and carers to report practitioners who are abusive or harmful to clients. Critical incidents such as acts of violence, aggression, seclusion as well as procedures and policies should be audited regularly and actions that are taken, if required, should be documented. The monitoring of care can be used to determine resources necessary for clients as well as to monitor performance of staff and to inform training.

Activity

Reflect on how you create an environment in which care is provided that balances safe observations and privacy. Indicate how you regularly and actively involve clients in identifying care that meets their safety needs.

Principles of self-care

Self-care is described as 'the choices people make and the actions people take on their own behalf in the interest of maintaining their health and wellbeing' (DoH, Self-care, 2003:1). Self-care can be categorised as:

a. Self-management of health (lifestyle)
b. Self-management of health status information (monitoring and diagnosis)
c. Self-management of care choices (decisions)
d. Self-management of illness (treatment, care and rehabilitation)' (DoH, Self-care, 2003:1).

Patients/clients should be able to make choices about self-care and those choices should be respected. Their self-care abilities should be continuously assessed and inform care management. As noted in the benchmark above, a comprehensive ongoing risk assessment should be undertaken and every individual that is involved in the management of self-care including patients/clients/carers must become aware of inherent risks and how these may be addressed most appropriately. Within the context of the aforementioned, patients/clients and/or carers and advocates must have the knowledge and skills to manage all aspects of self-care and patients/clients and carers must work in partnership to establish their individual responsibilities in meeting self-care needs.

Within the health care context, patients/clients and/or their carers and advocates must understand and be able to access the services that the organisation provides. The environment in which care takes place must promote the patient's/client's ability to self-care. Patients/clients/carers must be able to access resources that enable them to meet individual self-care needs. In addition, they should be involved in planning and evaluating services. Therefore, patients/clients/carers must be made aware of all the available self and provided care options; appropriate consistent information should be provided and discussed. Finally, monitoring should be undertaken to ensure that care does reflect patient choice.

Activity

Document how patients/clients and/or their carers and advocates understand how to access services that your Primary Care Trust provides.

Communication between patients, carers and health care professionals

Communication is 'a process that involves a meaningful exchange between at least two people to covey facts, needs, opinions, thoughts, feelings or other information through both verbal and non-verbal means, including face to face exchanges and the written word' (DoH, Communication between patients, carers and health care professionals, 2003:1). Patients and carers should experience effective communication that is sensitive to their individual needs and preferences and additionally that the communication promotes high-quality care for the patient. Therefore, all health care personnel should 'demonstrate effective interpersonal skills when communicating with patients and or carers' (DoH, Communication between patients, carers and health care professionals, 2003:3). Communication should take place at a time and place that is acceptable to the patient/client/carer(s) and health care personnel. 'All patients' and or carers' communication needs should be assessed on initial contact and then regularly reassessed' (DoH, Communication between patients, carers and health care professionals, 2003:3). Furthermore, additional communication support such as provision of a health advocate for interpretation purposes should be negotiated and provided when a need is identified. Information that is accessible, acceptable, up to date and meets the needs of individuals should be consistently and actively shared and widely promoted across communities. Appropriate and effective methods of communication should be 'used actively to promote understanding between patients and or carers and health care personnel' (DoH, Communication between patients, carers and health care professionals, 2003:3). Essential elements to consider are that all patients and/or their carers must be able to communicate their individual needs and preferences at all times and that their contribution to patient care is valued, recorded and informs both patient care and health care personnel education with ongoing review (DoH, Communication between patients, carers and health care professionals, 2003). Therefore, to communicate effectively, you must ensure that particular attention is paid to the patients' and/or carers' hearing, vision and other physical and cognitive abilities as well as their preferred language and possible need for an interpreter.

Activity

Reflect on the methods of communication you use to actively promote understanding between patients and/or carers and health care personnel.

Promoting health

This benchmark (DoH, Promoting health, 2006b) provides a framework for shifting the focus from treating ill health to ensuring the promotion of healthier life choices, and is firmly embedded in all good patient care. There is an agreed person-centred outcome in which nurses support everyone so that they will make healthier choices for themselves and others. Within this benchmark, indicators of best practice are that:

'Individuals, groups and communities are helped to make positive decisions on personal health and well-being

Practitioners have and use their knowledge and skills to promote health

Individuals, groups and communities are able to identify their health promotion needs

Every appropriate contact is used to enable individuals, groups and communities to find ways to maintain or improve their health and well being

Individuals, groups and communities are actively involved in health promotion planning and actions

Health promotion is undertaken in partnership with others using a variety of expertise and experiences

People have access to health promoting information, services and/or support which meets their individual needs and circumstances

Individuals, groups, communities and agencies influence and create environments which promote peoples health and well being

Health promoting activity has a sustainable effect that improves the public's health' (DoH, Promoting health, 2006b:2).

For example, if the first indicator – 'Individuals, groups and communities are helped to make positive decisions on personal health and well-being' – is considered, then we see that in a person-centred approach the nurse would ensure there is access to advocacy services and interpreting services and that there is a comprehensive directory of local health-promoting services for people in their care. Within the GP practice setting or WiC, there is sign-posting of information and services for people. As a nurse, you ensure that decisions made by the patient/client/carer are based on informed choices and opportunities. You ensure that there are opportunities to participate in relevant programmes such as the 'the expert patient' or stop smoking programme and finally that there is evidence of directed or self-referral to health-promoting services within the GP setting or WiC.

Your health-promoting competencies should be linked to the Knowledge and Skills Framework (KSF) (NHS, 2008). The KSF defines and describes the knowledge and skills that you need to apply in your practice in order to deliver quality services. It provides a single, consistent, comprehensive and explicit framework on which to base review and development and allows for the operation and implementation of the Agenda for Change (DoH, 2004). It is a generic competency framework developed from existing best practice. Within this context, you should have a personal development plan (PDP) and personal portfolio (PP) that reflects health promotion training. You should demonstrate within the PP how you have shared best practice and that you can demonstrate an understanding of diversity and its impact on health.

Activity

Demonstrate in your PP how you have and use your knowledge and skills to promote health and to reduce health inequalities (DoH, Promoting health, 2006b).

Consider how the advice that you give is evidence based when you are suggesting the use of health care products or services (NMC, 2008).

By drawing on the Essence of Care Framework (DoH, 2003, 2006b), you will have the opportunity to improve the delivery of nursing and health care that is provided by you and other health care practitioners.

Conclusion

In summary, this chapter has focused on some of the core attributes and knowledge that are required to provide high-quality care. It has provided an introduction to the art and science of nursing which is fundamental to the delivery of high-quality nursing care and described how to deliver care that is sensitive to the patient's/client's/carer's personal needs whilst understanding the related scientific knowledge. In addition, this chapter has delineated a framework for describing and providing high-quality care. The core message in this chapter is the importance of delivering care that is focused on the needs of your patients/clients/carers and their best interests.

References

Carper, B. (1978) Fundamental patterns of knowing in nursing. *Advances in Nursing Science*, 1(10); 13–23.

DoH (2000) *The NHS Plan: A Plan for Investment, A Plan for Reform*. London: The Stationary Office, Department of Health.

DoH (2001) *Essence of Care*. London: The Stationary Office, Department of Health.

DoH (2003) *Essence of Care*. London: NHS Modernisation Agency, Department of Health.

DoH (2004) *Agenda for Change Final Agreement*, http://www.dh.gov.uk/en/ Publicationsandstatistics/Publications/PublicationsPolicyAndGuidance/DH_ 4095943 (accessed 17 August 2008).

DoH (2006a) *Modernising Nursing Careers – Setting the Direction*, www.dh.gov. uk/cno (accessed 17 August 2008).

DoH (2006b) *Essence of Care: Benchmarks for promoting Health*, http://www. dh.gov.uk/en/Publicationsandstatistics/Publications/PublicationsPolicyAndGuid ance/DH_075613 (accessed 17 August 2008).

DPA (1998) *Data Protection Act 1998*, http://www.opsi.gov.uk/Acts/Acts1998/ ukpga_19980029_en_1 (accessed 17 August 2008).

NHS (2008) *Knowledge and Skills Framework*, http://www.nhsemployers.org/ pay-conditions/pay-conditions-782.cfm (accessed 17 August 2008).

NMC (2008) *Code of Conduct, Nursing and Midwifery Council*. London, advice@nmc-uk.org, www.nmc-uk.org (accessed 1 October 2008).

RCN (2008) *Competencies. Advanced Nurse Practitioners – An RCN Guide to the Advanced Nurse Practitioner Role, Competencies and Programme Accreditation*. London: Royal College of Nursing, https://www.rcn.org.uk/__data/assets/pdf_ file/0003/146478/003207.pdf (www.rcn.org.uk) (accessed 1 October 2008).

Watson, J. (1999) *Postmodern Nursing and Beyond*. Edinburgh: Churchill Livingstone.

Domain 7

Respecting Culture and Diversity

Meeting the cultural and spiritual needs of patients in general practice and WiCs

17

Anjoti Harrington

Introduction

The aim of this chapter is to consider some of the contextual issues related to the cultural and spiritual needs of clients. Besides, some of the key concepts that help to define the best ways of delivering care will be examined. Following this critical discussion, a recommended framework for communication is examined that demonstrates sensitivity and respect towards clients from different backgrounds. The chapter includes a number of activities for readers to reflect on their current knowledge relating to diversity.

Learning Outcomes

- To demonstrate respect for the dignity of every human being, irrespective of their age, gender, religion, socio-economic class, sexual orientation and ethnic or cultural group
- To recognise the client's right to choose their care provider, participate in their care and refuse their care
- To promote diversity and equality
- To respect the inherent work and dignity of each person and their right to express spiritual beliefs
- To assess and value the influence that a client's spirituality has on their health care behaviours and practices.

Background

Terhune (2004:199) defines diversity as:

> Diversity is an elusive concept with multiple definitions and approaches in both scholarship and practice. However, diversity is relational. It is about the

exploration of the "other" and the self-examination of the internalized effects of that exploration. It is about critical reflection, dialogue, change, growth, and maturation, as well as creativity in thinking, knowing, being, and engaging in the world.

Clearly, diversity is multi-faceted. In a world where the diversity of ethnic, cultural and personal beliefs, values and lifestyles has never been greater, such relationships that walk-in-centre (WiC) nurses or practice nurses (PN) form with their clients require special attention. Client encounters, especially those in WiCs, can be brief, so it is essential to establish a timely and effective rapport. Care then can be thought of as a culturally mediated negotiation of the best ways forward. It is not simply a consumption of services that nurses and others provide, but an exploration of what might make most sense and seem best value to clients within the realistic confines of health care resources.

Respectful care is not delivered in a vacuum; it works within a series of contexts that are practical, philosophical and political. WiCs, for example, have been conceived as a means to increase access to health care resources for clients, and also to make better use of the resources available. General practice has been challenged to work more efficiently and effectively, especially in the face of a growing number of patients dealing with long-term conditions (Baggot, 2004). The advent of the new General Medical Services (new GMS) contract (DoH, 2003) has been a significant catalyst for the increasing development of services aimed at clients with long-term conditions. PNs play a significant part in the delivery of these services, with long-term conditions now being an essential service that all practices must provide (Drennan and Goodman, 2007).

Respecting culture and diversity, as a part of respectful care, has to work equally efficiently and effectively. We need better, rather than more, ways to quickly determine the needs of clients. If we are, for example, to both accommodate the growing number of patients who use WiCs (Salisbury et al., 2002) and recognise the diversity of patients and their requirements, we have to increase our understanding of culture as a mediator of health and illness and find ways to work with patients that make best use of cultural practices that enhance independence.

Equally important as a context are the related matters of patient dignity and nursing's aspirations towards holistic care. The drive to protect patient dignity is enshrined within government and health care organisation policy (e.g. Billericay, Brentwood and Wickford Primary Care Trust, 2006), but we need to be aware that dignity is a concept itself mediated by culture (Matiti, 2005). Our efforts to assist others are culturally coded.

Populations of people from different ethnic cultures are not equally distributed across the UK. The Home Office's National Statistics Census released the 2001 population survey in February 2003 and it reported that 8% of the UK population, that is, over 4.6 million people, came from an ethnic minority community. Refer Table 17.1. The South Asian community is the largest ethnic minority group living in the UK; they represent just over 4% of the population (ONC, 2001). This ethnic group consists of four sub-groups, namely Indian: 1.8%, Pakistani: 1.3%,

Table 17.1 Major Population Groups in the UK (ONC, 2001)

Ethnic group	Number (to nearest 1,000)	Total % of UK population
Total population	58,790,000	100
White	54,150,000	92.1
All minorities	4,640,000	7.9
Indian	1,053,000	1.8
Pakistani	747,000	1.3
Black Caribbean	566,000	0.9
Black African	485,000	0.8
Bangladeshi	283,000	0.5
Chinese	247,000	0.4
Other	240,000	0.4

Bangladeshi: 0.5% and other Asians: 0.4%. The South Asian culture is very diverse and it encompasses many languages and dialects, religions, beliefs, histories and countries of origin (DoH, 1995).

According to Ethnic Diversity in the UK (www.ipa.co.uk, 2008), data from the 2001 Home Office Census show that ethnic minority groups are more likely to live in England than any other country in the UK. They make up 9% of the total population; 3% live in Scotland and Wales and 1% live in Northern Ireland. In London, ethnic minorities make up 29% of the population. The report also noted that ethnic minority communities are larger in the following areas of England where they make up a respectable percentage of the total population:

1. the West Midlands 13%;
2. the South East England 8%;
3. North West England 8%;
4. Yorkshire and the Humber 7%.

With regard to the South East, the London borough of Tower Hamlets has a multi-culturally diverse population; it includes Bangladeshi, Chinese, Somalis, Pakistanis, Africans, Caribbeans, Asians, mixed race and White Indigenous group (ONC, 2001).

The last context that we should consider concerns the confidence and the experience of the nurse, whether as a PN or WiC nurse. Nurses who come to practice from relatively homogenous communities will require a form of induction and professional development different to that required by nurses who come to practice from more heterogeneous communities. Staff development, therefore, needs to focus on related dialogues, such as: between the nurse and the health care system, and between the nursing care provided there and the nature of health care needs and situations presented by patients from different ethnic communities.

Key concepts

We have already made reference to some concepts that enable us to appreciate more respectful forms of care and it is now time to examine these in detail. Some of the concepts that we use daily are referenced against personal meanings and it is helpful to check whether we are all thinking in the same way. Some of the inequalities that exist within society and especially within health care are based on the different ways in which concepts are understood and used (Balarajan and Raleigh, 1995; Nazroo, 1998; Wanless, 2001; Aspinall and Jacobson, 2004).

Respect

Let us start with the concept of respect. Tschudin (2003:34) examined this concept and remarked that: 'we do not always like someone at first sight. However, in caring we respect a person first of all, and this may sometimes surprisingly lead to a mutual liking'. The Oxford Advanced Learner's Dictionary (1999:999) defines respect as: 'to show consideration or care for something'. Respect for a client's faith and culture is vital when one considers the ethics of care. Noddings (1984) reports that care is rooted in receptivity (a person is received or accepted as he or she is), relatedness (receiving someone and being aware of someone's presence or being) and responsiveness (a professional relationship is created to accommodate the other person's presence). However, the Nursing and Midwifery Council (NMC) makes it explicit in *The Code* that it is imperative for nurses and midwives to treat people as individuals and to respect their dignity (NMC, 2008). Therefore, unlike Noddings (1984), the person (i.e. the client) must be accepted as he or she is by the nurse or midwife.

From the concept of ethical care giving, it means that PNs and WiC nurses need to pay more attention by being willing to give 'diverse groups' time and be willing to understand their physical, emotional and spiritual needs; be sympathetically understanding about their concerns; and be aware of how their relationship or interaction with the client can hinder or promote health and well-being. In these terms, respect is not determined by the extent to which others are like us, but in terms of the diversity and richness they have been exposed to. Respect is based on a commitment to variety and the potential that this offers to the society.

Ethnicity

The following is an example on how an advanced nurse practitioner (ANP), based in a WiC, addresses meeting the needs of her diverse practice population:

> The Walk-in-Centre where I work is in the East End of London. Staff see people of a huge variety of ages, social situations, ethnicities and cultures. I find it an enormous challenge to manage the different consultations that result from seeing clients from such diverse backgrounds. Language is an obvious and immediate difficulty. Often clients will bring a friend or relative to translate, which is an enormous help. There are of course obvious drawbacks to this set up. I remember one time informing a lady (via her husband) that she was pregnant, only 8 months after the birth of her first child.

The husband was delighted, the lady clearly not. I wished I had been more sensitive to the situation and found a way to tell the lady alone. As there is a large Bangladeshi population, the reception staff were originally recruited largely from the same population as it was felt they would be able to help with translation. There are problems to this: Often, the receptionists are busy doing their work and unwilling or unable to come and assist in what may be a long and drawn out consultation. In addition, they may not have had much, if any training in medical translation. It is much easier to work with a professional advocate who can translate directly when this is needed and advocate when this is needed, and who knows which role they should take on and when. However, having someone in the room to translate is far preferable to having to use a service such as language line. This is an invaluable service, but I find it extremely difficult to remember what I want to ask and be succinct and to the point when I am handed the phone. Also, if I then want to do a physical examination, the conversation has to stop and then I either phone the language line again or try to have covered all eventualities before hanging up. Neither is ideal, and I do not feel often I have connected with the patient and really understood what is going in.

Another aspect is culture. I believe 'cultural competence' comes down to two things: never making assumptions and having the confidence to ask people what they mean, when as the other day, a patient said they had a 'normal Indian meal' for example. What does that mean? Probably, very different things to different individuals. I do not have a problem with asking any patient whether they drink alcohol or smoke or use other drugs, even if they 'appear' that they may be adhering to one religion or another. And I find patients do not mind answering the question. One interesting aspect of culture perhaps is people's description of symptoms. Certain groups of patients may complain of being 'hot in the head' which over time I find often means they have a headache. Another common one is 'total body pain' which is often it seems, synonymous with what I might call depression. But not always; it is essential to ask people what they mean. I find people do not mind being asked!

For me, the important aspect of ethnicity is that of propensity to disease. I know that for example, South Asian populations have a much greater risk of Type II Diabetes Mellitus than the Caucasian population. Therefore, in consultations with groups at higher risk I am careful to ask about family history of diabetes, to look at risk factors and symptoms closely and have a lower threshold for offering a random or fasting blood sugar test.

Similarly it is important to consider which drugs may be more effective in different groups: The British Hypertension Society guidelines for blood pressure management vary according to the person's ethnic origin. Certain groups are also at higher risk of complications: for example stroke and end stage renal failure as a result of diabetes are much more common among the black population than in non-blacks. Therefore, these patients need to be managed

110% in terms of their glycaemic control, their blood pressure control and renal function. In the WiC, of course, this is not an area we would manage ourselves; but we do have a responsibility to make sure the patient is aware of the need to manage their illness well, and it is our responsibility to try to ensure this happens.

In short, ethnicity where I work is very important, as it determines how a patient may be assessed and managed in terms of physical illness. This is I feel the major relevance of this Domain to nursing. Otherwise we are all individuals. (Vicky Lack, ANP/lecturer)

Race and culture

Having examined the issue of ethnicity, it is also necessary to explore other definitions such as race and culture. Johnson (2003) states that the term 'race' denotes a primary characteristic which is inherent, biological and physical; its origin is from genetic descent and it is a permanent feature. On the other hand, culture is a behavioural expression, written or spoken language and the style of dressing that people wear, type of food they eat and their home furnishing. It is hard to identify behavioural or personal culture because it is acquired unconsciously (Henley and Schott, 1999). Our own culture becomes noticeable when we meet other people from a different society or country. An outsider may have very little knowledge about a person's value system or custom. Therefore, part of treating other individuals with respect requires a person to be willing to enquire about their culture, values and norms.

Johnson (2003:3) suggests that in traditional anthropological terms, there are four major human 'races'. He categorises them as 'Caucasian' – White or European; 'Negroid' – Black or African; 'Mongoloid' – Asian, Chinese or Indic; and 'Australoid' – the Aboriginals. Race, therefore, is a concept that has no obvious purchase on health care unless we discuss conditions or risks that are inherently associated with a common genetic ancestry and where the understanding of race helps us to understand risk and formulate better treatments. Ethnic group or ethnicity is an identity; it is multi-faceted and 'political', socially constructed internally and externally, and also legal. It could also be situational and negotiated. Hillier (1991), cited in Henley and Schott (1999:xxi), defines an ethnic group as a social group with distinctive language, values, religion, customs and attitudes.

A sample of studies examining the role of ethnicity on health status demonstrates the importance of understanding the link between ethnicity and health. In the USA, the concept of ethnicity has been applied extensively to the study of hypertension amongst American Blacks in whom hypertension is more common and more aggressive than other ethnic groups (Amudha et al., 2003). A study in South Africa found that whilst coronary heart disease (CHD) is 'epidemic' in the White and Indian population, it is still uncommon in the Black community (Seedat, 1999).

Higher levels of cardiovascular disease are seen in the Southeast Asian population, which is often associated with higher levels of diabetes mellitus, familial hypercholesterolaemia and waist circumference. Johnson and Rawlings-Anderson (2007) further elaborate that whilst populations of African and Afro-Caribbean descent have lower levels of CHD, they have higher levels of hypertension and stroke. What these previous studies demonstrate is the relationship between ethnicity and health status. Therefore, it is imperative that a client's ethnicity is explored during a client consultation by a PN or a WiC nurse. The example provided by the ANP demonstrates how this practitioner is alerted to the predisposition of clients from some racial groups (i.e. South Asian) to diabetes mellitus compared to other racial groups.

Activity

Reflect on when you as a practitioner explore ethnicity during a client consultation.
   Once you have established a client's ethnicity, what research evidence do you use to individualise your consultation?

Nursing is usually more intimately associated with culture and ethnic lifestyles. The culture that individuals learn, that which has developed over generations, is something that we must work closely with as it influences definitions of wellness, progress, and desirable and undesirable behaviours. It influences not only the conception of health formed by an ethnic minority, but also the form that health care takes as conceived by the ethnic majority. It is in these terms that respectful care becomes complex, for we are all products of our culture and yet work with a nursing ethos that encourages us to understand and support others (NMC, 2008).

Religion

Religious beliefs can be influential in ethnic identity. Religious customs and beliefs may be the most important defining feature of an ethnic lifestyle and perhaps of an ethnic community. Religion is defined by Fulcher and Scott (2005) as a system of beliefs through which people organise and order their lives. Islam, for example, provides detailed guidance on how to conduct daily life and is not readily disaggregated into weekly religious services or periodic festivals, compared to Catholicism, for example.

However, regardless of the religious persuasion of clients, the NMC (2008) emphasises the importance of treating people as individuals and respecting their dignity. Surely, one of the cornerstones of treating individuals with respect and dignity is acknowledging their religious choice? However, there are some occasions when an individual's religious choice can have a negative impact on their health outcomes. Such an example can be where a Jehovah's Witness refuses to have a blood transfusion for themselves or for a child, when the condition is life threatening. In rare cases such as the previous, a court order may be obtained that overrides the wishes of the individual.

> ## Activity
>
> Consider the example of the Jehovah's Witness. Are there any examples you can reflect on in practice where religious and/or other preferences have shaped an individual's decision? What are your thoughts on this?

Henley and Schott (1999) discuss the positive influence of religion on an individual's life in providing meaning, spiritual support and moral guidance. Religion is also said to strongly affect people's health beliefs and ways in which health should therefore be sustained as can be seen in Table 17.2 (Spector, 2004).

The concepts of religion and spirituality become key when we consider nurses' aspirations to deliver holistic care. What, in practice, represents spiritual care and how can spiritual care be represented when the client encounters illness and health care? In some Western conceptions, the notion of spirituality is rather more loosely associated with a sense of purpose, of living with one's values and beliefs intact, those pertaining to a wide variety of life decisions (Galek et al., 2005). We can be 'spiritual' without being religious. In many ethnic minority communities though, the notion of spiritual health is closely bound with religion and the observance of religious customs and duties (Helman, 2001). For example, we may often see an Asian

Table 17.2 Examples of Traditional Health Maintenance.

	Physical	Mental	Spiritual
Maintain health	Wear proper clothing, eat a balanced diet, exercise and rest	Maintain family relationships to gain social support and respect the elders, develop some hobbies and pray to God	Faithfully pray daily or worship, meditate and adhere to religious rituals or requirement
Protect health	Eat special food and food combinations, for example, hot or cold food, rich or bland meals. Wear symbolic clothing such as a head scarf; wear warm clothes in winter or jewellery to ward off evil spirits. Practice sexual activity as per religious rituals, for example, no sex during menstruation as it is classed as dirty	Avoid certain people who can cause illness. Limit certain family activities, for example, pub and clubs. Consumption of alcohol. Attendance at family get-together parties, for example, weddings, celebrations of birthday's, etc.	Adhere to religious customs, for example, fasting. Wear symbolic amulets and other symbolic objects to prevent the 'Evil Eye' or defray other sources of harm. Practice magic – religious folk medicine, for example, use charm bracelets, waist bands and chant holy words to prevent and cure illnesses
Restore health	Use homeopathic medicine, take herbal medicine, eat special food, massage, acupuncture or colonic lavage	Relaxation, exorcism, see a faith healer	Pursue a pilgrimage, exorcism, meditation

Source: Modified and adapted from Spector (2004:77). Permission obtained from Pearson Prentice Hall.

man with a red spot on his forehead; this indicates to someone who understands the Asian religious customs of the individual that the man had been to the temple, he has prayed and the priest has put the spot on his forehead as an acknowledgement of praying and what might be called spiritual grace in Christian parlance.

Whilst religion and spirituality are closely bound up with ethnic culture, we should not assume that the relationship is static. Some people make choices early in life that they will practice their religious faith and others may take up their religion seriously in times of ill health or when they are reaching death as a final stage of life. Patel et al. (1998) have reported that many young Blacks and ethnic minority groups return to religion when they grow older and others may turn to new faiths or denominations. There are similarities to how health is viewed across the life span. Blaxter (2001) explored the concept of health and concluded that the way health is conceived differs over the life span. She found that younger men tended to speak about health in terms of physical strength and fitness, whilst younger women favoured ideas of energy, vitality and the ability to cope. In middle age, concepts of health were associated with total mental and physical wellbeing, whilst older people viewed health in terms of functionality, contentment and happiness. This demonstrates the importance that age can play on an individual's health beliefs.

Key concepts and diversity

We can now sum up the above key concepts in order to understand the final and overarching concept, which is diversity. Clients with certain shared, racial/genetic backgrounds may be more prone to having to deal with particular health care problems, as we have already discussed.

Association with an ethnic group and its values and practices might also serve to support the patient or to enhance the risks that they face, because the individual reasons, 'this is how we do things and this is what is normal'. An understanding of health belief models such as *The Health Belief Model* (HBM) (Becker, 1974) can assist the practitioner in developing an insight into the underpinning views and beliefs that can shape a client's behaviour.

Although the HBM was initially developed with reference to health promotion, it has been widely applied to the management of long-term diseases. The principal components of the HBM are:

- perceived susceptibility: a person's own view of their health risks which may arise from their condition;
- perceived severity: a person's own evaluation of the consequences (health and social) of contracting the disease or its side effects;
- perceived benefits: the benefits the person believes can be gained by following recommended advice;
- perceived barriers: the negative aspects associated with undertaking recommended health care (Becker, 1974).

What emerges within a health consultation whether with a PN or a WiC nurse can be a complex interaction considering the health beliefs that a client brings with them. However, much as practitioners might hope to offer to each a standard prescription for managing diabetes, asthma, heart disease, obesity or depression, they must acknowledge that whilst there may be a finite number of health problems, there are a diverse number of ways of experiencing and dealing with these because of a client's health beliefs. If we are to engage the client as a partner in care, someone whom we assist to take charge of their situation, then we need to engage them with a respect for the contexts in which they cope with the health issue. It is then necessary to work with the health beliefs, experiences and preferences that they bring with them.

A framework for care

In order to respect a client's health care decisions, practitioners must know how to communicate clearly with the client and the client's family to develop a mutual understanding of each other's cultures. Henley and Schott (1999) suggest that health professionals need to demonstrate a willingness to learn about each patient's beliefs and needs by saying that most people are happy to explain provided they are asked in a respectful way and at an appropriate time. Munoz and Luckman (2005:12) note that:

> to improve your interaction with patients from other cultures, you should assess each patient's level of understanding rather than assume that a patient understands what you are saying.

Culturally competent care involves attending to the total context of the patient's situation, and his/her physical, social, emotional and spiritual needs. Spector (2004) states it is necessary to view culture as a luggage that each of us carries around for our lifetime. Furthermore, Spector (2004) elaborates that culture is the sum of beliefs, practices, habits, likes, dislikes, norms, customs and rituals that we have learnt from our families during our socialisation.

What frames successful care then is a communication approach that helps us to explore preferences, needs and assumptions. Because our care encounters may be quite brief, it is important that this can be reduced to a useful aide-memoire that reminds us what we are doing (refer Figure 17.1).

This aide-memoire constructed for this chapter is: communicate, explore and sensitively ask (CESA). It has been developed from Munoz and Luckman's (2005) Chapter 11: *Eliciting Assessment Data from Patient, Family and Interpreters*.

The following describes how this framework (i.e. CESA) can be used in the clinical setting. Each of these sections will now be examined.

Communicate

Begin by approaching the patient slowly, greeting them respectfully and waiting for the patient to acknowledge your presence (Townsend, 2001 cited in Munoz

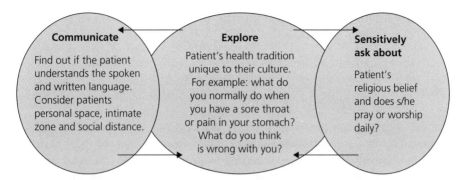

Figure 17.1 A CESA framework for assessment of needs (Munoz and Luckman, 2005)

and Luckman, 2005). Introduce yourself by name and your status. Explain to the client that they can speak freely to you about their symptoms and fears. Let them know that the information that they impart with you will be shared with other health professionals in order to provide them with a diagnosis and treatment.

Whilst we have yet to navigate what will seem pertinent and sensitively put questions, communicating in this way establishes that there is a supportive purpose for the communication. At best, it allows that others might be involved too if this is the client's preference.

We can describe this as the start of a therapeutic relationship. Munoz and Luckman (2005:143) state: 'therapeutic communication is goal oriented'; the goal is to help patients from different cultures. They suggest that we should explore:

- what the patient has experienced and in what ways their values and beliefs about their health, illness and type of treatment they expect affect this;
- with the patient what might represent realistic, specific, achievable, measurable and timely health goals;
- ways in which a recommended medical or nursing intervention might assist the patient with their physical, mental, social and spiritual well-being.

Next, inform the client of what you hope to do for him/her and offer the client opportunities when they can ask you questions. Nod occasionally and ask pertinent questions about them and their health problems. Be aware of your facial and bodily expressions when communicating with clients from a different culture. Touch, for example, is culturally important. You should avoid touching the patient as routine, even if it is an accepted norm in your own culture and a personal preference as a means of reassuring patients.

You will need to determine whether the client speaks, writes or understands the English language. Does he or she need a translator? Find out if the client is willing to disclose his/her signs and symptoms with you. Is the client able to listen to you and understand you? Minimise the use of medical jargon; consider voice tone and speed of speech, which can all affect a client's understanding and willingness to talk to health care professionals. Convey your willingness to assist the individual with his/her health problem. It is important to convey empathy and to acknowledge the client's fears or anxieties.

Explore

Offer the client a quiet place to sit where you will not be disturbed during your consultation, but remember that isolation could worry a client if their partner or other family member has not been invited to join you. Adopt a formal approach when taking a medical history or assessment. If the client has brought a companion, check out if s/he wishes the companion to be in attendance when you are going to ask about their health problem.

It may not be deemed respectful to address older patients by their first name. Using a formal term of address is especially important with older patients. Some Asian patients find it difficult to fully share their health problem and they could be hesitant to divulge all the signs and symptoms of their illness. For these reasons, you may have to approach sensitive subjects more slowly and then to offer a short rationale as to why you are making the particular enquiry. Munoz and Luckman (2005) suggest that establishing rapport is not difficult and they recommend health care professionals initially ask the client non-health-related questions, for example, 'where are you from? How long have you lived in the UK? Do you like living here? Is your family living with you?'. If the client feels comfortable with these initial questions, then they may be more comfortable in talking about their presenting complaint.

Active listening is vital when engaging in a dialogue with a client. It is important for the practitioner to consider the seating arrangements in the consultation room. If, for example, the client appears uneasy, pull up a chair and position yourself parallel to or lower than the patient. This position helps the client to feel more in control and you may appear more supportive (Munoz and Luckman, 2005). You might also mirror the client's use of eye contact, whether increasing or decreasing eye contact as appropriate for that culture.

Health professional staff can offer a little personal disclosure to help establish a rapport. For example, 'I get a bit of indigestion pain if I have eaten so much fatty food' or 'I have difficulty sleeping if I go to bed immediately after a big meal'. Remember to use minimum disclosure; this is only to establish a comfortable, engaging and reassuring way to put your patient at ease.

Sensitively ask

If you suspect that the health care problem could impact on or be influenced by religious customs or observances, you will need to make discrete enquiries in this area. For example, 'I wonder whether your problem (e.g., a client with diabetes mellitus) has affected the chance to conduct your religion as you would like?'

Alternatively, 'Can you tell me about your religious observances? I want to understand what might have been difficult for you here'.

Allow silence as a communication technique when appropriate. 'Silence gives your patient time to reflect and speak' (Munoz and Luckman, 2005:155). They also cite Davidhizar and Geiger (1994) who state that some patients who belong to religious groups are sometimes silent because they believe that they are listening to and communicating with God (Munoz and Luckman, 2005). Therefore:

- Do not interrupt short silences even if this temporarily makes you feel uncomfortable. If the patient looks lost, say gently: 'you seem quiet and you may wish to have a bit more time to think about what you want to say, do let me know what your feelings and thoughts are when you can'. Do not pressurise the patient to talk but encourage the client by saying: 'I can see you seem upset, perhaps we can talk about what is troubling you'.
- Some clients may choose to show fear and anxiety by crying. Provide support if the client expresses emotions of fear, anxiety or distress by saying: 'It is alright to cry. I can tell you don't like talking right now, so I'll just sit here with you for a few minutes'.
- Be silent yourself and let the client initiate conversation. Sitting quietly with a client may encourage the person to break the silence and communicate verbally with you.
- Pay attention to non-verbal communication. Touch the client only when you know that touching is permissible in that culture. Avoid touching a Vietnamese, Cambodian or Thai child on the head because the head is traditionally considered the site of the soul in these cultures.
- Do not touch any religious armlet or bracelet that a client is wearing and if you require it to be removed, ask the client if he/she can move it away so that you can examine that part of the body.

Within the above framework, it is important to give extra consideration to the matter of probing experiences of illness or treatment and understanding how the client interprets these. Discussing the ways in which we experience the body is an intimate matter. As you explore topics with the client, you need to be alert to the following expressions:

- that which is seen as stigmatising, lowering the status or honour of the individual or family;
- that which is best dealt with through a single sex conversation or perhaps even discussed with a representative of the client;
- that which explains the cause of illness or a problem (e.g. refuting the patient's sincere explanation of a cause of illness in terms of 'bad karma' would be extremely insensitive; it is better to discuss what additional factors may have been influential);

■ areas where your treatment or guidance competes with other preferred ways of proceeding (this may arise, for instance, where alternative medicines are taken with or instead of conventional medication);
■ concern regarding what you or others consider to be normal or acceptable (e.g. the acceptable means of disciplining children may vary from culture to culture).

In these instances, it may be more appropriate to make a note to return to the subject matter again after consulting on the best ways to proceed. Poorly handled communication in culturally sensitive areas can lead to the consultation being curtailed or terminated.

We have now reached the point where we can conclude the factors surrounding culture and diversity and how these impact on health care delivery as perceived by the client. If we set aside the traditional notion that culture, ethnicity, religion and spirituality are factors that can interfere with the real business of promoting health and treating injury or illness, we can then start to plan care that is respectful and sensitive to a client's needs. Instead of treating diabetes mellitus, we help a client from a particular cultural background to manage their illness. The emphasis on the client and their management of a problem is instructive. We can only achieve this if we are ready to re-examine our own understanding of some important concepts and to remember the contexts in which we deliver health care. Consultation times of a PN or a WiC nurse per client may be condensed into 10–15-min appointment times. Therefore, developing expertise in consultation skills is imperative to ensure a successful consultation.

Activity

This leads to some exercises that you can undertake to examine the communities that you come into contact with.

1. Investigate what ethnic communities are part of your practice population. Identify the strategies you have used to engage with these communities. Are there any concerns that these communities have expressed about their health care?
2. Complete a series of personal reflections and local discussions regarding the key contexts and concepts shared here. Have you, for instance, clarified what it really means to deliver holistic care as a WiC nurse or as a PN? What do we really know about dignity, other than what we would consider dignified ourselves? To what extent are we trapped by ethnocentric ideas of nursing care – that which is most acceptable or helpful? Have we clearly distinguished between race, culture and ethnicity?
3. Identify where you have gaps in your knowledge about culture and lifestyle. Ascertain whether there are study days or courses that you can go on, or better still, whether there are individuals from an ethnic community who might agree to act as a consultant to you and colleagues, explaining important points.
4. Examine the resources that are provided in your place of work. Are these sufficient? What improvements could you recommend here?

Conclusion

This chapter has examined meeting the cultural and spiritual needs of clients. The population of the UK is growing and becoming more ethnically diverse. The diversity of the population brings opportunities for all to gain a greater understanding of other cultures. Within the health care context, it is crucial for health care professionals to develop an understanding of the communities that they serve, so that consultations with clients from diverse groups are effective, particularly when research evidence has identified that certain ethnic groups have higher degrees of morbidity in relation to some long-term conditions. Therefore, the PN or WiC nurse needs to ensure that their consultation is both relevant and pertinent to that client. The CESA framework has been developed as an aide-memoire to use in a client consultation, which emphasises the importance of skilful communication.

Finally, although the chapter has specifically focused on meeting the cultural and spiritual needs of diverse populations, it also provides an opportunity for the reader to reflect on how they communicate with the communities that they serve.

References

Amudha, K., Wong, L., Choy, A. and Lang, C. (2003) Ethnicity and drug therapy for hypertension. *Current Pharmaceutical Design*, 9(21); 1691–1701.

Aspinall, P. and Jacobson, B. (2004). *Ethnic Disparities in Health and Health Care: A Focused Review of the Evidence and Selected Example of Good Practice*. London: Health Observatory.

Baggot, R. (2004). *Health and Health Care in Britain*. Basingstoke: Palgrave.

Balarajan, R. and Raleigh, S. (1995) *Ethnicity and Health in England*. London: HMSO.

Becker, M. (1974) *The Health Belief Model and Personal Health Behaviour*. New Jersey: Slack.

Billericay, Brentwood and Wickford Primary Care Trust (2006). *Policy for Privacy and Dignity* (TCP028), www.bbw-pct.nhs.uk/Policies (accessed 1 May 2008).

Blaxter, M. (2001) What is health? In Davey, B., Gray, A. and Seale, C. (Eds.) *Health and Disease: A Reader*. 3rd edn. Buckingham: Open University Press.

DoH (1995) *Delivering Race Equality in Mental Health Care*. London: Department of Health.

DoH (2003) *New General Medical Services Contract*. London: Department of Health, http://www.dh.gov.uk/en/Managingyourorganisation/Humanresourcesand training/Modernisingpay/GPcontracts/DH_072341 (accessed 27 April 2009).

Drennan, V. and Goodman, C. (2007). *Oxford Handbook of Primary Care and Community Nursing*. Oxford: Oxford University Press.

Fulcher, J. and Scott, J. (2005). *Sociology*. London: Oxford University Press.

Galek, K., Flannelly, K., Vane, A. and Galek, R. (2005). Assessing a patient's spiritual needs – A comprehensive instrument. *Holistic Nursing Practice*, 19(2); 62–69.

Helman, C. (2001). *Culture, Health and Illness*. London: Arnold.

Henley, A. and Schott, J. (1999). *Culture, Religion and Patient Care in a Multi-ethnic Society: A Handbook for Professionals*. London: Age Concern.

Hornby, A.S. and Wehmeier, S. (Eds) (2005) Oxford Advanced Learners Dictionary. 7th Ed. Oxford: Oxford University Press.

Johnson, M. (2003). Ethnic diversity in social context. In Kai, J. (Ed.) *Ethnicity, Health and Primary Care*. Oxford: University Press.

Johnson, K. and Rawlings-Anderson, K. (2007). *Oxford Handbook of Cardiac Nursing*. Oxford: Oxford University Press.

Matiti, M. (2005). Patient dignity: Everyone's business in healthcare. *Diversity in Health and Social Care*, 2(4); 259–261.

Munoz, C. and Luckman, J. (2005) *Transcultural Communication in Nursing*. New York: Thomson, Delamar Learning.

Nazroo, J. (1998) Genetic, cultural or socioeconomic vulnerability? Explaining ethnic inequalities in health. *Sociology of Health and Illness*, 20; 714–734.

NMC (2008). *The Code. Standards of Conduct, Performance and Ethics for Nurses and Midwives*. London: Nursing and Midwifery Council.

Noddings, N. (1984). *Caring: A Feminine Approach to Ethics and Moral Education*. Berkley, CA: University of California.

ONC (2001) *National Statistic Online*. UK: Office of National Census, www.statistics.gov.uk (accessed 1 December 2007).

Patel, N., Naik, D. and Humphrey, B. (1998) *Vision of Reality: Religion and Ethnicity in Social Work*. London: CCWETSW.

Salisbury, C., Chalder, M., Manku-Scott, T., Nicholas, R., Deave, T., Noble, S., Pope, C., Moore, L., Coast, J., Anderson, E., Weiss, M., Grant, C. and Sharp, D. (2002) *The National Evaluation of NHS Walk-in-centres*. Bristol: University of Bristol.

Seedat, Y. (1999). Ethnicity, hypertension, coronary heart disease and renal diseases in South Africa. *Ethnicity & Health*, 1(4); 349–357.

Spector, R. (2004) *Cultural Diversity in Health and Illness*. New Jersey: Pearson Prentice Hall.

Terhune, C. (2004) From desegregation to diversity: How far have we really come? *Journal of Nursing Education*, 43(5); 195–196.

Tschudin, V. (2003) *Ethics in Nursing – The Caring Relationship*. London: Butterworth.

Wanless, D. (2001). *Securing Our Future, taking a Long Term View, An Interim Report*. London: HM Treasury, www.hm-treasury.gov.uk. (accessed 1 April 2008).

Cultural diversity within the general practice and walk-in-centre settings

18

Maisie Allen

Introduction

"It is much more important to know what sort of a patient has a disease than what sort of disease a patient has" (William Osler, cited in Dubos, 1997:1).

The aim of this chapter is to take a pragmatic approach to help nurses understand the complex topic of multiculturalism in professional practice. Primary care nurses (PCNs) are frequently in the privileged position of introducing people to the National Health Service (NHS), seeing people for the first time as they register and remaining close to the community in which they practice. Nurses practicing in inner city areas constantly interact with richly diverse communities, presenting them with many opportunities to learn about other cultures and becoming culturally intelligent. Daily, they will come across people who are and act differently from themselves just as they too will appear different to others. They will come across people who react, in ways they do not understand, to seemingly ordinary situations. Nurses like others would have learnt intuitively, and sometimes backed up by cultural knowledge, how to negotiate the unchartered channels of multiculturalism and how to deal with the feelings that unfamiliar situations bring. Nurses as professionals in primary care can bridge the cultural gap and make the difference to patients from different cultures to tackle the health inequalities of ethnic minorities in the UK.

Learning Outcomes

- To understand the complex nature of multiculturalism in professional practice
- To become culturally aware of the diverse nature of cultures
- To comprehend the processes in becoming culturally competent
- To identify how multiculturalism and diversity impact on health.

Background

Culture is a 'soft' but dynamic concept, powerful and deeply rooted. We all exist within our own culture which we defend vehemently but yet we are unaware of the subtle ongoing changes within our own culture. In times of illness and when feeling vulnerable and confused, there is a tendency to cling to familiar surroundings, objects and rituals for comfort. By simply being aware, the professional nurse becomes more sensitive and more open to the emotional and cultural needs of patients, therefore gaining their trust and cooperation.

Cultural awareness and cultural knowledge training are poorly addressed in the NHS. Multiculturalism tends to get hijacked by the more dominant political 'diversity' agenda. In a developed society, diversity and multiculturalism should go together hand in hand. However, there is a slippery slope of being seen and heard to do the right thing paying lip service to a serious issue. Cultural knowledge and competency training are not well delivered and more often serve to categorise and reinforce stereotypical ideas of people within other cultures unifying their characteristics and highlighting differences. It is not easy for an individual alone to challenge dominant Western attitude of 'we know best'.

To understand multiculturalism and become culturally competent, it is important for nurses to first understand their own individual, professional and organisational culture. When we understand our own culture and its rituals, it becomes easier to understand the other cultural layers we take on through life and other people's cultures.

Nature, nurture, culture

Culture can be described as the collective mix of how different groups of people think, feel and act. These can be recognised in the way particular groups of people greet each other, eat, demonstrate feelings and observe social boundaries. Hofstede (2003) describes culture on two levels. In his view, culture in its narrow sense is described in Western languages as 'civilisation' such as education, art and literature. At a deeper level, culture is considered to be a collective programming of the mind which distinguishes members of one group or category of people from another. Culture is different from human nature. It comes from the individual's social environment and is learned rather than inherited.

In health care, the diverse racial, ethnic and socio-cultural backgrounds of nurses and their patients present daily challenges to how quality care is provided in all NHS settings. Cultural and language differences are likely to cause misunderstanding which can lead to perceived misuse of services and lack of compliance by patients which in turn can impact on the patient's health outcome (NHS, 2008a).

Culture is complex and is more often described in narrow terms such as *people being different and doing things differently*. If patients are 'doing things differently', it means nurses are also 'doing things differently'. This means that nurses must consider the impact of their own culture during their interactions with patients, how their own culture has shaped their values and their thinking and how these may influence their conversations with patients and subsequently the decisions they will make.

If, as Hofstede (2003) says culture is learnt and human nature inherited, this means that there are aspects of culture we learn and others that are intrinsic to our being which makes us unique. He suggests there are close links between what is referred to as human nature – what are inherited through our genes; culture – what is learned; and our mental programming – our personality which is each individual's unique way of perceiving and interpreting the world. These are the attributes that make us individual, unique and diverse. Multiculturalism is the many layers of culture within our own society with additional cultures from different parts of the world which we absorb, adopt or distance ourselves from.

The terms 'multiculturalism and diversity' tend to be used interchangeably referring to race and ethnicity, that is, to groups of people who can mainly be recognised as being visibly or not so visibly different, for example, Black and minority ethnics (BME) regardless of whether they were born and raised in the UK. However, diversity, cultural awareness and cultural knowledge have different approaches.

Compliance with Equal Opportunities and Human Rights legislation has tended to drive NHS organisations to take political and bureaucratic approaches when dealing with a diverse workforce and communities. Despite the growth in the number of policies, equality schemes and diversity committees, there is still no real shift on the health inequality agenda. Legislation shifts behaviour but rarely beliefs, that is, the lens through which we see situations. The diversity agenda focuses heavily on risk avoidance, meeting risks and monitoring standards. At best, the policies can demonstrate a process and at worst they can further polarise the views of decision-makers and confuse an issue to be managed or a problem to be solved (Wood et al., 2006). However, it is important to acknowledge that Equal Opportunities and Human Rights legislation in the UK is ahead of other European countries.

Activity

How do you understand the terms 'multiculturalism and diversity'?
How are diversity, cultural awareness and cultural knowledge approached in your practice setting?

Nursing in a diverse and multicultural NHS

The NHS is the largest employer in the UK with more then 1.2 million employees with approximately 400,000 nurses of which 8% are from BME backgrounds. The numbers are higher in larger urban areas, for example, London, than in rural areas. The NHS is also the largest employer of BME staff, making up 14% of the overall workforce (NHS, 2006).

This is a significant number of the workforce who comes from diverse backgrounds and cultures bringing with them their unique perspective and personal experiences of health, illness and health care delivery. The different ethnic groups that make up the NHS are in themselves diverse. There are age differences, established immigrant communities and new arrivals, and cultural and religious differences which do not make them homogenous groups. We cannot assume one understanding of what it means to be Asian or Chinese. However, they all share a common experience of discrimination which influences how they view the NHS and those who provide health services (Coker, 1999). As the largest employer in Europe, and the third largest employer in the world, it can be assumed that the organisation represents the multicultural society that is the UK. However, the NHS persistently fails to meet the needs of its ethnic population. This failure on the part of the NHS is recognised by the Department of Health (DoH, 1998).

The NHS is a huge and remote body responsible for organising and delivering health care in different local settings by a diverse group of diverse professionals of which nurses are the largest group. Nurses as frontline professionals must possess the ability to make the service appear local and personal to each and every patient who interacts with the service. This demands that nurses are socially and culturally savvy as well as technical masters in their chosen field of practice. They must avoid retreating behind the anonymity of the wider NHS. In primary care, nurses must demonstrate the ability to respond and deal flexibly with the many health problems they are likely to encounter from the community and possess the cultural and emotional intelligence to deal with the owners of these problems.

Dealing with people's multicultural needs begins with empathy, which is a fundamental competence of social awareness. Social awareness in turn is an important dimension of emotional intelligence. Goleman et al. (2002) make the point that empathy is not 'I'm okay, you're okay mushiness', but it is being able to take other people's feelings into thoughtful consideration and making intelligent decisions that still pay attention to those feelings in the response. Goleman et al. (2002) indicate that crucially, empathy makes resonance possible for people. Professionals who lack empathy act in ways that create dissonance. Empathy is a necessary skill for getting along with people from diverse cultures regardless of whether they are patients or colleagues. Empathy creates openness and removes misconceptions which occur in cross-cultural dialogue. It lets people tune in to the subtleties in the conversation, for example, body language and tone, so that the emotional messages can be heard. As the dominant culture, most White British people would not have experienced discrimination and may find it difficult to understand the feeling. In simple terms, to encompass multiculturalism, nurses must be receptive to different needs, even those that do not resonate with theirs, and listen empathically, and be authentic and congruent.

Probably all nurses in care settings will have received 'diversity' training often described as 'the sheep dip' approach to training. Diversity training addresses the key areas of equality and human rights legislation which the NHS and organisations must comply with. It demonstrates legal compliance and meets risk management standards. Through their impact assessments, organisations must take into account the positive and negative impact of policies across the board. Whilst the idea is laudable, the focus remains on output rather than outcome, creating another misconception that equal means same.

Diversity training takes a broad brush approach. It recognises the equal value we must place on contributions from all the different social groups. However, when poorly delivered, it can point out aspects that differentiate cultures such as race, religion, language and accent which serves to reinforce stereotypes.

Nurses have a duty to ensure they at least attend diversity training in their organisations. There is a dual responsibility, on the organisation to make such training available and on nurses to attend. The nurses must be aware of the legislative frameworks. Furthermore, they have a duty to request further training to broaden their knowledge of multiculturalism especially if they are practicing in an area of high ethnicity. Training must go beyond gestures of offering translation and interpretation in many languages, different foods and a quiet area for prayer. They must not be seen as 'Saris, steel bands and samosas', the tokenistic gestures that should now belong in another era. Getting to grips with multiculturalism involves understanding why translation and interpretation is important and where should the prayer room be located. There is still anecdotal evidence of health professionals still using family members and young children as interpreters. The question nurses need to ask is how would they feel if intimate details of their condition were discussed with their child?

At the heart of multiculturalism and diversity is preservation of self-respect and personal dignity. This is demonstrated in the way people sensitively deal with different issues rather than trying to 'normalise' the issue. Is it alright for someone else to accept the things that we would not accept for ourselves and our family? Are the practices we consider 'normal' to us acceptable to others? Living in a multicultural society means acknowledging the different cultures and practices and in a civilised society giving people the freedom to live in their respective cultures and practice their faith.

Experienced nurses have increased capacity to tolerate ambiguity and handle difficult situations and stress. They are in the special position of seeing human beings in their most vulnerable state and how people in those times become strongly attached to their faith, cultures and rituals. This places nurses in the unique position of being able to witness and participate in the diverse faiths, beliefs and cultures of their patients. Learning self-management will make them aware of their own emotions when they too might be feeling vulnerable.

Activity

Reflect on the diversity training you have received in your organisation. Has it met your needs? Is there something more that is needed in order to improve the care you provide within a multicultural health service?

How does multiculturalism and diversity impact on health?

The previous paragraphs explained how our thinking and our interactions can be influenced by culture which in turn is reflected in our behaviours and attitudes. Intelligence does not prevent people from having prejudiced views; rather they are more likely to think before they speak and act. Cultural intelligence is not beyond the realms of nurses' intellectual capacity. They can acquire the skills to challenge their own thinking and that of others to ensure they do not unconsciously collude with policies and decisions that will maintain the status quo and perpetuate the vicious cycle of health disadvantage for BME people. Whilst there needs to be real organisational commitment to the agenda, nurses should feel sufficiently empowered to take responsibility for their own personal and emotional development.

The NHS recognises that BME communities have worse health than the overall population and that the pattern of disease and poor health can also vary from one community to the next. For example, the incidence of a relatively common condition like diabetes can greatly differ. Asians have a 5–6-fold higher incidence of getting diabetes compared to Mauritians who have a 6–10-fold higher incidence despite sharing similar physical characteristics (NHS, 2008b).

The causes of ethnic health inequalities are multifaceted. Apart from being more socio-economically disadvantaged compared to the White population, there are other complex issues that impact on the health of the ethnic population. Nurses need to understand how racism and discrimination together with differences in cultures, lifestyle and biological susceptibility contribute to poor health (Platt, 2002).

Access to health services for the BME population is patchy across the country although access to primary care seems to be on the same level as the White British population. However, South Asian men report lower access to other treatment and services following diagnosis, for example, access to smoking cessation and post-coronary care (Postnote, 2007).

The NHS is committed through many initiatives to tackle lack of access to health care for the Black and ethnic minority population. Access refers not only to physical access to the building of services being provided in a manner that is culturally acceptable, but also to the invisible barriers that are attitudes and communication styles once over the threshold. Language, customs, rituals, dress and the environment can appear offensive. A lack of empathy towards how different ethnic groups view illness and disease and use conventional medicine can lead to lack of concordance and exacerbation of a chronic condition.

Race for Health is an initiative funded by the Department of Health working with PCTs and NHS Trusts to improve the health of people from BME backgrounds. The following stark statistics quoted by Race for Life (Hally, 2008) must strengthen the business case for commissioning the right services:

- male life expectancy in Church St, Westminster, is 67 years compared with 83 years in Belgravia, 1 mile away;
- the prevalence of stroke amongst African Caribbean and South Asian men is 70% higher than the average;
- men and women of Indian origin are three times more likely than most people to have diabetes;
- South Asian people are 50% more likely to die prematurely from coronary heart disease than the general population;

- infant mortality in England and Wales for children born to mothers from Pakistan is double the average;
- young Asian women are more than twice as likely to commit suicide as young White women.

What can nurses in primary care do to improve health care in a multicultural society?

Nurses in primary care have a vital role to play in first understanding the ethnic make-up of the community they serve. The poor quality of ethnicity data remains problematic. The Department of Health Quality and Outcomes Framework (QOF) (DoH, 2008) provides a small financial incentive for general practitioners to collect ethnicity data. However, this remains patchy and undermines planning. If nurses in primary care want to seriously address health inequalities in the ethnic population, collecting this simple but effective data is a good place to start. It will provide nurses with a clear and meaningful picture of the health profile of the ethnic population. It will also provide the necessary ammunition to influence health care policy, commissioning and deliver better outcomes.

Commissioning services that are targeted to Black and ethnic minority groups is vital. Profiling the population of the practice is important and can be kept relatively simple provided the important information is collected. Practices in one PCT have been trained in data collection, cross-matching key data on obesity, coronary heart disease and diabetes which can show if patients are falling through the net.

Nurses need to develop an appetite to tackle and lead change. Absence of significant data or training should not induce passivity. There is an imperative need for nurses to act as leaders and seek the support they need to make changes even if these are small and incremental. Forming small networks to share knowledge and having a mentor to develop leadership qualities are the first steps that can start to make the difference. On another practical and human level, nurses need to develop self-awareness and explore the various types of problems that occur in cross-cultural encounters and learn to deal with them as they arise. Listening to their own intuition, nurses will be aware when there has been missed communication, when they are being bureaucratic and when they are making decisions based on a limited amount or flawed information. This should prompt the nurse to become more curious and ask further questions. Regardless of culture, people would rather be asked about their beliefs and preferences rather than having others guessing and assuming. Questions, framed with curiosity and sensitivity, should not cause embarrassment to the nurse or the patient. Political correctness should not be used as a reason for not asking questions about country of origin, language, literacy, economic status, social networks and acceptability of treatment if the information will help decision-making.

On a practical note, nurses need to make sure patients from different cultures have access to independent language facilitation so that they can effectively express their health needs. Privacy and dignity and cultural preferences in clinical consultations must be respected.

Activity

Here are some simple questions and actions to facilitate cross-cultural discovery dialogue.

▨ What do you think has caused your problem? What do you call it?
▨ Have you seen anyone else about this problem apart from a doctor?
▨ Have you used other treatments?
▨ Who else gives you health advice?
▨ What language do you speak at home?
▨ Determine the patient's priorities (Carillo et al., 1999).

The questions in the activity box above are indeed simple but the answers may be surprisingly different when the respondent is White British or newly arrived Somalian. Focusing on the individual rather than their illness is more likely to create empathy. Ultimately the owner of the illness is the individual who has to make sense of the problem.

Conclusion

This chapter has taken a pragmatic approach to help nurses understand the complex topic of multiculturalism in professional practice. It has indicated that PCNs are frequently in the privileged position of introducing people to the NHS, seeing people for the first time as they register and remaining close to the community in which they practice. It was identified in the narrative that nurses practicing in inner city areas constantly interact with richly diverse communities, presenting them with many opportunities to learn about other cultures and becoming culturally intelligent. Daily, they come across people who are and act differently from themselves and they too appear different to those from other cultures than their own. This chapter has provided tools for understanding multiculturalism and demonstrated how to bridge the cultural gap and make the difference to patients from different cultures in order to tackle the health inequalities experienced by ethnic minorities in the UK.

References

Carillo, E., Green, R. and Betancourt, J. (1999) Cross cultural primary care: A patient-based approach. *Annals of Internal Medicine*, 130(10); 829–834.

Coker, N. (June 1999) *Is the NHS sensitive to its Diverse Communities?* London: Kings Fund News.

DoH (1998) *They look after their Own, don't they?* Report of an Inspection of Community Care Services for Black and Minority Ethnic Older People.

London: Department of Health, http://www.dh.gov.uk/en/Publicationsandstatistics/Lettersandcirculars/Chiefinspectorletters/DH_4004608 (accessed 26 April 2009).

DoH (2008) *Quality and Outcomes Framework (QOF)*. London: Department of Health, http://www.dh.gov.uk/en/Healthcare/Primarycare/Primarycarecontracting/QOF/index.htm (accessed 26 April 2009).

Dubos, R. (1997) *Mirage of Health Utopias, Progress and Biological Change*. New Brunswick, NJ: Rutgers University Press.

Goleman, D., Boyatzis, R. and McKee, A. (2002) *The New Leaders. Transforming the Art of Leadership into the Science of Results*. London: Little Brown (an imprint of Time Warner).

Hally, H. (2008) *Race Equality in Health – The Key to World Class Commissioning*. Manchester: National Health Service, www.raceforhealth.org (accessed 22 April 2009).

Hofstede, G. (2003). *Cultures and Organizations*. London: Profile Books Ltd.

NHS (2006) *Breaking through Programme*. London: National Health Service Institute for Innovation and Improvement.

NHS (2008a) *Equality and Diversity*. London: London Deanery.

NHS (2008b) *NHS Diabetes (National Diabetes Support Team)*, www.diabetes.nhs.uk (accessed 22 April 2009).

Platt, L. (2002). *Parallel Lives? Poverty among Ethnic Minority Groups in Britain*. London: CPAG.

Postnote (January 2007) *Ethnicity & Health*. No. 276. London: Parliamentary Office of Science and Technology.

Wood, P., Landry, C. and Bloomfield, J. (2006) *Cultural Diversity in Britain. A Tool Kit for Cross Cultural Co-operation*. York: Rowntree Foundation.

Index